Advance Praise for *The Informed Parent*

"Clear, comprehensive, and resolutely evidence-based, *The Informed Parent* is a fabulous resource for science-minded parents. Haelle and Willingham have tirelessly compiled the evidence on so many questions that cause parents to worry and wonder, and with all of this science at their fingertips, they'll be able to make confident and informed choices for their families. From pre-conception to preschool, you'll find yourself returning to this book again and again."

—Alice Callahan, PhD, author of *The Science of Mom: A Research-Based Guide to Your Baby's First Year*

"*The Informed Parent* is a beacon of science-based sanity for new parents caught in a blizzard of dubious child-rearing advice. Tara Haelle and Emily Willingham are sure-handed guides, distilling the most up-to-date, reliable research into sensible advice that neither patronizes nor terrorizes. Circumcision? Television? Nipple confusion? Relax, Tara and Emily have got you covered."

—Dan Fagin, director of the Science, Health, and Environmental Reporting Program at NYU, and Pulitzer Prize–winning author of *Toms River: A Story of Science and Salvation*

"In *The Informed Parent*, Emily Willingham and Tara Haelle, two widely respected science writers (and parents), explore key questions about child health, beginning with fetal development and continuing into toddlerhood. The result is engaging, conversational, deeply researched, and smart, a book that should be considered a necessary resource for all twenty-first-century parents."

—Deborah Blum, director of the Knight Science Journalism Program at MIT, and Pulitzer Prize–winning author of *Love at Goon Park: Harry Harlow and the Science of Affection*

"Finally! An amazing, informed, evidence-based tour through the most common questions and concerns of parenthood that I can recommend without hesitation. A must for any science-minded new parent, or for anyone who thinks Google doesn't replace expertly curated information."

—Yoni Freedhoff, MD, assistant professor of family medicine, University of Ottawa, and creator of the *Weighty Matters* blog

"Parents in the Internet age have to navigate their way through a maze of confusing information and misinformation. Tara Haelle and Emily Willingham are the perfect guides to what's fact and fiction when it comes to the science of parenting."

—Seth Mnookin, associate director of MIT's Graduate Program in Science Writing, and author of *The Panic Virus*

"Science-based. Judgment free. A perfect guide for evidence-based parenting!"
—Ari Brown, MD, pediatrician and author of the Baby 411 book series

"In *The Informed Parent*, journalists Tara Haelle and Emily Willingham manage to answer everything a parent could possibly be worried about during pregnancy, birth, infancy, and toddlerhood. What makes this book different from every other book on this subject (and there are many) is that the authors take on not only the science of what concerns us, but encourage us to think along with them—giving us the tools to answer other questions in the future. It was like reading the answer sheet before the test."
—Paul Offit, MD, chief of the Division of Infectious Diseases,
Children's Hospital of Philadelphia

"With *The Informed Parent*, Tara Haelle and Emily Willingham have gifted today's neurotic parents with fuel—and ultimately antidote—for their obsessive researching. Unlike most parenting books, the authors never preach, condone, or praise. Instead, they report the science on all possible parenting controversies in a lay-friendly (and often pithy) style, allowing the reader to come to her/his own conclusions. Well-written, impeccably researched, and brilliantly suited for millennial parents, *The Informed Parent* should be on the top of everyone's baby shower list."
—Suzanne Barston, the "Fearless Formula Feeder" and author of
*Bottled Up: How the Way We Feed Babies Has Come to Define Motherhood,
and Why It Shouldn't*

"Is it confirmation bias to say that anyone who decides to look at scientific facts instead of hectoring parents is doing the world a service? If so, consider my opinion biased: This book will help a lot of folks!"
—Lenore Skenazy, founder of the book, blog, and movement *Free-Range Kids*

"As a mom, I can confidently say that *The Informed Parent* will be a lifesaver for all moms and dads going through the anxiety and excitement of raising a young child. From autism to organic food, the authors demystify modern parents' most prevalent fears for the first four years, and effectively arm them with a critical thinking cap for years to come. If you're tired of the mommy (and daddy) wars, or simply need help separating the credible wheat from the misinformation chaff on the Internet, look no further."
—Kavin Senapathy, science advocate and author of *The Fear Babe*

THE INFORMED PARENT

A SCIENCE-BASED RESOURCE
FOR YOUR CHILD'S FIRST FOUR YEARS

TARA HAELLE
AND EMILY WILLINGHAM, PhD

A TARCHERPERIGEE BOOK

tarcherperigee

An imprint of Penguin Random House LLC
375 Hudson Street
New York, New York 10014

Most TarcherPerigee books are available at special quantity discounts for bulk purchase for sales promotions, premiums, fund-raising, and educational needs. Special books or book excerpts also can be created to fit specific needs. For details, write: SpecialMarkets@penguinrandomhouse.com.

LIBRARY OF CONGRESS CATALOGING-IN-PUBLICATION DATA

Names: Haelle, Tara, author. | Willingham, Emily Jane, 1968– author.
Title: The informed parent : a science-based resource for your child's first
four years / Tara Haelle and Emily Willingham, Ph.D.
Description: First edition. | New York, NY : Perigee, [2016] | Includes index.
Identifiers: LCCN 2015046759 | ISBN 9780399171062 (paperback)
Subjects: LCSH: Child rearing. | Parenthood. | Pregnancy. | Child
development. | Families—Health and hygiene. | BISAC: FAMILY &
RELATIONSHIPS / Parenting / General. | HEALTH & FITNESS / Pregnancy &
Childbirth. | FAMILY & RELATIONSHIPS / Life Stages / Infants & Toddlers.
Classification: LCC HQ769 .H228 2016 | DDC 649/.1—dc23

PRINTED IN THE UNITED STATES OF AMERICA
1 3 5 7 9 10 8 6 4 2

Book design by Elke Sigal

We dedicate this book to our sons.

Contents

Introduction

Based on persistent headlines about the "mommy wars," you could conclude that a visit to your local playground or a mom's group outing might require decking yourself out head to toe in Kevlar. But the reality on the ground is different. There is no war, and we'd like to see that metaphor retired entirely for anything but, well, war.

There is, however, a whole lot of bias and judgment. All the time, every second, judging is the background noise of our social interactions. In the parenting arena, that judgment feels—and is—very, very personal. Of all the judgy noise around us, parenting criticism comes through loudly and clearly, a painful signal that elicits defensiveness and anger. Passing judgment on another parent, especially when that judgment is grounded in a "philosophy" of some kind, is a rude and nosy and even hostile thing to do. It's one reason that some of us rarely do it in our face-to-face interactions. But that doesn't mean we're not *thinking* it. And a lot of the time, what we are thinking or another parent is thinking has little to do with what the latest research says.

Of course, it's not a war. It's human . . . humans raising other humans. Not one thing we do nor one philosophy we follow will guarantee the outcome we intend. We don't even need science, for once, to tell us that.

But science is useful, because the practice of science produces data instead of anecdote—data we can use for evidence-based decision-making as parents. In this book, we look at what science has to say at the various crossroads parents encounter, from vaccines to attachment parenting to circumcision to screen time. We don't dole out a lot of advice—after all, we don't know you or your family and can't say which route would be best for you and your child. But we give you the scientific information you need to map your own path. And here and there, we divulge what we ended up doing, which may not have been terribly scientific at the time.

We take on questions like: Should we circumcise our son? Is any sleep-training approach okay? Should I buy conventional or organic food? Is formula all right, because breastfeeding is just not for me? Is home birth ever a safe option? Does too much screen time harm children, and what is "too much" anyway? This book gives you the tools you need to decide, not within the framework of a parenting philosophy but within the framework of interpreting science for your family's unique situation.

Perhaps the most important of these tools is understanding how to decipher the evidence. We don't tell you what to do, because how you use the evidence depends on your specific circumstances. We work hard to limit or expose bias—yours, ours, theirs. As humans, we commonly overlook gaps in logic and ignore evidence that counters our existing beliefs and expectations. No one, including scientists, is immune to the mistakes in interpretation that all of us make when assessing evidence. As we dig into data, we note the traps to watch out for as you weigh research findings in the context of your personal needs.

Mistaking correlation for causation is one of the most common cognitive errors because the human mind seeks patterns and sees relationships in coincidence. That tendency is useful when your friend goes missing at the same time a lion is sighted near your village, and you then are on alert for lions. But it can mislead when the apparent associations are more subtle. Just because organic food purchases have increased at a similar rate as autism diagnoses over the past decade, for example, doesn't mean they're related.

Another common thinking trap is confirmation bias, which leads us toward information confirming what we already think and turns us away from what contradicts our beliefs. Countering this bias requires playing devil's advocate with yourself and fighting your natural defensive reaction when evidence goes against a deeply held belief. Be on the lookout: confirmation bias might take hold as you read this book, often taking the form of cherry-picking data that conforms to what you believe. Even if you acknowledge the data, you might be inclined to diminish its relevance or ignore a larger consensus of data. We try to help by representing the entire cherry tree, if you will, in each chapter. We also focus on evidence from research, not anecdotes (even though we share a few from our own lives). As a common saying goes, the plural of "anecdote" is not data.

Some kinds of research carry greater weight than others. The gold standard is the randomized controlled trial, in which neither researchers nor patients know who's receiving what intervention. This study design is intended to erase many of the problems of bias. Other kinds of clinical research include retrospective studies, taking a look back at already collected data and seeing what patterns emerge. But because these investigations weren't controlled or planned ahead of time, the evidence they yield will be subject to caveats. And then some scientific publications aren't based on original work at all but instead synthesize existing findings in a subject area. These systematic reviews and meta-analyses are great for getting a perspective of the state of the science, but because the authors select what to search for and include, they can be subject to bias too. The best ones give an assessment of the bias in the studies they evaluate and rate the evidence on a standardized scale. For this reason, we frequently describe the types of studies we're discussing.

> The plural of "anecdote" is not data.

Finally, accept the fact that you (and we) probably are overestimating how much you (and we) know and understand. No matter how nice and unassuming you might be or how supersmart you are, you and the rest of us are all subject to superiority bias, known as the Dunning–Kruger effect. In short, it's our tendency to overrate ourselves while underrating others. Remember how we find ourselves making comparisons to the Joneses and judging each other's parenting styles, our own most favorably? We're Dunning–Kruger-ing all over the place when we do that. If most of us are average parents, then most of us are not superior to other parents. What most of us *are*, though, is hoping to be the best parent we can be in the only situation that matters: for our children. You're the only parent you need to worry about, and we want this book to help you be the best evidence-based parent you can be.

We hope this book will save you from the danger of Dunning–Kruger, but we also hope it helps you navigate some of the knottiest parenting questions we face today. Our goal is to place the strongest evidence in front of you, explained in a way you can understand, so that you can accurately decide what's best for you and your family.

A Note on Terminology

We are aware of the developmental distinctions between the embryo and the fetus. In some cases, we use both terms when both stages are relevant, but in others, for brevity and to avoid repetition, we default to "fetus" or "fetal." The word "data" is treated as a plural noun because it represents two or more pieces of information from a study. The term "birth defect" carries obvious negative connotations, and we have sought to diminish the possibility of adding stigma by instead using the term "congenital anomaly."

CHAPTER 1

Parenting Begins Before Pregnancy

The Parental Age Effect

Obviously, women reach an age at which they no longer can have children. Why do women become unable to conceive, and what effects can age have when women do conceive?

First, some interesting findings from 2014 suggest that the longer women are naturally fertile—whether they conceive a child or not—the longer women tend to live. This beneficial effect of persistent reproductive capacity into, say, one's forties can be offset, though, by having three or more children. So there's a balance for women between some sort of as-yet-unknown health effects of reproductive capacity into middle age and having a limited number of offspring.

Males of our species make reproductive cells their entire adult lives. The belief once was that a man's age didn't influence outcomes for children he fathered, but recent findings call that into question. Some developmental conditions—including autism and schizophrenia—have been linked to having an older father, or even an older grandfather. The grandpa link is just math, but the older fathers association goes beyond that to findings of accumulating DNA changes with age in men that result in conditions like autism in their children. Having a young father (age 20 to 24) has also been linked to increased risks of bipolar disorder, and being an older father (over age 45) is associated with increased risk of bipolar disorder, attention-deficit disorder, or autism in the child. These findings do not mean that an especially young or an older man will unquestionably father a child with psychiatric or developmental conditions, given that many of these conditions carry a genetic component, and there is certainly the potential for other factors to play a role.

Women, of course, have a different way of doing things, gametically speaking. After many rounds of hormone stimulation and hormone and ovum release over the decades, women eventually have their last menstrual cycle (menopause). Once the process of ovarian hormone waning begins, a woman is in perimenopause, which can last for several years. During this time, a woman can conceive, but doing so becomes increasingly difficult. Even for a woman who's been regularly ovulating on a classic 28-day calendar her entire reproductive life (if you find her, please let us know), ovulation and hormone cycling become unpredictable until they just don't happen at all.

With increasing maternal age comes an increase in various negative outcomes. Norway, Sweden, and Denmark happen to be countries that track their residents' health data in careful and complete ways. These registries of information are good sources for researchers trying to tease out links between factors, such as maternal age when giving birth, and outcomes, such as prematurity. Studies from Norway and Sweden covering more than 1 million women have found increased risks of fetal or neonatal death with increasing maternal age, starting at age 30. For women age 40 or older who delivered, there was a link between this "advanced maternal age" and risk for miscarriage, preeclampsia, and gestational diabetes but not for stillbirth or spontaneous preterm delivery. A few other studies, though, have confirmed an increased risk for stillbirth and preterm delivery for women age 40 or over, and an increased risk of cesarean delivery.

Do these findings mean that once you reach a certain age, you shouldn't conceive? Not necessarily; and don't forget the recent findings that the ability to do so without much trouble can signal overall health and longevity. But if age increases risks for certain unwanted outcomes—and studies in the aggregate agree on that—that's a consideration to add into your calculations about your behaviors and choices around pregnancy and birth. For example, if you're over 40, the increased risks of complications in pregnancy and birth might guide your choice of healthcare provider to ensure access to appropriate and expert medical care if interventions are needed.

The Most Important Prenatal Vitamin

Folic Acid

Prenatal vitamins vary in their offerings, but do you actually need what they offer? In fact, most nutrient recommendations that health organizations issue are not based on firm evidence. About the only thing we're sure of is that the most important nutrient in pregnancy is folate (also known as folic acid or vitamin B9), from conception through the first trimester. After that, the benefit-to-harm ratio for supplements gets fuzzier, partly because women in the developed world generally get the bulk of what they need from their diet.

Folate, which occurs naturally in foods like oranges, nuts, and beans and is available as a supplement, plays a starring role in the forming nervous system. Sufficient folic acid in the first month of embryonic development prevents defects in the neural tube, which forms by the 28th day after fertilization and develops into the brain and spinal column. Insufficient amounts of folic acid can contribute to neural tube defects such as spina bifida and anencephaly.

The problem is that many women—especially those with unplanned pregnancies (about half of all pregnancies each year)—don't know they're pregnant in that first month. By the time they know, it's usually too late to affect neural tube formation. Therefore, the US Preventive Services Task Force recommends that women who could become pregnant take a daily supplement of 400–800 micrograms above and beyond the folate they get from food. To address potential deficiencies in women not getting enough, folic acid has been added to enriched bread, cereal, flour, cornmeal, pasta, rice, and other grain products since 1998. Within a year or two of this federally mandated fortification of grain products, births with neural tube defects declined approximately 20% to 30%.

So far, a high intake of dietary folate has not proved to be harmful. However, 1,000 micrograms is considered the safe upper limit for taking folic acid supplements because too much may mask symptoms of vitamin B12 deficiency, which, ironically, can cause brain, spinal cord, and nerve damage to the person taking it. A balanced diet and supplements of 600 micrograms should get you within range. Women on a special diet should consider how that affects intake.

Iron and Iodine

Iron is a critical part of functioning hemoglobin, which carries oxygen in red blood cells, and myoglobin, which carries oxygen in muscle cells. Insufficient iron can lead to fatigue and anemia, which has been linked to low birth weight, preterm birth, and prenatal depression. Because women have a greater blood volume while pregnant, they need more iron, a recommended 27 milligrams instead of 18 milligrams, the standard recommendation for adult women between the ages of 19 and 50. Most people are aware that red meat, such as beef, is rich in iron, as are poultry, liver, tuna, and salmon. But iron is also present in whole grains, iron-fortified cereals, dried beans, dried fruits, and egg yolks. The research consensus is that iron supplements reduce the risk of anemia, iron deficiency, and low birth weight. However, side effects of too much iron include constipation, nausea, vomiting, diarrhea, and pregnancy complications due to high hemoglobin, and taking vitamin C increases iron absorption. Most routine prenatal care involves checking iron levels.

Iodine is essential for both thyroid hormone production and normal fetal brain development. Pregnant women need about 50% more iodine than non-pregnant women to prevent problems with fetal neurological development. Since the 1920s, when iodized salt arrived in many parts of the world, iodine deficiency hasn't typically been a problem; but pregnant women may not get enough if they eat a lot of processed foods, which don't contain iodized salt, or if they don't use much iodized salt themselves. Other dietary sources include seafood, seaweed, and dairy and grain products. Supplemental iodine—which more than half of all prenatal vitamins don't include—improves birth weight, infant mortality, and cognitive development in children, but only in regions with moderate to high iodine deficiencies.

A 2014 statement from the American Academy of Pediatrics (AAP) noted concerns about insufficient iodine levels in pregnant women in the United States, based on recent data that some pregnant women aren't getting enough, especially those eating little dairy. Although the evidence doesn't indicate supplementation for all women, guidelines supported by the American Thyroid Association, the National Academy of Sciences, and the Institute of Medicine (IOM) suggest considering supplements if a pregnant woman gets less than the recommended 220–250 micrograms. Excess iodine intake can cause thyroid problems for the developing fetus, leading to the question of how much is too much. The upper limit might be about 500 micrograms a day, though even that guideline is based on weak evidence.

The Enigma of Vitamin D

Everyone has something to say about this nutrient that we can manufacture ourselves with sufficient sun exposure or take as a supplement, but we lack much reliable evidence about it. Even the daily recommendation of 5 micrograms (200 IU) or 400–600 IU, depending on whom you ask, and the IOM's safe upper-level intake of 4,000 IU per day aren't based on clear evidence. Vitamin D helps maintain bone health and calcium levels, and severe deficiencies can cause rickets, but what constitutes inadequate levels or deficiency during pregnancy is not known. (The IOM says levels less than 12 ng/mL, or 30 nmol/L, put someone at risk for deficiency.)

Some systematic reviews have linked blood levels below 50 nmol/L to an increased risk of preeclampsia, gestational diabetes, preterm birth, small-for-gestational-age babies, bacterial vaginosis, and, to a lesser extent, an increased risk of cesarean birth, slightly shorter gestations, and postpartum depression; others found too little evidence for any of this, and no studies establish that too little vitamin D causes anything. In fact, a Cochrane Review (see the appendix for more about Cochrane Reviews) found that vitamin D supplements during pregnancy—despite increasing vitamin D levels in women—did not prevent any poor maternal or newborn outcomes. So women's levels increased, but what difference did it make?

Whether women should take vitamin D supplements during pregnancy is unclear and may depend on skin pigmentation, sunlight exposure, and physiology. You can bump intake through your diet with fatty fish, liver, mushrooms, egg yolks, some cheeses, and fortified milk, yogurt, cereals, and fruit juices. It doesn't take much sun to boost your levels either: 5 to 30 minutes anytime midmorning to midafternoon, but as always, consult with your medical professional about what's right for you. Sunscreen does allow some vitamin D synthesis in the skin.

The Rest of the Alphabet

Again, most of the evidence isn't there to recommend most other nutrients. Calcium supplements may help reduce the risk of preeclampsia if women are not getting enough through dairy products (see also the discussion of preeclampsia on page 57), and zinc supplements might very slightly reduce preterm birth risk if women are deficient. Vegetarians may be at risk for vitamin B12 deficiency.

Most Americans already get sufficient selenium daily through meats, fish, grains, cottage cheese, and eggs, and too much extra selenium can increase the risk of type 2 diabetes. Vitamin A supplements reduce anemia in women in regions where deficiency is common (or in HIV-positive women), but too much vitamin A during pregnancy (more than 10,000 IU a day) can cause congenital anomalies (and most prenatals have 4,000 to 5,000 IU).

So Pop a Prenatal or What?

Should you take a prenatal multivitamin? Unfortunately—other than the recommendation to take folic acid—there is no general recommendation that can be made for all women on this question. Deficiencies don't tend to occur in high-income countries where balanced diets fulfill the needs of healthy individuals without special medical conditions.

The only benefit seen in the research for prenatal vitamins is a moderately reduced risk of low birth weight and underweight babies, again only for women in low-income countries where known nutrient deficiencies exist. We don't have studies showing improved birth outcomes for women in high-income countries taking prenatals, and most women in the United States probably don't need them.

Then why do clinicians recommend them? They are likely working off a better-safe-than-sorry mind-set given that women's diets vary so dramatically. In addition to the vitamin A risks noted above (watch out for other supplements with high levels of vitamin A, such as cod liver oil), the biggest other risk for a combined prenatal supplement is nausea. Taking them at night can reduce nausea.

If you decide to take a prenatal multivitamin, look at how much of each nutrient it contains and think about what you do and don't get from your diet. Most prenatal vitamins are pretty similar, but about half lack iodine. Because vitamins are not regulated as strictly as medications, brands containing a "USP Verified Mark" have met key quality requirements.

Whether to Worry About Weight During Pregnancy

The guidelines for how much weight a woman should gain during pregnancy have changed over the years. A few decades ago, women were advised that more than 20 pounds of weight gain was too much. These days, when the average pregnant woman gains 30 pounds or so with a full-term pregnancy, the weight-gain recommendations are based on the woman's pre-pregnancy weight in terms of body mass index (BMI), a ratio of her height to weight. For example, a woman who is underweight pre-pregnancy (BMI <18.5, Western world) is recommended to gain from 28 to 40 pounds. But a woman who is obese before pregnancy (BMI 30+) is recommended to gain only 11 to 20 pounds. The IOM decided on these recommendations in 2009, but according to the American College of Obstetricians and Gynecologists, some physicians think the limits for overweight and obese women are too high.

Studies suggest, however, that women who adhere to the IOM ranges have the least risk of adverse outcomes. Gaining too much or too little for your pre-pregnancy weight class (normal, overweight, or obese) can affect newborn weight (too large or too small) and increase your risk for pregnancy complications like preeclampsia.

Your weight before you conceive is also a factor in the size of the baby—being underweight is a risk for having a low-birth-weight baby while being overweight or obese increases the odds for a very large baby. Furthermore, the child's odds of later being overweight or obese are greatly increased if the mother is either overweight or obese prior to pregnancy, though it's difficult to tease out how much of this association is actually related to the mother's weight versus other factors, such as household practices and the family and social environment, which play a role in the weight of both mother and child.

One study has suggested that weight gain during pregnancy carries greater risks compared to those associated with pre-pregnancy weight status. That long-term study looked at relationships between adult weight status and gestational weight gain of the mothers. The results indicated that the key factor in offspring BMI at any age was how much weight the mother gained *during* pregnancy. Even women who had lower weights before pregnancy but gained a lot during pregnancy had children with higher BMIs. That leaves us unsure about which factor is more important for offspring weight status: maternal pre-pregnancy weight, as some studies suggest, or maternal weight gain per se.

One way to address both head-on, presumably, would be to not be overweight or obese before pregnancy and then to gain not too much and not too little weight during pregnancy (both so simple, right?), although no one seems quite sure what the sweet spot is. For an overweight or obese pregnant woman who might want to limit her pregnancy weight gain, how much can interventions positively affect the mother and her child? One analysis of multiple studies suggested that dietary and lifestyle interventions help limit weight gain and might reduce the risk for gestational diabetes but don't affect infant birth weight. Another analysis of trials involving 182,130 women found a reduced risk of high blood pressure and preeclampsia and diabetes during pregnancy with just an average weight loss of 2 pounds. A good diet and appropriate exercise probably aren't going to be bad things, regardless, but as always, consult with a medical professional about your personal situation.

What comes through pretty clearly from many studies is that maternal obesity before pregnancy is associated with increased risk for mother and baby in several ways, including preterm birth, cesarean, neural tube defects, and gestational diabetes. The risks aren't all confined to women who are overweight to obese, however. Having a low BMI or low pregnancy weight gain could be a risk factor for first trimester miscarriage, and preterm delivery has also been linked to low pre-pregnancy BMI.

Selecting a Maternity Healthcare Provider

Much of this section has to do with where you live and what options you have. Some women have only one option: a local hospital or medical care center with a handful of obstetrician-gynecologists (ob-gyns) who handle all maternity care in the area. Sometimes, in such situations, there might be non-nurse midwives available, but as far as a spectrum of choices, the larger and more diverse your local area, the greater and more diverse your options will be.

This section is US-centric and thus focuses on the uneven availability of choices in the United States. Some countries, such as those in Europe, have a much more integrated model of obstetric care that looks to safety, empowerment, and comfort by including midwifery and availability of critical interventions, features that ideally would become the gold standard for maternal and infant care around the world. At least one large US center, Boston Medical Center, has given a trial to what is called collaborative care, which integrates the services of obstetricians, midwives, and family doctors, based on the fact that obstetricians can be in short supply and the benefits midwifery care has to offer. But such programs have yet to take off nationally, even as increasing numbers of women receive care from midwives, nurse practitioners, and physician assistants. Indeed, they may take longer to gain a foothold in rural areas, where cultural collisions between midwives and economics play a role in limiting efforts at such collaborations.

Thus, women face uneven choices in the United States. If you have no choices in terms of provider, you still have options for how you can express your hopes and expectations to your provider.

Types of Providers

The typical choices for a maternity care provider are an ob-gyn, who is a medical doctor, or a midwife, or both. Midwifery in the United States is wildly variable, and different states have different laws regulating its practice. Midwives can be certified in one of three ways, according to the Midwives Alliance of North America: certified midwives (CMs); certified professional midwives (CPMs), who are certified through a nationally based program established in the 1980s; or certified-nurse midwives (CNMs). The last group consists of people who have a nursing degree in addition to midwife training. Midwives who attend home births are called direct-entry midwives (DEs), regardless of their certification or qualifications.

As of this writing, CPMs can practice legally in 28 states. Because the states determine the legality of CPM practices, where you live can have a big effect on whether such midwives will be available to you.

Birth Facility

Where you live affects not only your choice of healthcare provider category but also your choice of facilities. Women in rural areas often have only one option for birth when it comes to a medical facility: the local hospital or the hospital in the nearest city.

Most women give birth in the hospital, a trend that began in the 1940s and continues today. A small but growing population of women have become more interested in birth options outside of the hospital, including free-standing birth clinics and planned home births. We address the pros and cons of home birth on page 60.

The science on where women give birth and what the best setting might be is problematic because much of the commentary and research are published in journals of organizations committed to selling women on a specific way of birthing, what it references as "normal childbirth." Normal is not, however, a good metric for real life and the human condition, and the use of the term has the effect of making any woman feel abnormal if her experience doesn't conform to this ideal of "normal." The goal is safe birth, with a healthy baby and a mother who is as comfortable and empowered as possible.

Communicate Your Personal Considerations and Factors

If you already have a provider whom you trust, you're good to go except for one question: Who is the backup? One human being can't be available 365 days a year to attend deliveries. So one thing you need to ensure is that you know who the backup attendant is and that you have met and talked with that person about how you feel.

Many women have had the experience of handing over a "birth plan" to an obstetrician or the attendants at the hospital only to find that it's treated with about as much respect as a used tissue. From the perspective of the mother, this plan is intended to communicate beforehand—at a time when she can communicate as opposed to later, when it might be more difficult—what her choices would be under various circumstances. From the perspective of a seasoned birth attendant, even the word "plan" is misapplied when it comes to giving birth, because they've seen exactly how unpredictable it all can be, how no one can predetermine what will happen and which actions might be critical. It might be better to consider it a communication of preferences and hopes or choices than a plan.

But a woman still has some choices to make, and she has the right to request certain courses of action and to communicate her wishes. She can control some factors involved in delivery. Short of an emergency situation, she ought to be able to say who should be allowed in the room. She ought to be able to request available things that make her comfortable. She ought to be able to communicate how she feels about interventions used without emergency indications, such as induction or breaking the amniotic sac. You might think that you have preferences about pain interventions, but pain is notoriously personal and unpredictable, and at least one study indicates that 90% of women with a birth plan who receive an epidural for pain, whether or not they had determined not to have one, were satisfied with its effects. The same study found that the women surveyed felt having the birth plan helped them clarify their thoughts and facilitate communication with the people providing their healthcare. We note that the women most likely to have a plan like this tend to be white and college educated. Not everyone has the luxury of staking a claim to choice or planning when it comes to childbirth options.

Even though nature always has its own "plan," it's still wise to identify and communicate your needs. Clinicians may have seen it all, but you haven't. The best you can do is let them know how you feel, what you'd like when the choice is available, and what will help alleviate any fear or anxiety you're feeling.

The level of detail of a birth plan will vary. If you're comfortable and on good communication terms with your provider, you might just need to talk about it in person. If you're the kind of person who makes to-do lists, creating a document might be more your style. Sure, some of this is just a crutch or a way to work through mentally what awaits you. But it also is a way for you to become familiar with and state your preferences about the various medical turning points that can arise during birth. But remember the perspective of the people with whom you're sharing this plan: they can tell you a hundred stories for each preference you share of women with that preference who had to abandon it.

That abandonment of the plan can be an issue. Some women may feel that if they create the plan and the plan doesn't happen, somehow this shift from their preferences or hopes means failure. It doesn't. It just means you're a parent.

The Conception Calendar

The way we learn about conception in sex ed, you might come away thinking that it's just a matter of sperm meets egg following sexual congress, sperm and egg fuse, and voilà!—conception achievement unlocked. But the reality is more complex, and the timing is more delicate than the presence of 7-plus billion people on earth might indicate.

In fact, for some women, conception can be so difficult that they never conceive at all. We address some of these issues and the science around them in the section on in vitro fertilization on page 14, but here, we'll explain nature's calendar of conception, how you might be able to tell if you've conceived without even looking at a calendar, and the biology that underlies all of the constructs we've built around dates and menstrual cycles and thermometers and ovulation.

The average menstrual cycle lasts 28 days, with the midway point marking ovulation, aka "egg pops into fallopian tube, ready to meet the right sperm." Hormones drive this "popping" event, all spiking in a synchronized way after spending some time nurturing the little gamete to this point. For the average cycle, ovulation happens on day 14. The window of time for fertilization begins at that point and lasts, according to the stereotype, about 24 hours. Then, it's progesterone's time to shine as the casing the egg left behind in the ovary gets busy pumping out the hormone to support the uterine lining for a couple of weeks in case an embryo shows up to implant. A no-show means a progesterone plunge and with that, the shedding of the uterine lining, aka menstruation, your period, Aunt Flo, etc. That shedding takes us back to day 1 of the cycle, which, for the average woman, happens every month for approximately 30 or 40 years, pregnancies not included.

So now that you know all of that, toss it. Odds are good that your body doesn't adhere to this schedule.

Given these vagaries and unpredictables of being a real human instead of a robot following a predetermined time line, how do we know when that critical moment—ovulation—is about to happen, is happening, or has happened? It would be useful to have a skin-color signal to alert us to the Right Moment, but we don't. What we do have is body temperature.

Body Temperature

Our body temperature follows our hormones. Estrogen cools us down during the follicular, egg-developing, uterine-lining-building phase, and progesterone heats us up during the waiting, luteal phase. Right before we pop off an egg from ovary to fallopian tube, we release a burst of hormones, including estrogen, that causes a pretty decent drop in body temperature, as much as a half degree. If you measure your temperature in the morning over the course of a cycle, you'll see for yourself the way temperature changes course. During the follicular phase, before ovulation, estrogen builds. Your temperature upon waking—and the usual advice is to measure it at the same time every morning, before you even sit up—will be relatively low, perhaps 97.9 degrees Fahrenheit. Then, often, there's a drop and ovulation. Following ovulation, the temps can spike up a half degree or more. At that point, the egg's out of the ovarian barn, and if there's not already some sperm there to meet it, fertilization likely will have to wait for the next cycle.

The standard advice is to use a special basal body temperature thermometer to chart this temperature change, which can require increments of a tenth of a degree to follow accurately. Because your temperature doesn't go up until after you've ovulated, charting these fluctuations can tell you more about your general cycle rather than serving as an ovulation indicator for a specific cycle. It can also tell you when ovulation has already happened so that you can just have sex for fun, instead of with the added stress of wondering if this time is *it*.

If you're not pregnant, that temperature bump you get after ovulation—brought to you by the hormone progesterone—will drop dramatically right when your period begins following the progesterone plunge.

What does temperature do when you're pregnant? If your temperature stays up and no period arrives, then you might want to consider taking a pregnancy test.

Cervical Changes

Another option is to track the activity of your cervix. The way it feels and the secretions it emits can tell the knowing and experienced woman a whole lot about what's going on in her ovaries and fallopian tubes.

While estrogen's lowering your body temperature, it's also causing an increase in the amount of cervical mucus you're producing. As you approach ovulation, the mucus becomes pretty abundant, and if you can get ahold of enough, you'll find that you can stretch it between two fingers in a mucous string. This clear, slippery stuff facilitates the entry of sperm into the cervix at just the right time.

So when ovulation has happened and you've got no reason to let sperm or anything else into your cervix, the mucus thickens and becomes sparse and sticky, producing a tacky feeling as you tap it between your index finger and thumb. This barrier is not at all a fail-safe way of keeping sperm *out*, but it certainly inhibits their ease of passage *in* at a time when they're not going to do anything but get lost and die anyway.

If sperm do get in at the right time, and one does find its way to the egg and fuse with it, your cervix gets pretty interesting. Within days of this event, your cervix, which hardens and drops during the luteal (progesterone) phase, will become notably higher and soft and squishy. When Emily was pregnant with her third child, she discovered this fact for herself. Not everyone will have the same experience, but to think that one could identify pregnancy with the simple touch of a finger seems remarkable indeed.

The In Vitro Effect

There is so much science to parse through when a couple or individuals are considering assisted reproductive technology (ART) to become pregnant that they will need to consider all the evidence and their particular circumstances with a fertility specialist. But while they remain so focused on getting pregnant, they may think less about what happens after they get pregnant . . . or years down the line. Fortunately, the prospects for both look pretty good as far as researchers can tell. A 2015 study involving more than 1.35 million ART cycles found very low rates for the most serious possible complications: infection, hemorrhages requiring transfusion, moderate or severe ovarian hyperstimulation syndrome, hospitalizations, complications with anesthesia or a medication, or a mother's death within 12 weeks of the cycle. The most common of these was ovarian hyperstimulation syndrome (154 cases per 10,000 cycles over the decade studied), followed by hospitalizations (35 per 10,000 cycles).

As far as the developing fetus, the evidence has shown a small higher risk of congenital anomalies in children conceived through ART, but this risk appears more associated with what contributed to the fertility problems in the first place. Even so, the absolute risk of congenital anomalies remains very small. The baseline risk across all pregnancies for a congenital anomaly is approximately 3%, so the increased risk identified in one review of 20% translates to an adjusted risk of 3.6%—not even a full percentage point higher than the risk any pregnant woman faces for a baby carried to term.

And what about after the baby arrives? A number of studies have assessed children's mental, psychological, motor, cognitive, emotional, and social development up through at least 8 years old and found that children born following an IVF pregnancy fell within the normal range, with no significant differences compared to their non-IVF-born peers. Researchers have also identified positive family relationships among those born by IVF, and one review found that mothers of children born by IVF reported less parenting stress and more positive mother–child and father–child interactions than mothers of children conceived through sexual intercourse.

The Facts About Genetic Anomalies and Inheritance

Genes might be one of the most misunderstood concepts in biology. Perceived as discrete units or packets passed from parent to child as is, they are instead fluid structures consisting of small and large modules that can be changed and interchanged and even internally altered to produce a variety of possible outcomes from the same material.

The molecules that make up genes can be removed, added in, and substituted. These changes, which we call mutations, can have effects ranging from nothing at all to alterations big and small, good and bad.

The tiniest possible change in DNA is called a single nucleotide polymorphism, or SNP (pronounced "snip"). This kind of change consists of a removal or addition or substitution of a single alphabet letter, or base, in the DNA string. We're walking around with thousands of these little changes in our DNA that have no effect on us—that we know of. But some can be linked to phenotypes, including those for disorders and disease. These alterations might not themselves cause a disorder or disease, but researchers can look at these SNPs in hundreds or thousands of individuals and evaluate how many people with a specific letter in a particular spot have a specific condition. If more people with G than A in a given location on the DNA have condition X, then a researcher might say that a G there is associated with an increased risk of X.

In fact, if you've done the "mail your spit in a vial" thing with one of the companies that give you information about your risk for various health conditions, that's how they generate your risk profile. They take the studies that have reported an association between specific SNPs and increased or reduced risk for a condition, like lupus or heart disease. Based on your own sequence, these companies use this information to give you a risk value relative to the general population. So when you read something about "gene variants" or SNPs and a "link" to a condition, often it's these small variations between individuals that constitute the "variant" in the gene sequence.

The Relevance of Parental Gender

Many people think of biological sex in the animal kingdom as binary—male or female. But in fact, even anatomical sex can be a continuum. Sometimes both sexes exist in the same individual, and sometimes an individual starts as one sex and then morphs into another, whether for genetic or environmental reasons. The concept of gender, referring to the level of socially defined masculinity or femininity in one's identity—and which may or may not correspond with one's anatomical sex—similarly occurs along a spectrum and is even more fluid than sex. A person's gender identity arises from the extent to which they identify with masculine and feminine traits, or neither.

And how much does an individual's gender influence one's ability to parent? It doesn't. Credible studies suggest, for example, that the difference between having two same-sex parents or two opposite-sex parents, regardless of gender identity, has no effect on the quality of a child's upbringing. In 2013, the AAP stated that "children need secure and enduring relationships with committed and nurturing adults to enhance their life experiences for optimal social-emotional and cognitive development. Scientific evidence affirms that children have similar developmental and emotional needs and receive similar parenting whether they are raised by parents of the same or different genders."

Adoption

One of the first issues affecting the science around adoption is how personal and different every scenario is. Is it an international adoption? What is the child's birth country? Where did the child live before the adoption? Is it a cross-ethnic adoption? How old is the child? Is open adoption planned, or even a possibility? All these factors and many, many more play into adoption outcomes, including those related to the child's health and well-being.

Researchers urge that when considering the health and well-being of an adopted child, clinicians and parents have to be aware that some developmental outcomes may be different for the child, especially if the child experienced deprivation, isolation, instability, or other negative and stressful exposures before the adoption. Paying careful attention to any signs that a child is not developing typically allows for earlier support or intervention. Most children in international adoptions have spent their lives in orphanages, rather than in anything approximating a family home. According to studies of children adopted from Guatemala and China, younger children from foster care tend to fare better in terms of growth and cognitive testing than do children from orphanages. The longer a child spends in orphanage conditions, missing the early childhood window of forming strong family attachments, the greater the risk of struggles with attachment to the adoptive family. Indeed, age at adoption is a critical factor in general for the overall outcomes of an adoption. A UK study of more than 37,000 adoptions found that children who are age 4 years or older when adopted are at greater risk of experiencing a "disruption" of that adoption, researcher-speak for a premature separation from the adoptive family.

For younger children who are adopted, as with any major transition with an infant or young child, issues can arise around sleeping and eating. Developmental delays in internationally adopted children are not uncommon but generally don't tend to persist. Children whose early years are spent in institutional care do have delays in growth and head circumference but tend to catch up, especially the younger they are when adopted. Another consideration is that in open adoptions, parents can have some awareness of the mother's overall health, behaviors during pregnancy, and even family history, but for closed adoptions or international adoptions, these factors are unknown. Research suggests that a large number of internationally adopted children were born to mothers who received no prenatal care, and some of these children are exposed to a gamut of prenatal potential disruptors, including smoking, drugs, and alcohol. Given the conditions of care for many of these children, malnutrition or growth and developmental delays also are all common, and children can struggle with sensory integration problems from their early lack of attachment forming and of help with self-regulation.

As children make transitions, they will have emotional and physical responses, and there may be no transition as powerful as joining their new parents for the first time, no matter how that happens. A roller coaster may be the norm at first, with intense behaviors, sleep changes, bowel changes, and other shifts that need to be sorted out. And as with any experience involving all unfamiliar people, food, language, and surroundings, that sorting out and settling down takes time.

One of the features of a child who has spent time in an orphanage is what is known as "orphanage behaviors." Children who are left to their own devices to soothe can turn to some specific behaviors for self-soothing. These can include rocking, flapping, head banging, tooth grinding, and sensory seeking that seems atypical, such as smelling things closely. Generally, these behaviors resolve over time as a child, in the family setting, learns other ways of soothing, but his persistence warrants attention.

The developmental delays that are common in international adoptions are present in children from almost all countries. The long-term outcomes of these delays are not quite nailed down, but it is critical to let all your child's clinicians know about the adoption so that they can watch specifically for some delays and other manifestations that are common to this population of children. According to one review, motor delays tend to resolve pretty quickly while language and cognitive delays will require a longer catch-up time. A useful bit of US-based information is that community-based early intervention programs are typically available for internationally adopted children because of the frequency of such delays in this population.

And what about the parents? Not surprisingly, if the parent—or, at least for the existing studies, the mother—has preexisting symptoms of depression or if the child has fairly intense behavioral or emotional problems, stress on the mother in an international adoption is relatively high at 6 months post-adoption. Having more children in the family before the adoption also increases the risk for stress at this time point.

One thing that doesn't appear to have a negative influence on the adopted child and family is the gender of the adoptive parents, at least according to one study of 82 high-risk children adopted from US foster care into heterosexual or homosexual households. On a positive note, the children on average showed gains in cognitive development, regardless of household category. On another positive note, even though the gay and lesbian parents adopted children who had the highest biological and environmental risks, gains were similar between the household categories.

CHAPTER 2

Bun in the Oven

The Benefits and Risks of Embryonic and Fetal Screening and Tests

From the first peed-on stick to the fetal tracking during labor, modern-day pregnancy can seem like one long string of tests. In the first weeks, there's the pregnancy test itself, relying on detection in the urine or blood of a hormone (human chorionic gonadotropin, or hCG) that is present only if an embryo is implanted. There are the maternal tests for blood pressure, protein in the urine (a potential sign of preeclampsia), and gestational diabetes. And then there's the prenatal or fetal testing, designed to screen for or diagnose significant anomalies, such as chromosome conditions called aneuploidies (for example, trisomy 21, aka Down syndrome), or other conditions. Screenings can rely on blood tests and involve specialized ultrasounds to look for hints of developmental derailments. The consequences of these test results depend on individual decision-making.

What any expectant parents must understand about such testing is that the vast majority of initial tests, no matter how much they promise near 100% accuracy, are screening tests. They are not diagnostic. Screening determines how *likely* it is that a certain condition exists by relying on probabilities based on combinations of factors. Only diagnostic testing can *diagnose* that the condition certainly exists. The only tests that are truly diagnostic of a chromosome-based or other genetic condition involve direct sampling of fetal cells, such as amniocentesis. Thus, any result from prenatal screening tests that suggests an elevated risk for a developmental condition should always be followed up with diagnostic testing.

Although people often talk about screening results as "positive" or "negative," and we use those terms here, they are not very precise. A better framing would be "risk score," with a higher score implying a higher probability or risk. If someone uses "positive" or "negative" when talking about screening tests, keep in mind that those are inaccurate ways of characterizing any screening. As an example, a routine mammogram, which is a screening test, can help identify areas in the breast with visual risk factors for cancer, but a biopsy is used to give a definitive diagnosis. In the case of prenatal screening tests, rather than identifying a visual risk factor, most of them provide a statistical estimate of risk or probability that a certain condition is present.

> Screening determines how *likely* it is that a certain condition exists.

Many of these tests are now available for first- and early-second-trimester testing so that expectant women can find out about these probabilities early and pursue diagnostic testing, if needed. Initial tests involve blood draws to assess parental genetic factors, such as being a carrier for cystic fibrosis or other recessively inherited conditions. This testing is not diagnostic and gives parents only the probability of having a child with the genetic condition.

Cell-Free DNA Testing

At the cusp of the first and second trimesters, testing that screens the fetus itself for anomalies becomes possible. These noninvasive screenings, called cell-free DNA testing, involve detection and analysis of fetal DNA in the mother's blood. The DNA gets there because placental cells that undergo cell death during the normal course of development release these DNA fragments, which enter into the maternal blood. They are present in the mother's blood in much greater quantities than complete fetal cells and with advances in DNA sequencing, serve as a source for detecting fetal genetic anomalies.

This approach may seem foolproof at first because it uses DNA from an implanted embryo. But many variables can affect the outcome. The methods used to perform the sequencing include sequencing the entire genome, sequencing only targeted portions of the genome, or identifying single changes in the sequence that are associated with disease.

These tests basically add up the DNA present from specific chromosomes. If the amount for fetal chromosome 21 DNA exceeds the expected fetal-to-maternal ratio, extra copies of fetal chromosome 21 might be present. All these tests rely on properly done lab techniques and statistical analyses. And there's just the smallest chance that the cells that contributed to the placenta from the implanted embryo differ genetically from those that make up the embryo. For these reasons, these tests are still considered to be screening tests, with results that tell you only about risk and probability, not a diagnosis. In fact, these tests have yielded false-positives, suggesting a chromosomal abnormality when there isn't one.

For example, in a study of 5,974 samples applying one such commercially available test, false-positives were detected for Down (trisomy 21), Edwards (trisomy 18), and Patau (trisomy 13) syndromes. In a small number of cases, the test indicated a very strong probability of these conditions, but the fetal chromosome numbers were actually normal. The false-positive rate in some studies is about 0.5% for high-risk pregnancies, the population in which these tests were initially evaluated. The positive predictive value—meaning the probability that a positive result predicts an actual chromosomal abnormality—in high-risk pregnancies is 97.9%, which looks like a great number if you're talking about lottery tickets but leaves sufficient uncertainty for concern if you're talking about a fetus. That rate is even lower—less than 50%—in evaluations of some of these tests in low-risk patients.

In addition, there's also a fairly high rate of "non-reportable" results (meaning, not usable) of 1% to 5%, which vary depending on the type of pregnancy (high risk or not) and which methods are used. In one of these studies evaluating the test, for example, 3 of 1,471 samples were false-positive for Down syndrome (indicating trisomy 21 when the chromosome number was normal), and in 13 pregnancies, the testing failed; all those also had a normal chromosome number. In fact, non-reportable results occur more often among women whose fetus does have a chromosomal anomaly because the anomaly can affect placental size and the ratio of maternal-to-fetal DNA in the mother's blood, with the maternal DNA drowning out the fetal signal.

False-negatives are also possible; in studies evaluating the same test mentioned above, 3 of 212 fetal cases of Down syndrome were missed. Other reports suggest that some of these tests are more accurate for some trisomies (trisomy 21 and sometimes trisomy 18) than others (trisomy 13). One 2014 review notes that these tests are best validated in high-risk pregnancies (older women, family history) and for trisomies 21 and 18. Groups that represent genetic counselors and ob-gyns collectively have said that genomic prenatal testing could be appropriate in high-risk pregnancies in the context of appropriate counseling. There is still debate about whether these tests are appropriate in low-risk pregnancies, however, because the overall likelihood of these conditions is so low. Furthermore, the rate of false-positives in low-risk pregnancies may cause excess worry or more pregnancy losses because the diagnostic tests carry a tiny risk of miscarriage.

For these reasons, any woman having cell-free DNA testing done should understand that these screens report mathematical results, not diagnoses. If the screening shows concerning results, diagnostic testing would follow. Amniocentesis and chorionic villus sampling (CVS) are considered the gold standard for fetal diagnosis.

Amniocentesis and Chorionic Villus Sampling

These diagnostic tests aren't simply done in the first place because they are very invasive and carry their own, if relatively minimal, risks. In addition, amniocentesis is a second-trimester test, done between weeks 15 and 18 of the pregnancy. For women who might consider termination in the case of fetal abnormalities, that's after the first trimester abortion window. Amniocentesis has an extremely high diagnostic accuracy of 99.4% but carries a risk of miscarriage of approximately 1 in 350, although those values include procedures done using older techniques. CVS can be done as early as 10 weeks but also carries risks, including introducing defects in fetal fingers and toes; however, risk lessens the later the test is performed. CVS also carries a risk of miscarriage of approximately 1% (though the rate varies based on a woman's risk profile). Diagnostically, CVS is less accurate than amniocentesis, about 98% for chromosomal conditions. The chorionic villi arise from different cells (placental cells) than the rest of the embryo, and any changes that arose in these very early cells separately from the embryo or vice versa would not reflect the fetal condition accurately.

Ultrasound Screening

Ultrasound can also serve as a noninvasive screening tool for fetal anomalies. One such test is the nuchal ultrasound, which measures the thickness of a fluid-filled space on the back of the fetal neck. This space is a normal feature in every fetus, but in the presence of trisomy 21 and some other chromosomal conditions, it can be thickened, with a measurement of 3.5 millimeters or higher being an indication for diagnostic testing. The nuchal measurement is done toward the end of the first trimester. On its own, this measure isn't that great and has a 5% false-positive rate, but it is typically combined with blood values for human chorionic gonadotropin and pregnancy-associated plasma protein A to yield yet another statistically derived risk measure for these conditions. Specialized ultrasounds can also be used to screen for structural and other anomalies that might point the way to the diagnostic tests for chromosomal abnormalities. Ultrasound is not very accurate, however, as a stand-alone screening for chromosomal abnormalities.

Neural Tube Defect Screening and Other Biomarkers

With the exception of ultrasound, most of these screenings and diagnostic tests focus on identifying genetic and chromosomal anomalies. They do not address another major fetal development concern: neural tube defects, which are an incomplete development of the central nervous system, with outcomes that vary from no brain development at all (anencephaly) to gaps somewhere along the spinal cord (meningomyelocele, encephalocele, open spina bifida). Ultrasound late in the second trimester (18 to 20 weeks) will detect the vast majority of neural tube defects, but earlier detection is usually desired. In the second trimester, from 15 to 20 weeks, women undergoing standard prenatal care will find themselves offered the quad screen. The four measures in the quad are alpha-fetoprotein, human chorionic gonadotropin, a form of estriol (an estrogen), and inhibin-A. The results for each measure are considered along with gestational age to arrive at a probability score (for example, 1 in 500) for different conditions, including Down, trisomy 18, and neural tube defects.

Elevated alpha-fetoprotein is the critical biomarker for screening for neural tube defects, but the relevant values depend on ethnicity, maternal weight, and maternal diabetes, among other factors. For trisomies, this protein is usually lower than normal.

These tests require an accurate measure of gestational age, or the results can be off, and the sensitivity is not that impressive. Even when done with precision, these screenings still have a 5% false-positive rate. That means about 5 in every 100 pregnant women will experience unnecessary anxiety and further testing. In addition, this testing misses about 20 in every 100 cases of Down syndrome.

Things to consider in deciding whether to do these tests and which ones to do include your own particular risk factors for the conditions in the first place, how the testing might affect you emotionally (such as triggering anxiety), the risks of the diagnostic tests, and whether the results of the screenings or diagnostic tests will change any decisions you might make. Some women may want to pursue a termination while others may want to prepare for a birth differently, such as reaching out to support organizations. Regardless of how these individual factors differ for each woman, it's important that women ask their providers to explain the risks and benefits of any screening or test they might take and that they seek out more information regarding any possible fetal conditions before making further decisions.

What We Did: Emily had a specialized ultrasound screening with each pregnancy and what at the time was a triple screen in her third pregnancy. The results indicated no reason to pursue diagnostic testing. She declined amniocentesis, which was recommended during her pregnancy with her third son because she was high risk, a "geriatric" over age 35. Tara did all the prenatal screenings included with standard prenatal care, including ultrasounds. She also did the MaterniT21 test with her second, but for the two weeks it took for the results to return, she experienced high levels of anxiety, including a couple of anxiety attacks and crying bouts, due largely to how predictive the test can be.

AUTISM: WHAT WE KNOW ABOUT CAUSES

Autism research is an ever-changing landscape that features much speculation and misinformation. The evidence for the involvement of genetics in autism is strong. Scores of candidate gene changes have been identified. Identical twins, whose DNA sequences are the same, show the strength of the gene connection—if one twin is autistic, the other one has a 60% to 90% chance of also being autistic. (The studies vary, and no one study trumps another sufficiently to nail down the numbers.)

Autism is thought to begin during embryonic and fetal development. It may be that when the genes involved in brain development kick in, those with autism-related changes result in the development of an autistic brain—and person. Another possibility is that events during these critical periods of brain development, such as a maternal infection, might influence these pathways that lead to autism. The genetic changes involved generally trace to genes associated with brain development, nerve cell communication, and nerve cell connectivity, not unexpectedly.

No single study or group of studies unequivocally demonstrates that a set of gene changes or environmental factors or both leads to autism. And we have no rational reason to expect that it will be a single set. Rather, we will likely find many interactions of different gene variants under different environmental inputs—from the cell nucleus outward—that result in the varied manifestations of the condition we call autism.

Morning Sickness Management

Having nausea and vomiting during pregnancy is the norm for 80% to 90% of women and almost always starts in the first trimester. Although it lasts a little over a month on average, it can stretch all the way into the third trimester for up to half of women. It's also something of a misnomer: only about 2%

of women experience nausea and vomiting only in the morning. Yet for such a common malady, we understand little about it. The exact cause is unknown, though it may have to do with placental products because it correlates with a mother's placental mass and her hCG levels. Other possibilities include causes arising from estrogen and progesterone, thyroid problems, serotonin imbalances, and *Helicobacter pylori* infections.

But there is some good news that comes with all the retching. The common belief that having more nausea and vomiting is associated with a reduced risk of a miscarriage is backed by pretty good evidence. In one fairly large study, women with no nausea or vomiting at all were about 3 times more likely to have a miscarriage than those with any nausea or vomiting, and other studies found similar results. But once you're out of the miscarriage danger zone of the first trimester, it's less clear whether all that misery influences any other outcomes, such as birth weight, preterm delivery, or congenital anomalies. Preemies and stillbirths may be less likely, but the evidence isn't strong—unless it's a severe condition called hyperemesis gravidarum (HG), which we'll get to in a moment.

Younger women, first-time moms, and those with major depression or a history of migraines or motion sickness are more likely to experience nausea and vomiting. So what do you do about it? A recent Cochrane Review discussed several moderately effective treatments but ultimately concluded that we just don't have very much good information about what works. The evidence clearly shows that acupressure, acustimulation, and acupuncture don't work any better than placebo, and the evidence on chamomile, lemon, and mint oils is too sparse to parse.

The best evidence is for vitamin B6 and, if that doesn't help on its own, adding doxylamine (found in Unisom SleepTabs) can reduce symptoms by 70%. The newest drug approved by the FDA for nausea and vomiting in pregnancy, Diclegis, a combination of B6 and doxylamine, is considered safe.

The support for ginger isn't great, but a couple of trials have shown that it works almost as well as B6, whether it's ginger extract, ginger tea, or ginger ale. Ginger tended to help nausea the most without really changing how often women threw up and was not associated with an increased risk of miscarriage, heartburn, or drowsiness.

If vitamin B6 with doxylamine or ginger aren't cutting it, there are other pharmaceutical options, but these tend to be used only for those suffering from HG. HG affects about 1% of pregnant women, but it's serious. If you're vomiting more than 3 times a day or well past the first trimester and you're at risk for dehydration, it could be HG, which means seeking medical attention to rule out other possibilities (gastrointestinal illnesses, migraines, or liver or pancreatic diseases). HG can be life-threatening to a mother and her embryo or fetus because the severe dehydration can lead to electrolyte imbalance, severe weight loss, and excess ketones. Babies born to moms with HG are more likely to arrive early, have a low birth weight, and have a 5-minute Apgar score (see page 120) below 7 if their mothers also gained little weight (or lost weight). HG in a first pregnancy increases its likelihood in later pregnancies, and overall risk is 50% greater if the embryo or fetus is female.

A couple of drug options are available for HG. The most common, ondansetron (Zofran), isn't approved for treating nausea and vomiting in pregnancy but was designed for the nausea and vomiting from surgery, chemotherapy, or radiation therapy. One large study from Denmark (more than 600,000 women) found no increased risk for stillbirth, preterm birth, congenital anomalies, or underweight or low-birth-weight babies with this drug. The same researchers similarly found no increased risk of congenital anomalies, miscarriage, or stillbirth with metoclopramide, another common drug prescribed for HG. Aside from these, chlorpromazine, prochlorperazine, and promethazine are anti-nausea drugs considered sufficiently safe for pregnancy so far. Several antihistamines—diphenhydramine (Benadryl), meclizine (Antivert), and dimenhydrinate (Dramamine)—may (safely) help with nausea and vomiting, but scopolamine (an anti-nausea drug) and corticosteroids used in the first trimester are linked to congenital anomalies.

Pregnancy and Mood

While expecting her second child, Tara knew that the "baby blues," which affect up to 4 out of every 5 women, were largely the cruel effects of plummeting estrogen and progesterone while her body tried to remember what it was like not to incubate a baby. But postpartum changes hit her hard all the same. She couldn't focus on something as simple as a TV sitcom. She walked into the bathroom and forgot why she was there. She tried to ask her son's pediatrician a question and instead randomly started bawling.

These symptoms—the irritability, mood swings, crying, concentration problems—often fade quickly. Most baby blues resolve by the tenth day postpartum. But Tara remained vigilant about monitoring how she was feeling: her mental health history put her at higher risk for any of the more serious mental health conditions that can accompany pregnancy and the postpartum period. As it turned out, even after feeling better for a while, she did develop postpartum depression a few months later and knew to make an appointment right away.

Most women have heard of postpartum depression, though it may evoke for them the horror stories of women drowning their children or driving them off a bridge. Such severe, extreme cases of postpartum psychosis occur in about 1 in 1,000 women. But postpartum depression without psychosis is much more common; it's the most common complication with pregnancy, in fact. And it's not the only mental disorder associated with pregnancy; others include prenatal depression, postpartum anxiety (or panic) disorder, and, though rarer, postpartum obsessive-compulsive disorder. Fathers can experience prenatal and postpartum depression too.

These are genuine medical conditions that require treatment. It makes no more sense to say depression is "all in your head" than it does to say diabetes is "all in your kidneys." Pregnancy-related mental health conditions affect about 1 in 10 women (and men), and the risk factors are similar across the conditions. A personal or family history of depression, anxiety, bipolar disorder, or other mental disorders is an obvious risk factor: about half of all women with postpartum depression have a history of a previous depressive episode, and about a quarter to half of all women who experience postpartum depression once will experience it again. Unsurprisingly, women who have experienced domestic violence are at a higher risk for these disorders as well as post-traumatic stress disorder. Overweight and obese women may have a slightly elevated risk also: one study found that obese women have 1.4 times greater odds of prenatal depression and 1.3 times greater odds of postpartum depression.

A number of things might increase your risk of a mood disorder, though not all of these are agreed-upon risk factors: anxiety in pregnancy, gestational diabetes, having multiples (twins, etc.), being young and/or a first-time mom, experiencing relationship or financial problems, having an unplanned or unwanted pregnancy, lacking a support system, recent stressful life events or stressful events during the pregnancy or delivery, having unrealistic expectations of parenthood, a history of severe premenstrual syndrome, and, for those with a history of depression, insomnia during pregnancy. We discuss postpartum depression in further detail on page 149.

Prenatal Depression and/or Anxiety

Although most people have heard of postpartum depression, many may not have heard of prenatal depression even though it's about as common (7% to 14% of pregnant women). Tara experienced it, in part because of first trimester anxiety—the wait to progress to that critical second trimester—and in part because of concurrent circumstances and her mental health history. All-day morning sickness and the conflict of how she was "supposed" to feel (happy) about her planned pregnancy with how she felt (anxious) didn't help.

Having an unwanted pregnancy is one risk factor for prenatal depression. Even women who desperately wanted their pregnancy, however, can experience related depression without recognizing it because they haven't heard of it. Several of the symptoms, such as sleep disturbances, appetite changes, fatigue, and decreased sex drive, are common in pregnancy anyway, but in depression, they will usually be accompanied by feelings of guilt and hopelessness, poor self-esteem, an inability to enjoy oneself, and suicidal thoughts.

An additional challenge is the uneasiness many women have about taking antidepressants while pregnant even though many women's prenatal depression might actually be a relapse if they discontinued antidepressants before becoming pregnant, as Tara tried to do. Eventually, Tara decided that her inability to function wasn't worth the trade-off. And she likely would have returned to her medications anyway: one study found that women who stopped taking antidepressants before pregnancy were 5 times more likely to relapse while pregnant compared to women who continued taking them.

Even among women who continue taking antidepressants while pregnant, about a quarter of them will relapse. Changes in a woman's blood volume, liver metabolism, and kidney functioning while pregnant might affect drug concentrations in the blood. Indeed, blood levels of tricyclic antidepressants drop as much as 65% during pregnancy. Some women may therefore need to increase or otherwise tweak their dosage of tricyclic antidepressants or selective serotonin reuptake inhibitors (SSRIs) while pregnant—always under the guidance of their doctors.

In deciding whether taking medication is worth the risk, women also have to consider the risks posed by untreated depression and anxiety, such as poor nutrition, inadequate or excessive weight gain, poor prenatal care, and substance use—all of which can negatively impact the fetus. Further, prenatal depression can greatly increase the likelihood that a woman will experience postpartum depression and all the consequences for her and her family that come with it. Even the depression and anxiety itself—without other factors—can have a negative impact on a fetus.

For women without a history of previous depression or with mild to moderate depression or anxiety, medication may not be necessary, at least not right away. Cognitive behavioral therapy, interpersonal therapy, or other individual or group therapy is equally as or more effective than medication if you have the resources (time and money) to try therapy first. Some research has looked at estrogen therapy as a treatment, but the findings have been inconclusive, and estrogen can affect breast milk production and increase the risk of blood clots. Light therapy has not shown success, and the jury is still out on acupuncture, yoga, and exercise (there's simply not enough data). However, in conjunction with therapy and/or medication, exercise, sunlight, yoga, sufficient hydration, and a balanced diet may all help.

Stress in Pregnancy: It's Complicated

Studying stress in pregnancy is challenging because of the many interacting factors in the lives of women with major stressors and the many ways to measure stress. In fact, one review of 138 studies found that 85 different instruments were used to measure stress. With so many different ways to assess stress—and classifying it as acute or chronic, since there can be overlap—it's incredibly difficult to look at collective findings and reach any definitive conclusions.

If looking at stress and pregnancy outcomes has many interacting factors, assessing children's long-term outcomes has even more curve balls. The two biggest are disentangling prenatal exposures and early life experiences and teasing apart a shared genetic background. If a child has behavioral or cognitive difficulties, is that because of exposure to stress in the womb, conflict in the home after the birth, or inherited maternal gene variants that contributed to the mother's stress? For example, one study found higher levels of depression in 11-year-olds whose mothers had more stress during pregnancy—but the same study found having a younger mom, having a lower IQ, or experiencing recent bullying were also related to depression. It's hard to control for all those contributing factors to pinpoint the role of mom's pregnancy stress.

Still, one recent review suggested that up to 15% of a child's emotional or behavioral problems might be related to stress and anxiety a mother experienced while pregnant, even after taking into account all the other contributing factors. And we're starting to learn more about chemical and hormonal changes during pregnancy that might explain that. We know a mother's cortisol levels correlate with a fetus's cortisol levels, for example, but that link is weaker earlier in pregnancy and strengthens with each trimester, so perhaps stress earlier in pregnancy has less impact. It's not clear. We also don't know how much mom's diet might play a role. Another study found poorer cognitive outcomes and greater "fearfulness" in children of mothers under chronic stress while pregnant, especially stress involving a partner. But there is no reliable way to completely disentangle prenatal stress effects from how those mothers might influence their children after birth—especially if the stress is still a part of that family's life.

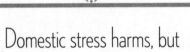

Domestic stress harms, but support networks help.

What we do know, however, is that the most detrimental stress is relationship stress with a partner and that a strong social support system reduces the risk of preterm birth or low birth weight. A large body of research shows that domestic stress harms, but support networks help. The big takeaway, then, is not to stress over stress—especially stress you cannot control—but that seeking out a support network, particularly with relationship stress, can improve outcomes for you and your child.

Prescription Drugs in Pregnancy

The first thing to recognize when it comes to taking medications during pregnancy or while breastfeeding is that every question is based on assessing the risks and benefits of taking and of not taking the medication. It is virtually impossible to find a medication that would be considered 100% safe to take while pregnant. Some women might still need to take medications with known negative side effects during pregnancy because *not* treating their condition can cause more serious problems for the mother, fetus, or both. For example, antiepileptic drugs that are taken for epilepsy or bipolar disorder, such as valproate or valproic acid (Depakote), can have serious negative effects for the embryo or fetus, including neural tube defects. Although many women would be best off discontinuing these medications during pregnancy because of fetal risk, for some women, the frequent seizures valproate prevents would put them or their fetus at greater risk than the medication would.

Obtaining reliable data about pregnant women is difficult because they are rarely participants in clinical drug trials, for good reason: it often would be unethical to test a drug on a pregnant woman without knowing whether it might harm the baby. However, excluding pregnant women from most clinical trials also largely leaves women and doctors in the dark about what drugs can be used relatively safely—or not.

So where do we get any safety data about medications in pregnancy? Some come from women in clinical trials who didn't know they were pregnant initially, but most evidence comes from case–control studies (comparing women who did and didn't take a medication after the fact), which involve a lot of uncontrolled confounding factors (explained on page 306), and animal studies, which don't involve people.

These limitations have led to conflicting or inconclusive findings, something especially seen with antidepressants. Sometimes, even when it appears that a small risk to the embryo or fetus may exist, it's so small that it's tough to rule out all the other possibilities that could have explained that risk. About 3% of all newborns in the general population have congenital anomalies (about 10% of these are caused by drug exposures), so a drug that results in 3.5% of newborns with defects increases the risk only a tiny amount, and that tiny amount may be related to other factors that a study doesn't adequately account for. A drug might also present different risks at different points during the pregnancy, making measurement even tougher. Aspirin products, for example, are riskier in the third trimester than earlier in pregnancy. At present, for more than 80% of the 400 to 500 drugs approved by the US Food and Drug Administration (FDA) in the past 20 years, doctors do not have enough evidence to clearly know the risks to the baby of the mother's taking these drugs while pregnant.

Despite all these challenges, the FDA had attempted to provide some guidance regarding medications during pregnancy with a classification system beginning in the 1970s. Five categories—A, B, C, D, and X—represented levels of safety and evidence for different drugs, and any number of websites found through a search could tell women what category a particular drug was in. However, at the end of 2014, the FDA abandoned this system in lieu of a new one . . . with no categorization at all. Over the next several years, the FDA will phase in a new system in which all drugs approved since 2001 will include pregnancy and lactation subheadings of "Risk summary, Clinical considerations, and Data" in the prescribing information healthcare professionals receive from manufacturers.

The FDA's reasoning is sound: consumer feedback had conveyed that the categories were overly simplistic and confusing, and we agree. But the change introduces new problems: it's not clear where this information will be on over-the-counter medications, whether patients will be able to easily find it for prescription medications, what this means for any medications approved before 2001, or how frequently the new labels will be updated with new data. Regardless, it will take several years for the changes to occur, so for now, we are banking on the assumption that most women, and even clinicians, will continue to rely at least in part on the ABCDX classifications. The labyrinthine FDA website will include updates as the new system is implemented, but we've described the older system here since it will likely live on for years to come on websites and on labels.

Unfortunately, very few medications are in Category A, composed of drugs that well-controlled studies have shown do not pose a risk to the embryo or fetus. Category B includes most of the medications your obstetrician or midwife would approve of, such as Benadryl, Zyrtec, Pepcid, and Zantac. For these drugs, animal studies have not shown a risk in utero, and observational studies in pregnant women so far have not shown risks, though not enough evidence from well-controlled studies in pregnant women exists.

Category D includes drugs that we know carry fetal risks based on past studies but which also may offer enough of a benefit to some women that they may still be taken. Most antiepileptics, as mentioned previously, are Category D. Ibuprofen is Category B up until the last trimester, when it becomes Category D. Category X medications are those that absolutely should *not* be taken during pregnancy under any circumstances. These include thalidomide, the acne medication Accutane (isotretinoin), the class of antibiotics known as tetracyclines, the antifungal drug fluconazole (name brand Diflucan), and blood pressure drugs known as ACE (angiotensin-converting enzyme) inhibitors.

Vitamins, minerals, and compounds in herbs are biologically active, so it's also important to check on the safety of these before using them during pregnancy. A more complete list of all the drugs that are known to cause minor or significant congenital anomalies or complications can be found on the FDA website. The term to search for is "teratogen," which describes substances known to cause harm to a fetus.

That leaves the great big Category C, a problematic category (and probably the reason for the FDA's shift to a new system): either studies have shown negative effects in animal studies but we have no good human data, or we have no good data from animal or human studies and we just don't know. It's usually Category C drugs, including several antidepressants, that send women in circles trying to decide whether the benefit the medication offers is worth hints in the limited data of some kind of risk.

Of course, drugs may be miscategorized. Some medications, such as tricyclic antidepressants, are labeled as Category D even though available data so far appear to show that these medications are safe for pregnancy. Most drugs are classified before extensive animal or human data are available, making the information less reliable, and classifications rarely change even after more data become available.

Because we cannot cover all drugs, we address some common classes of drugs, such as antiepileptics and stimulants for ADHD, on our website, TheInformedParentBook.com, and only briefly touch on pain-killers and antidepressants here. For medications that treat chronic conditions we don't address, including allergies, high blood pressure, diabetes, acid reflux, and high cholesterol, there are usually Category B or sometimes widely used, considered-safe-enough Category C medications available. (Exceptions are the most common medications used for high cholesterol, the Category X drugs Lipitor and Zocor.) You can check a drug's (former) category on the website SafeFetus.com. We cover marijuana during pregnancy in the section relating to alcohol, since both drugs are used recreationally (see page 48).

Important Note: We address vaccines during pregnancy—specifically the flu and pertussis vaccines—in the vaccines section on page 115.

Pain-killers

Pregnancy can sometimes be a nonstop ride through Painville. Back pain, aching hips, swelling ankles, headaches, burning sensations . . . sometimes you just want some relief. But because we lack a convenient selection of Category A pain meds, we're left sifting through the evidence to decide what we can take without harming that little creature we're incubating.

First, realize that the condition causing pain can sometimes cause adverse effects for the fetus too, requiring a balancing of risks. Despite what you may have heard about the epidemic of prescription narcotic use during pregnancy, for example, these medications can be safely taken when truly medically necessary and under a doctor's supervision. But most women will reach for over-the-counter meds, usually nonsteroidal anti-inflammatory drugs, or NSAIDs (aspirin, ibuprofen, and naproxen) or acetaminophen (Tylenol). The data on NSAIDs are mixed for early pregnancy, but not for the third trimester, when these meds can wreak all kinds of havoc: delaying labor, increasing maternal blood loss during birth, and causing maternal anemia, fetal hypertension, fetal kidney problems, and premature closure of a blood vessel that diverts blood away from a fetus's underdeveloped lungs until birth.

But tried-and-true acetaminophen offers good news: in pretty solid studies, there's no evidence that it causes congenital anomalies, including in one recent one with more than 88,000 women. In fact, some research shows serious congenital anomalies to be a higher risk among those with fever or infection who don't treat it with acetaminophen. Although researchers had once linked prenatal exposure to acetaminophen with asthma in childhood, later research has shown that other factors explain the association (usually the reason mom is taking the medication). So there's no convincing evidence at present that using acetaminophen as directed during pregnancy is something to worry about, and using it to treat a serious condition might reduce the risk of congenital anomalies. The only concern with acetaminophen is overdose, and the best way to avoid an overdose is to take it as directed and to check the labels of other medications used in combination, such as cold medicines, which often include acetaminophen as an ingredient.

Antidepressants

By the time we know how—if at all—antidepressants affect a fetus, we'll probably be growing babies outside the human body and the whole question will be moot. But until then, we must grapple with an incomplete risk–benefit equation because we lack sufficient information to make a truly informed choice—though it's not for lack of trying. Few drugs have been studied for use during pregnancy as much as antidepressants, especially the most commonly prescribed ones, SSRIs. But the mountains of evidence are inconclusive, contradictory, and sometimes rife with bias, leading to an unending controversy over whether antidepressants actually negatively affect a fetus.

In exploring those mountains, we found a small but statistically significant increased risk does exist for a few conditions: low birth weight, preterm birth, or some congenital anomalies, including several heart defects. The absolute risk of these is very low—less than 1% for congenital anomalies—and the increase in risk is so small that it's hard to tease out whether it's from the medication, the underlying condition being treated, or another factor. But a whole other solid body of research has found similar increased risks with untreated depression and anxiety in the mother, and it's impossible to control for the very condition being treated. Further, untreated mood disorders can be life-threatening—the fetus rarely makes it if the mom doesn't.

So here's the nutshell: presently, there is not convincing evidence that SSRIs cause miscarriages. There's not much convincing evidence that SSRIs cause more congenital anomalies than untreated depression, anxiety, and similar conditions. Up to a third of newborns exposed to antidepressants during pregnancy will experience neonatal withdrawal, which is usually mild, doesn't require treatment, fades within a week, and may be lessened with breastfeeding. Not much evidence exists on long-term outcomes, but what does exist suggests that a mother's present mood affects children's mood and behavior more than prenatal antidepressant exposure does. But the confusion will continue here because the interacting factors and the potential for bias are high. If there were major concerns about treating mood or anxiety disorders with antidepressants, however, it would have shown up in the thousands of existing studies (see page 33).

Sex During Pregnancy: Can You Do It? Do You Want To?

Let's take the second question first: Do you want to? Obviously, the answer will vary from woman to woman. But studies addressing this question largely indicate that women feel the influence of a lot of factors weighing on, and against, their sexual urges during pregnancy. These factors appear to be cross-cultural and often linked to the physically evident changes of pregnancy. Studies suggest that sex is more frequent earlier in pregnancy, and a growing belly as a physical impediment might be an obvious explanation for, say, less inventive couples as the third trimester progresses. But it's not as simple as "there's a belly between us."

Couples tend to fear harming the baby (you won't, unless you've got a condition that expressly requires you to abstain, something to discuss with your clinician). Just being aware of a pregnancy, according to one cross-sectional study of 130 married pregnant women in the first trimester, can affect how often a woman has sex. That report, relying on responses to a questionnaire and a sexual function assessment scale, suggested that simply knowing of the pregnancy led to reduced arousal, lubrication, and satisfaction scores for these women in early pregnancy. In other words, women who didn't know they were pregnant had more sex and thought it was better than women who did know, even though all the women were in the first trimester.

Nevertheless, while sex might be more frequent in the first trimester, women who can get around barriers related to mechanics, physical appearance, and concerns about urinary incontinence report having greater satisfaction with third-trimester sex compared to first-trimester sex. So there's that to look forward to, as long as those awareness factors don't get you down.

A popular scale used in these studies is the Female Sexual Function Index. One study that applied this scale also addressed intercourse patterns across trimesters and found again that frequency declined as the pregnancy progressed. Almost 40% of the women in that study expressed concern that sex would be harmful in some way, and more than a third of their male partners had the same concern. When both partners have this fear, it's no surprise that sex takes a backseat, and not in the fun "with a blanket under the stars" way. The authors of this study note the low rate of women who talked about sex and sexuality with their healthcare providers, a common theme across investigations that address that question. And that takes us to question two . . .

Is It Safe?

The short answer is yes, unless you have a specific medical reason to avoid it. Always talk to your clinician about this important aspect of quality of life and relationships.

One reason to engage with your healthcare practitioner about these issues is that the factors driving your choice to abstain might be related to your mental health. One study that found a link between number of pregnancies and sex-related outcomes also found that having high scores for depression symptoms on a depression scale, especially early and late in pregnancy, was a strong predictor of struggles with sexual function in pregnancy.

What About That Semen–Cervix Thing?

You might have heard somewhere in the mommy-to-be rumor mill that semen contains factors that prime the cervix, soften it, bring on labor, or achieve other outcomes that can seem miraculous to the very-late-third-trimester woman with the weight of a bowling ball straining her lumbar spine. Unfortunately for the hopeful out there, a Cochrane Review from 2001 concluded that sexual intercourse as a way to induce labor remains an area of uncertainty.

Because how often women have sex is apparently more interesting than how they get the baby out, little research is even available on this subject. A 2006 study also found no effect of intercourse on labor induction or cervical ripening. The specific question of semen was not addressed, but another study from the same year did find that women having self-reported sex at term had reduced rates of induction at 41 weeks and an earlier onset of labor. If this were a Cochrane Review, we'd still have to conclude that having sex as a labor-induction method still lacks a solid evidence base, but, hey . . . why not try it?

Alcohol and Caffeine: To Drink or Not to Drink

Caffeine

For most women, abstaining from drinking alcohol during pregnancy should not be a big ask. Most people don't need alcohol to get them through the day, and if they do, that's indicative of a much bigger problem. But coffee? Are such drastic measures necessary to assure a healthy pregnancy?

Current recommendations suggest that pregnant women limit caffeine to 200 milligrams a day. Various sites will help you figure out how much that is for your preferred caffeine source, but it generally averages out to one of the following: about two 8-ounce cups of coffee, three to four 8-ounce cups of black tea, four cups of green tea, six cans of caffeinated soda, or a single 5-hour energy shot. Other sources of caffeine you might not think about include some prescription medications (such as pain relievers) and chocolate (about 100 milligrams in a cup of semisweet chocolate chips, for example). However, this recommendation seems a bit arbitrary and based on the precautionary principle when considering the evidence.

Caffeine and alcohol studies have some factors in common. Data collection is often based on women's reports, which can be subject to forgetfulness, misreporting, and intentional and unintentional bias. Many studies don't ask women about taking pain relievers or their chocolate intake, neglecting a possible source of caffeine that could affect the results. Alcohol and coffee drinkers tend to smoke more and share a variety of other health behaviors that nondrinkers don't share, behaviors that often aren't considered in studies. Furthermore, a majority of women change their intake after they find out they're pregnant, and those who make no changes may share behaviors that others don't.

The biggest confounding factor for caffeine–pregnancy studies is nausea and vomiting from pregnancy. Despite Tara's passionate, lifelong love affair with coffee, even smelling java risked making her vomit for the first half of her pregnancy. (Emily didn't drink caffeine during pregnancy.) It's difficult to figure out what role coffee and caffeine might play with miscarriage because even hard-core coffeeholics will forgo their favorite drink if they feel too sick to drink it. Because first-trimester nausea is associated with reduced miscarriage risk, nausea-wracked, now-caffeine-abstinent moms may be more likely to carry a healthy pregnancy to term—but is it because of quitting caffeine or is the nausea the real factor in the healthy pregnancy? Although the majority of findings from early studies found a higher risk of miscarriage with increased caffeine intake, the big nausea confounder makes their conclusions unreliable.

A pair of studies in 2008 that tried to account for the nausea problem and correct for other confounders came to opposing conclusions. One study of more than 1,000 women found a dose-related increased miscarriage risk with caffeine intake, but several research letters criticized the weaknesses of this study related to its confounders. The other study involved more than twice as many women, but adjusted for many of the same factors, and found no evidence of an increased risk of pregnancy loss at any point for any amount of caffeine.

A 2014 meta-analysis of 53 studies found a small increased risk of miscarriage—an extra 14% per 100 milligrams of caffeine—but the authors concluded that this finding and other already pretty modest risk increases for stillbirth, preterm birth, and low birth weight were most likely a result of confounders and bias in study designs. Another meta-analysis and a separate study of almost 60,000 women likewise found nothing to support a link to preterm birth.

That latter study did, however, find that lower birth weight is linked to caffeine intake: each 100 milligrams of caffeine per day was associated with a birth-weight reduction of 21 to 28 grams (around 0.05 pounds), and drinking more than 200 milligrams of caffeine per day increased the risk of an underweight baby by almost 50% compared to drinking 50 milligrams or fewer. These results are supported by those of another meta-analysis and a randomized controlled trial. These studies had the same limitations as the caffeine–miscarriage research, but their findings are a little more reliable because there's no known link between nausea and birth weight.

Alcohol

Few pregnancy restrictions are more debated than how much—if at all—a woman can drink during pregnancy. Despite tens of thousands of studies on the subject, the question for many women remains: Can I have a glass of wine with dinner? Can I have one glass a week? One glass a day? A beer at a weekend conference and that's it? The problem in trying to answer these questions is that the state of scientific research, as it is currently, is not (yet) equipped to answer such finely specific questions for each individual woman. The variables— genetic, environmental, psychological, etc.—are almost endless. But the evidence base does provide us with enough to lay out what we know and allow women to make their own decisions about whether to have a sip or a half glass or a glass of wine, or not. And we have to emphasize, perhaps more than in any other section of the book, we are not making any recommendations about what women should do. We'll relate what scientists have found to date and the limitations and considerations relevant to that knowledge.

When we discuss drinks, we use what most researchers use: one drink is about 0.6 ounces or 14 grams of absolute alcohol, which translates to about one beer, one 5-ounce glass of wine, or 1.5 ounces of liquor.

Alcohol supersedes tobacco, marijuana, cocaine, heroin, and pretty much any other non-pharmaceutical substance you can dream of in terms of how it can damage a developing baby in the womb. Fetal alcohol spectrum disorders, first identified in the 1970s, now comprise approximately 1% of all births in the United States, and the range of disabilities resulting from heavy, binge, or even moderate drinking during pregnancy can be devastating. While many people recognize the physical characteristics associated with Fetal Alcohol Syndrome (FAS), somewhere around 85% of individuals with prenatal alcohol exposure lack these physical features but have neurological, cognitive, developmental, or behavioral problems.

A developing embryo or fetus cannot metabolize alcohol—the organs aren't developed enough—and in both animal and Petri dish studies, alcohol interferes with cell function and normal brain development. All this cell hijacking manifests through attention, memory, and behavior difficulties in kids exposed in the womb to one-half to three drinks a day.

> A developing embryo or fetus cannot metabolize alcohol.

But maybe all you want is two or three glasses a week, or heck, one glass on Saturday nights. What effect would that have?

More than a dozen studies, some quite large and well conducted, have found no association between light drinking in pregnancy, such as a couple of glasses or fewer a week, and various negative outcomes. But each of these studies had some significant limitations. As with caffeine intake, alcohol intake is usually self-reported because no biomarkers are available to track ethanol intake. Self-report involves several limitations, including concern about stigma, knowledge of how much ethanol an alcoholic beverage contains, or how much was in a drink (mixed drinks, for example, can be quite variable in ethanol content), and when the mothers were asked (during or after pregnancy).

These studies typically use child behavior as an end point, which carries three main disadvantages. First, the measures usually are done in young children, which can be too soon for some behaviors to show up. (One study found 60% of 10-year-olds with FAS had attention problems, but only 10% of them showed those problems at age 5.) Second is the same old self-report issue, except in this case its parent report, which is subject to bias and other problems. (In one large study, teacher data showed a link between poor behavior and drinking during pregnancy, but parent data did not.) And finally, multiple studies found dose-response effects—the more mothers drank, the greater the impact on their kids—but it requires very sensitive tests to detect small effects.

Finally, we're all different, from person to person, with genetic and other background factors interacting by the hundreds to affect outcomes. Demographics and lifestyle can be huge confounders. As we already noted, heavy drinkers also tend to smoke more. Light drinkers tend to exercise more. How do we tease apart these and other factors and isolate ethanol intake only? As an example, of the hundreds of abstracts and dozens of studies we read on this topic, the most important paper, in 2013, did not involve children at all: it looked exclusively at mothers and illustrated the ultimate limitations for all other studies (and of course had limitations itself). More than 63,000 Danish mothers reported their drinks while pregnant, which were totaled across their whole pregnancy: 0, 0 to 10, 10–30, 30–90, and more than 90. Then they reported a huge range of other factors: their age, the child's father's age, marriage status, owning a home, their education, the father's education, various psychological and psychiatric measures and diagnoses, their pre-pregnancy weight, any diabetes or asthma or anemia they suffered in pregnancy, and how much they smoked cigarettes, ate fish, drank coffee, drank cola, watched TV, exercised, binge drank, or took vitamins, iron supplements, fish oil, pain relievers, or sleeping medications during pregnancy. Among a host of fascinating factors, owning a home was linked to less drinking, yet none of the other studies we assessed included this as a confounding factor. In addition, compared to the whole group, all-time abstainers were less likely to eat fish or exercise, more likely to watch TV and drink cola, and more likely to be overweight, have asthma or diabetes, or have a mental health condition. Pregnancy-only abstainers were more likely to pop vitamins and less likely to have anemia. Yet pregnancy-only abstainers and all-time teetotalers are often collapsed into a single group in studies on alcohol and pregnancy. It's easy to see how teetotalers' higher rate of psychological problems—a known risk factor for increased behavioral problems in children—might cancel out the ability to detect any possible behavioral effects among the children of light drinkers in pregnancy, especially when light drinkers typically have more education, higher incomes, healthier weights, and more fish on the dinner table. In fact, without exception, every single study that included women who drank just 1 to 3 or 4 drinks a week during pregnancy found that those women were wealthier, healthier (physically and mentally, when assessed), and better educated. Math is only so good, so statistical modeling cannot erase all that influence. "Residual confounding" will remain after adjusting for those factors.

Let's pretend for a moment that we have a magical mathematical formula that considers everything that could possibly differ among women's lifestyles, circumstances, or environments. Enter the final monkey wrench: a study in 2012 that looked at how both mom's and her child's genetics play a role in alcohol's possible effects during pregnancy. Twin studies had long ago found that alcohol does not reach both fetuses equally, perhaps related to where they are situated relative to the placenta. But how alcohol affects a fetus depends on the length of exposure, which depends on how well the mother and fetus each metabolize ethanol, which depends partly on four genetic variants identified in this study of more than 4,000 children. Some variants lead the body to metabolize the alcohol more quickly and some more slowly. The researchers looked at these genes in both mothers and their children and measured the children's IQ at age 8. For each of the four variants the children had, their IQ dropped almost two points on average—but only if their mothers drank 1 to 6 drinks a week. The children of mothers who abstained during pregnancy, even if they had all four variants, showed no difference in IQ.

Because this is the first study of its kind, it's impossible to know what the lowest threshold of alcohol is that interacts with these genetic variants. Because they deal specifically with metabolism, it may not require much alcohol if the problem relates to how long that small amount sticks around.

What do other studies on light drinking show? We know that the two most harmful kinds of drinking—aside from ongoing heavy drinking throughout a pregnancy—are binge drinking (even one episode of at least 4 to 5 drinks in one sitting) and any drinking during the first trimester, both of which show worse outcomes compared to occasional drinking during the second and third trimesters. In terms of pregnancy outcomes, women who had at least 1 drink a day had more miscarriages, especially during the second trimester, than women who drank less. There aren't enough data to determine definitely when the miscarriage risk increase vanishes, but one study found that 2 to 3 drinks a week increased the risk of miscarriage 66% in the first trimester and 57% in the early second trimester. Similarly, 10 or more drinks a week increased the risk of preterm birth, but the findings are inconsistent regarding drinking less than this.

A 2014 meta-analysis of 34 studies found some evidence that less than daily drinking might still influence child behavior. Among the issues identified were children having difficulty with self-regulation, interactive play, and needing more attention. The study found nothing consistent, however, to show mild or moderate drinking affected children's attention, cognition, language skills, or visual or motor development. One tiny study actually looked directly at the brains of 11 individuals exposed to alcohol in the womb. In the four mothers who drank between 0.1 and 0.49 ounces of pure alcohol a day (0.6 ounces is a single drink) and never binge drank, neuroimaging showed reduced gray matter in six parts of the fetal brain.

Then there are the studies finding no effects on children of mothers who had as little as 1 drink a week during pregnancy. We'll look at three of the best conducted and most cited ones.

The first, involving more than 10,500 children in the UK, compared women who have never drunk, who didn't drink only during pregnancy, who drank lightly during pregnancy (no more than 1 to 2 drinks per week or per occasion), who drank moderately (no more than 3 to 6 drinks per week or 3 to 5 per occasion), and who drank heavily (at least 7 drinks a week). The researchers accounted for a wide range of factors, even including parents' mental health and discipline strategies and mothers' attachment with their children. They measured kids' behavioral and cognitive outcomes when the kids were 3, 5, and 7 years old. About a quarter of the moms were light drinkers, and as in other studies, were more socioeconomically advantaged than mothers in all other categories. The researchers identified hyperactivity and behavioral and emotional problems in children of the heavy drinkers but found no difference in cognitive, behavioral, or developmental concerns between the kids of light drinkers and mothers who normally drank but were abstinent in pregnancy (they separated these from those who were always abstinent).

Sounds great, right? Here are the problems: the kids have been tracked to only 7 years old, well before many problems in alcohol-affected children develop. The data on children's behavior are based on mothers' reporting, and the tests may not be sensitive enough to pick up differences. The children of light drinkers were born into the most financially stable households with the most resources and the most capable parents—statistical modeling cannot adequately fully account for that. Finally, drinking was based on maternal self-report when the babies were 9 months old. The moms might have underreported, misremembered (insert "mom brain" joke here), or subconsciously misreported, since 9-month-olds already show individuality in their temperaments.

The second study often cited by those who contend light, occasional drinking during pregnancy is low risk followed the children of 2,900 mothers in Australia from pregnancy through age 14, with five assessments over the years. Occasional drinking meant up to a single standard drink a week, and light drinking meant 2 to 6 drinks a week. Similarly, the researchers found no effects on children's behavior among occasional and light drinkers.

Ready for the problems? One-third of the originally enrolled mothers were lost to follow-up—and these mothers mostly had lower income and education levels, the exact population in which you would be more likely to see any effects from small alcohol exposure. The authors also did not control for mothers' mental health. Since nondrinkers tend to have poorer mental health as a group, it's possible any effect in the occasional drinking group was cancelled out by the effects on children of mothers with mental health conditions. Finally, again, mothers reported both their own drinking and their children's behavior. But the biggest red flag? This study also did not find more behavior problems among children of heavy drinkers (11 or more drinks a week). Since behavioral problems in children of heavy drinkers is pretty well established, this result calls into question all the other findings in this study.

Finally, a group of five studies involved 1,628 Danish 5-year-olds who underwent a battery of tests for IQ, attention, executive function, and behavior. The researchers focused on mothers who had 1 to 4 drinks a week and controlled for mothers' smoking, number of children, education, pre-pregnancy weight, marital status, and IQ, plus the family home environment (including childcare situation, regularity of eating breakfast, and mothers' depression), children's health, and children's hearing and vision on the day of the assessment. As with the other two studies, they found no effects in the kids of light drinkers, though the authors themselves suggested their methods might have simply failed to find an effect that actually exists. But again, the kids were tested at 5 years old, before many effects may show up. And again, the authors found no association with binge drinking either. If they missed problems resulting from binge drinking, what else did they miss?

We could spend all day looking at every single study that found no link between behavior problems and light drinking, however it is defined (in fact, we spent several days doing exactly that with more than a dozen studies). But despite how large and well conducted many of these studies are, we find that every study detecting effects shows a linear association between the effect and alcohol exposure with no flattening out at lower levels. The greatest effects are seen with drinking in the first trimester, but they're still seen all the way until the end of the last trimester.

If you're freaking out right now because you had a few drinks before you knew you were pregnant, hang on. The three studies above and others like them can reassure moms who already drank before they knew they were pregnant that effects in their children until that point would be so negligible that they won't be easily detectable. Whatever negative consequences might exist would be subtle and potentially offset by the positive influence of other factors.

It's a tricky balance to say these studies can provide reassurance but perhaps might need to stop short of providing justification for a weekly drink, but there's also a problem with saying that any amount of alcohol during pregnancy, no matter how little, is serious cause for concern. That is, the stigma, stress, and blame it places on those who drank alcohol before they knew they were pregnant can have its own harms. One of Tara's friends found out she was pregnant a few weeks after New Year's, when she had downed a couple of glasses of wine. Her next several weeks were filled with anxiety attacks and stress about the damage she might have caused the embryo. In reality, the negative effects of that stress and anxiety may have exceeded whatever possible negative effects the 3 drinks over 5 hours on New Year's Eve caused.

It is possible to acknowledge that even small amounts of alcohol might harm a fetus while not heaping shame and blame on mothers who have already drunk while pregnant. It's likewise possible to recognize that a small or moderate amount of alcohol exposure before you knew you were pregnant may not have any significant clinical effects in your child while not presuming that a couple more drinks will have no effect at all.

Bottom line: no lower threshold of alcohol consumption has been shown to be "safe" or "no risk" to a developing fetus, and any amount of alcohol consumed by a pregnant woman will cross the placenta. If you're exposed, your baby is. But it's also not clear at what levels and with what timing of exposure we start to see clinical evidence of a risk in differences that we can actually detect. Just because we can't detect them doesn't mean they're not there; it just means we can't see them. Given the known effects of alcohol on developing cells, any amount of alcohol almost certainly has some effect, but the extent of it is uncertain. Few people, for example, would probably claim that a woman ingesting a teaspoon of wine would have any real impact on a fetus. Or 2 teaspoons. But what about a tablespoon? Or 5 tablespoons? Furthermore, some women, despite intending to drink only a half glass of wine, may actually pour more than a "half" glass if they're using a large glass—it's easy to overpour and not realize it. Ultimately, if there is a "safe" lower threshold of how much alcohol a pregnant woman can drink and have absolutely no effect on her embryo or fetus, we may never know what it is.

Marijuana

At the time of this book's writing, 23 states had legalized medical marijuana, including 4 where recreational use is legal. Unfortunately, it's difficult to determine the possible effects of cannabis during pregnancy since so many pot users also drink and smoke and are less likely to get prenatal care. Aside from two small, poorly conducted Jamaican studies suggesting no effect, better quality research has identified several patterns linked to cannabis exposure before birth: hyperactivity, impulsivity, and attention problems are more common past age 3, and verbal, memory, problem-solving, and math skills showed up later, after accounting for other factors, in children of moms who smoked marijuana in pregnancy. Although no studies look at marijuana use outside of smoking it, recent research on tetrahydrocannabinol (THC), the active ingredient in marijuana, strongly suggests it could interfere with fetal brain development in the exact spots you'd expect for future attention and hyperactivity problems. And since most research focuses on kids born several decades ago, before the potency of pot picked up, the findings may actually underestimate the effects today's Mary Jane might have on little Mary or little Jane.

Kitty Litter, Sushi, and Brie: Understanding Environmental Exposure Risks

One of the most frustrating things for Tara about pregnancy was forgoing some of her most cherished activities. Her favorite way to relax is a superhot bath with a healthy glass of red wine and a plate of crackers with Brie or Camembert cheese. Let's see: hot bath, red wine, soft cheese. If the guidelines frequently passed out to pregnant women are taken at face value, about the only thing she could do while pregnant was to take a warm shower and then have some crackers. Emily only had to give up soft cheese, but that was no fun, either. So we looked at what the evidence shows for risks of everything from hot tubs to hot dogs to hair dye during pregnancy. And it's a mixed bag.

It's Getting Hot in Here
When it comes to being overheated during pregnancy, a significant amount of animal research shows that higher body temperature increases congenital anomaly risk, but the handful of human studies are small case–control studies yielding limited evidence. Limited evidence doesn't mean "safe"—there's a slightly increased risk of certain congenital anomalies with sustained heat exposure above a normal body temperature, particularly in the first trimester—but rather that the question hasn't been studied enough. Bottom line: we lack quality evidence, but the tiny amount we have weakly points to a small increased risk of congenital anomalies when a pregnant

woman's core temperature is raised in the first trimester, whether through hot baths, hot temperature, or heating blankets. Evidence from animal studies shows a similar risk. We couldn't find studies looking at later trimesters in humans.

Leaving on a Jet Plane

Airline policies vary but most have some sort of limitation on flying while pregnant, ranging from a week before your due date to a month before if you're flying over water. Yet these have more to do with flight attendants preferring to serve drinks rather than deliver babies in midair. No studies have found reliable evidence to link pregnancy or fetal complications to casual or infrequent business air travel, but the data look a little different for flight attendants, pilots, and high-volume business travelers. The main safety issues for pregnancy and casual flight are cosmic radiation exposure and deep vein thrombosis risk.

Cosmic radiation—which our atmosphere usually protects us from—increases as altitude increases, so a trip to the moon while pregnant is probably a bad idea. We don't know definitively the radiation threshold at which miscarriage, congenital anomalies, developmental conditions, or childhood cancer become concerns, but it's generally thought to be above 20 millisievert (mSv), and a typical transcontinental trip exposes a person to only 0.3% of this amount. Without getting too far into the weeds, the average person shouldn't exceed 1 mSv per year, which goes for fetuses as well. (If that level can cause fatal cancer—a big theoretical "if"—the lifetime risk for the fetus would be about 1 in 10,000.) The longest intercontinental flight reaches only 15% of this limit. The best estimate is that it would take 80,000 miles to reach 1 mSv, well above a typical casual flier's annual miles but something for flight attendants and pilots to consider. Another consideration is brief increases in radiation during sun storms, but the radiation bursts from these last only a couple of hours, and the National Oceanic and Atmospheric Administration (NOAA) already monitors radiation bursts for airlines specifically for the sake of traveling pregnant women.

The risk of deep vein thrombosis, a blood clot that usually starts in the legs and can lodge in the heart or lungs and cause death, is about 1 in 4,500 within 8 weeks of a long-haul flight. Another study estimated a 26% increased risk for every 2 hours in the air. (The same study found an extra 18% risk for every 2 hours of any travel, since travel usually means sitting for long periods of time.) But pregnancy (until about 6 to 12 weeks postpartum) increases the overall risk of blood clots, and one study found that flying while pregnant increases the risk 14 times over not being pregnant and staying grounded—based on just three women with thrombosis. Overall, those authors estimated the risk of thrombosis to be 1 in 109 flights for a pregnant woman (or 1 in 109 pregnant women on a single flight). Without flying, the risk of deep vein thrombosis is about 17 incidents (with 1 death) per 10,000 deliveries, and it's about a third higher for women over 35. Exercise, frequent walks during the flight, not sleeping for long periods, and skipping window seats all reduce risk.

No strong evidence shows a risk of miscarriage, preterm birth, preeclampsia, or low birth weight among pregnant flight attendants or high-volume fliers. Though less studied, greater possible exposure to infectious diseases in airports and planes is a general concern for flying. Conscientious hygiene and getting recommended vaccines are the most effective prevention. And finally, noise levels above 85 decibels may be hazardous to a fetus, but this would be a concern only with some military flights, not commercial flights.

To Dye or Not to Dye

One of the more persistent admonitions out there is to avoid dying your hair while pregnant, but the evidence doesn't actually support this one at all. If you want to find out how much risk a particular compound poses, study the people exposed to it the most—in this case, hairdressers. Researchers did that and found no evidence that congenital anomalies, poor pregnancy outcomes, or children's developmental problems were linked to hair products. That said, emerging evidence suggests that the risks associated with a different beauty establishment—nail salons—may not be so low, at least for the employees, partly due to a class of chemicals called phthalates found in the products. This research was too new to assess in time for this book.

Toxoplasmosis: Cats, Gardens, Meat, Sandboxes, and Other Parasite Reservoirs

You've probably heard that you shouldn't change cat litter while you're pregnant, but statistically, the parasite you're trying to avoid is more likely to find you on a sand volleyball court or the local park's sandbox than in your cat's litter box. The critter is called *Toxoplasma gondii*, and it can cause an infection called toxoplasmosis. In most healthy individuals, toxoplasmosis symptoms may go unnoticed. They can resemble the flu, with muscle aches, but many people never experience even this. In fact, about 60 million people in the United States are infected and don't know it. The danger of the infection is for fetuses: among the 500 to 5,000 babies born with congenital toxoplasmosis in the United States each year, anywhere from 12% to 30% will develop eye diseases. More severe but rarer effects include miscarriage, stillbirth, smaller heads, cerebrospinal fluid buildup in the brain, and slowed motor or mental development.

To understand the risks of toxoplasmosis, it helps to understand the parasite's life cycle, which requires a cat for the parasite to develop the eggs, called oocysts because they're actually cysts containing the zygote. It takes a day for the spores to develop before a cat (who experiences no symptoms) can excrete them, and then they're released in the cat's feces for 1 to 2 weeks—up to 55 million oocysts a day. Once in the environment, it takes 1 to 5 days before the spores can infect another host. Those intermediate hosts could be humans, cows, pigs, birds, rodents, or any other warm-blooded animal. Infected birds and rodents then become the source for more cats that hunt and eat them and become infected. But cats can be infected just once, so infection is a concern for only early or first-time feline hunters. In fact, only about 1% of cats are shedding oocysts at any particular time.

Meanwhile, sheep, cows, or pigs pick up oocysts from soil, grass, water, or even animal feed, and their infected tissue can transmit the parasite to humans if the meat is uncooked. But humans (and other animals) can also become infected any time they ingest or inhale the oocysts. Sand or soil that feral cats use as their litter box is likely loaded with oocysts, which are remarkably resilient, remaining viable in varying temperatures for more than 4 years. Now, ready to be really freaked out? Cats deposit an estimated 1.2 million metric tons of poop in the United States each year. Community surveys have shown anywhere from 3 to 434 oocysts are in each square foot of earth—and it takes only 1 oocyst to infect a host. Flies and cockroaches can carry the oocysts to food, and even your puppy rolling around in cat poop can bring it in the house. Several studies have also found millions of them in uncovered children's sandboxes. When the oocysts dry out, they can become aerosolized (your child throwing sand at the park just became even more disturbing, didn't it?), so it's possible to inhale them. And this is the reason for the restrictions on changing the kitty litter: it's possible to breathe in oocysts if any are present.

But here's the good news: just like cats, humans can become infected only once, and about a quarter to almost a third of the US population has been there, done that. Furthermore, indoor cats who don't hunt or otherwise eat raw meat pose no threat. Or, if your kitty's heyday of rodent slaughter was in his youth, he's also probably been there, done that, and poses no threat to you, which is why the kitty litter guidelines are pretty insignificant. The US Centers for Disease Control and Prevention (CDC) estimates about 15% of women of childbearing age are immune to toxoplasmosis, so if you were to get tested and find you've already hosted the parasite, all the risk factors we're about to describe become moot.

And those risk factors? The biggest one is not sandboxes or sand volley-ball pits (the oocysts in a given place depend on the local feral cat popula-tion). It's uncooked meat. A study looking at risk factors in the United States found raw ground beef consumption had a sixfold risk and rare lamb had an eightfold risk. Working with meat, drinking unpasteurized goat's milk, and eating raw oysters, clams, or mussels were also risk factors. Owning three or more kittens is too, so maybe you shouldn't be gestating at the same time as your cat if the new litter will be learning to hunt before you give birth. Another study of 6 European cities found an increased risk of infection from gardening, but the biggest risks in that study also came from consum-ing undercooked lamb, beef, or wild game and from unpasteurized milk products. No risk showed up for contact with cats, cleaning their litter, or their diet or hunting habits. About half to two-thirds of the infections came from eating undercooked or cured meats, and up to 17% came from soil con-tact. In other studies throughout the world, owning a cat is almost never a risk factor, but contact with soil frequently is.

Thanks for All the Fish!

Raw oysters, clams, and mussels are responsible for a percentage of pregnancy-related toxoplasmosis infections each year (the number varies) because they feed by filtering ocean water—potentially taking up whatever is in that water in the process. Any filter feeder, including sardines or other shellfish, poses a risk because of the millions of pounds of contaminants that end up in the ocean from runoff. But what about sushi and ceviche? Both of these usually involve raw fish, though ceviche involves "cooking" the fish with the acidity of lime or another citrus. A variety of parasites live in raw fish as well, but pretty much none of them can survive deep-freezing, which the FDA requires for all "fresh" fish served raw except tuna (though it's local health authorities who enforce that regulation). So whether it comes from the grocery store or a good-quality sushi restaurant, the fish used to make sushi and ceviche should have been frozen first, which should kill any parasites. Still, about 10% to 20% of annual food poisoning cases in the United States involve seafood, usually raw or undercooked, so it's probably worth asking a restaurant if their fish was frozen.

The other big concern associated with fish is mercury content. Mercury collects in rivers, lakes, and oceans where microbes convert it into methylmercury, a neurotoxin at high doses (not to be confused with ethylmercury, a low-risk preservative used in some flu vaccines). Fish absorb the mercury, which then accumulates in their bodies, so the amount increases up the food chain: little fish are eaten by big fish that are eaten by bigger fish that are eaten by the biggest fish, and it's the biggest fish that are chock-full of mercury. Those biggest fish include sharks, tilefish (from the Gulf of Mexico only), swordfish, and king mackerel, followed by bigeye tuna, orange roughy, marlin, Spanish mackerel, and grouper. However, if swordfish is your favorite dish, what kind of risks are we talking about with mercury exposure?

A recent assessment by the FDA reviewed all the research to date on the effects of mercury consumption through fish. They begin with a horrific situation that put mercury's effect on our radar: the 20th-century mercury poisoning of the fishing town of Minamata, Japan, following an unrecognized industrial discharge of mercury into the adjacent bay, where it accumulated in the fish the villagers regularly consumed. That event and another in Iraq revealed that extremely high exposure to mercury could have disastrous effects, including paralysis and severe cognitive disability. But these episodes resulted from large-scale industrial contamination, not average consumption of fish from relatively uncontaminated waters. Since then, studies from New Zealand, the Faroe Islands, and the Seychelles have looked for effects at lower levels, generally reporting mercury exposure as parts per million (ppm) detected in human hair. One study found lower test scores among 4- and 6-year-olds with hair levels over 6 ppm, primarily from eating shark, and other studies in the 1990s found similar results.

But then enter one of the longest running, most solidly designed studies from the Seychelles, an island chain in the middle of the Indian Ocean where the staple diet is, unsurprisingly, fish. Women eat fish about 12 times a week there, with almost no other source of environmental mercury. Researchers have been testing pregnant women and their children there for several decades and have so far found virtually no cognitive, neurological, or developmental effects in children, up to age 19, whose mothers consumed mercury from fish. One study of more than 500 teenagers found no neurodevelopmental or behavioral concerns even though their mothers' mercury levels were about 6.9 ppm. A dozen other studies over the years found no consistent patterns related to mercury intake from fish, although they periodically have reported an uptick in some outcome here and there that barely reaches statistical significance. One reason for these anomalies, and the overall findings, may be that fish also contain omega-3s, a fatty acid linked to all kinds of benefits, from better heart health to better cognitive function to a lower risk of asthma, arthritis, ADHD, and Alzheimer's. Some of the data, when analyzed to account for effects from omega-3s, suggest there may be some small effects from the mercury that are offset by the positive effects of the omega-3s.

Meanwhile, another review of 20 mostly high-quality studies on mercury's effects yielded . . . confusion. Effects from mercury showed up in some studies but not in others, probably depending on what other factors they considered and how they measured the effects. So what's a fish-loving pregnant lady to do?

Well, a fish-loving pregnant lady can consider eating fish. A diet of 12 ounces of fish a week is linked to a lower risk of postpartum depression for the mother and higher IQs, better fine-motor coordination, and good communication and social skills in the child, benefits that continue for up to 18 ounces a week (4.5 servings). These benefits may be from the omega-3s and docosahexaenoic acid (DHA) but are likely from other nutrients as well, especially since omega-3 and DHA supplements have not shown the same positive cardiovascular, cognitive, motor, and language effects when taken on their own. (It's not clear why—perhaps the manufacturing process strips out antioxidants or as-yet-unidentified nutrients. We also don't know what an ideal intake of omega-3s and DHA might be, even from natural sources.)

The FDA officially recommends that pregnant women eat one to three 4-ounce servings a week. The US Environmental Protection Agency (EPA) recommends not exceeding a very conservative 42–64 micrograms of mercury per week, and the top four—shark, tilefish, swordfish, and king mackerel—contain about 100–220 micrograms per 4-ounce serving. Lobster and bluefin, skipjack, and yellowfin tuna have about 30–60 micrograms of mercury per 4-ounce serving. Shrimp has virtually no mercury, but it's low in omega-3s too. Other fish low in mercury include salmon, tilapia, canned light tuna, cod, and catfish. Salmon, sardines, pollack, squid, and Pacific and Jack mackerel are rich in omega-3s.

Listeriosis: The Culprit in Soft Cheeses, Deli Meats . . . and Almost Anything Else You Eat

Of the seven listeriosis species, nearly all human infections come from just one, *L. monocytogenes*, and three serotypes are responsible for 95% of those infections. The good news is that in the big scheme of things, listeriosis is rare, and incidence has dropped since the CDC implemented aggressive surveillance procedures. The disease affects about 7 per million US residents, but it's about 18 times more common in pregnancy, affecting an estimated 12 of every 100,000 pregnancies.

The bad news is that it's very destructive, hard to detect (some people show no symptoms at all), and hard to guard against. Symptoms are flu-like: fever, backache, headache, and muscle pains, sometimes with vomiting or diarrhea, so it's often initially mistaken for other conditions. Early diagnosis means better outcomes, since antibiotics can treat it. But listeriosis can fell full-grown, healthy adults, and the bacteria can cross the blood–brain barrier, the intestinal wall, and the placenta, so it poses serious risks to a developing fetus. Miscarriage or fetal death occurs about 20% to 30% of the time and preterm birth half the time. Among babies born with listeriosis, about a third have meningitis and/or bacteria in their blood and 90% require hospitalization. Fewer than 10% show no symptoms at all.

The recommendations against cheese come from a major epidemic in 1985, when two-thirds of 142 cases occurred in pregnant women, and the source was a Mexican-style cheese, queso fresco, made from unpasteurized milk. This outbreak led to the US *Listeria* surveillance system, which has reduced perinatal listeriosis by 44%. That surveillance system identified the following top food items implicated in pregnancy-related listeriosis between 2004 and 2007: turkey breast deli meat, pasta salad, butter, hot dogs, bologna, and queso fresco cheese. Another common carrier is refrigerated smoked seafood, including lox. But other sources could include ice cream (how cruel!), yogurt, pastrami, coleslaw, honeydew melon, and cantaloupe. In fact, one of the biggest outbreaks of listeriosis in the past decade involved cantaloupes in 2011, with 147 infections across 28 states resulting in 33 deaths and 1 miscarriage.

The problem with listeriosis is that it can show up anywhere, even in processed, mass-produced food. As we were writing this book, *Listeria* outbreaks occurred because of contamination of commercially produced, prepackaged caramel apples and ice cream. Although the bacteria can live in very high and low temperatures and high-salt environments, they can't survive pasteurization, which is why pasteurized soft cheese poses far less risk than unpasteurized cheese. So even though common pregnancy restrictions include hot dogs, deli meats, and soft cheeses, these items rarely pose more risk than any other food as long as they're pasteurized and if the meats are reheated until piping hot.

Aside from toxoplasmosis and listeriosis, the other big culprits annually giving 1 in 6 Americans food poisoning include *E. coli, Campylobacter, Clostridium perfringens,* and norovirus. These pathogens don't cross the placenta and pose risks to a fetus that are similar to any other illness, such as influenza.

Maternal Hypertension and Preeclampsia

We each had preeclampsia in two pregnancies, naturally leading to the question of whether it can be prevented after the first episode. Spending your last trimester of pregnancy desperately trying to reduce fluid buildup and taking your blood pressure every 10 seconds is not fun. Preeclampsia can also be fatal to the mother or the baby, and it's one of the developments obstetricians worry about most because it can come on hard and fast. It hits between 2% and 8% of women, and the triad that characterizes it consists of a bump in blood pressure, protein in the urine, and, sometimes, swelling, although that can be hard to distinguish from the usual Flintstone feet many women develop by the third trimester. Except for the swelling, these signs are hidden—you can't just tell that you have protein in your urine or that your systolic blood pressure has kicked up 20 points.

Physiologically, preeclampsia constricts the placental blood vessels, which restricts nutrients and oxygen to the fetus and puts the fetus at risk for growth retardation or preterm birth. But the "cure" for preeclampsia is often delivery induction before full term since the risks to the mother range from organ damage to death.

A handful of studies have found a higher BMI before pregnancy to be one risk factor for preeclampsia, and one reported that low levels of blood flow in the uterine arteries and low levels of placental growth increase the risk, but measuring these is rarely part of standard prenatal care. More obvious but less specific risk factors are having a first pregnancy, being obese, being over age 40, having a personal or family history of preeclampsia, and having preexisting conditions like hypertension, migraines, or diabetes that are associated with the circulatory system.

Bed rest has commonly been suggested as a way to prevent or at least delay the development of preeclampsia in at-risk women, but a Cochrane Review of the limited legitimate studies available—only two—found very little evidence on either side of the question. They also found no strong evidence to support limiting activity. In fact, the Cochrane Review authors literally say that "in the meantime, women will be guided by their own beliefs and reasoning, as well as those of their caregivers"—not terribly helpful given the goal of this book.

So what do we know? Briefly, Cochrane Reviews have identified no good evidence for Chinese herbal medicine, garlic, diuretics (which just cause nausea and vomiting), nitric oxide, exercise, or progesterone. One possible treatment under consideration is statins, since preeclampsia resembles cardiovascular disease and shares risk factors, but real evidence supporting this intervention remains on the horizon with studies still ongoing.

A 2014 systematic review of observational studies found that hypertension in pregnancy is linked to low magnesium and calcium; women with high calcium were especially less likely to develop hypertension. A separate Cochrane Review of 13 studies with more than 15,000 women suggested that daily calcium supplementation of 500 to 1,000 milligrams decreased the risk of preeclampsia (as well as preterm birth). However, several studies were small, negative findings (no effect) are less likely to be published in the first place, and the results likely apply primarily to women already not getting enough calcium in their diet. Consuming a lot of calories did not influence risk, but some studies indicated that eating a lot of fruits and vegetables is a good thing. Then again . . . when isn't it? A 2005 review looked at low salt intake in pregnancy since excess salt might boost blood pressure, but the only two trials they found had no evidence of benefit.

Meanwhile, aspirin has become a contender for preeclampsia prevention after a 2014 systematic review found that aspirin might possibly be helpful. However, most trials were small, so it's hard to know how real the risk reductions are (up to 5%). Another review of 59 trials (more than 37,000 women) found a 17% drop in risk with 75-milligram doses, but no one is quite sure about the possible long-term harms from regularly taking aspirin during pregnancy.

Ultimately, interventions targeting the circulatory system might help prevent and treat preeclampsia, but even established interventions like aspirin and statins need further evaluation for safety and real efficacy. The authors of the 59-trial Cochrane Review state in an online reply to feedback at the Cochrane site that "aspirin is the best we have to offer for prevention of preeclampsia." That's something for a woman at risk and her clinician to decide.

CHAPTER 3

⟿⟆

Delivery Day Around the Corner

Home Truths About Home Birth

Based on available evidence at the time of her first pregnancy (2000), Emily's choice of a birthing center with a certified-nurse midwife was a safe one for a woman having a healthy pregnancy, and her midwife and OB made the right decision to transfer care completely to the OB when her pregnancy became risky. In the interval since that time, however, there has been much debate over the safety of home birth. On one side are strident voices urging home birth not only in the interest of fewer interventions and overall comfort of care but also as a philosophical stance against medicalized birth. This faction makes home birth into a statement of womanhood itself and expends considerable energy on what amounts to shaming women who choose otherwise. On the other side are those who see home birth as a selfish, abusive, child-endangering choice made by controlling women who are too self-involved to consider the interests and safety of the child. In the midst of all the shouting sits the pregnant woman and the baby she will birth . . . somewhere.

The nirvana of complementary support and state-of-the-art specialty care is a rare thing in the United States; in the meantime, many women still seek the best evidence they can find for what constitutes the most personally appropriate, safe, and suitable choice for childbirth. But chasing down the evidence about the safest and most suitable choice for birth can prove confusing. Predictably, the conclusions and interpretations vary based on whether or not studies were done by groups of obstetricians or by midwives. Using language that barely conceals their contempt for the other's philosophies, behaviors, and interpretations, not unexpectedly, the studies the two groups produce tend to cancel each other out.

Complicating this issue more is that the best evidence around in-home birth or birth-center birth with midwives comes from nations that, compared to the United States, have a much more consistent system of midwifery licensing and oversight, along with consistent hospital-affiliated birth-center alternatives for expectant mothers. As we note on page 9, midwifery as practiced in the United States has no common credentialing body. Some midwives have no credentialing at all. Some are certified professional midwives, meaning they have professional certification but are not obstetric nurses or required otherwise to have related nursing training. And then there are the certified-nurse midwives who are trained registered nurses who also have midwifery certification. This last category of midwives, not surprisingly, has the best safety profile, likely in part because of the interaction between their training and their clientele. Thus, when Britain's National Health Service (NHS) announced in December 2014 that their latest guidance for healthy pregnant women is that it is safer to have their babies at home or in a birth center than in a hospital, that decision was very UK specific. The NHS based its conclusion on evidence suggesting that women with low-risk pregnancies fare better giving birth outside of a hospital maternity ward because they avoid surgical intervention, such as cesarean sections and episiotomies, and related infections.

The messiness around the way data are collected in the United States and interpreted through the filter of bias on either side of the discussion makes it almost impossible to perform trustworthy comparisons across studies or across practitioners.

Here's what we can say with certainty about the choice of birth attendant and facility: do your research on your home ground. What are the accreditations for the person (obstetrician, midwife, both?) and the facility (hospital, birth center)? What are the rates of maternal and neonatal mortality (if they're not readily available, ask)? What kind of care do you want for yourself and your child, and how does the attendant and facility you're considering manage that care? What level of risk are you willing to accept in terms of emergencies when minutes count (having emergency care available in the facility, 5 minutes away, 15 minutes away—because distance from a hospital seems to be a factor in neonatal mortality associated with home births)? What is the potential for backup care providers and communication and partnering in care between them, whether you're choosing a midwife or an obstetrician? And finally, two evidence-based bits of information arising collectively from the current studies, as much as we could discern the signal from the noise: (1) Women delivering for the first time with midwives in birth centers have a slightly higher risk of problems compared to women having a second or later child. (2) Labor and birth outside of a hospital, if it is an option, is not the safer choice for high-risk pregnancies.

What We Did: Emily planned in her first pregnancy to give birth at a freestanding birth center with a certified-nurse midwife and OB backup; however, because of pregnancy complications in the last trimester, she gave birth at a hospital, where practices had not yet transitioned into the family-focused, compassionate care some medical centers offer today. She had her second son at home with a midwife and OB backup; he was born on his due date, 4 hours after her water broke. She had planned another home birth with a certified-nurse midwife and OB backup for her third child but was again transferred to OB care with midwife backup. This birth occurred 5 years after her first experience, in a facility that had made considerable family-friendly adjustments to birth practices, including a quiet birthing room with only the OB and nurse (and any requested family members), and with labor, delivery, and recovery all in the same room. Tara had multiple risk factors for pregnancy complications and gave birth to both children in hospitals equipped to handle higher-risk births and with robust neonatal ICU departments. Both experiences were positive, but she was especially grateful for a hospital birth for her first child because a retained placenta required manual surgical extraction, and both her children required some NICU care.

The Placenta: Take It or Leave It

The list of seemingly magical properties the placenta allegedly confers if mom eats it is long, and heralded on an ever-growing number of websites.

But the evidence to support these claims is pretty much nonexistent. The studies on websites promoting placentophagy are a collection of distantly relevant findings that falls short of showing any benefits of maternal placental consumption.

The often-cited "Placenta as Lactagagon" was a poorly conducted study in 1954 that has never been replicated. The authors recruited women who were suspected to have difficulties with milk production and gave them "Lactofer," the name given to the dried and ground-up placenta "preparation," within 2 days after giving birth. The women began producing more milk within a few days . . . except that it's natural for a woman's milk to come in and then increase at about that time after birth. The study's procedure is so poorly described that it's not even clear if each woman received her own placenta or a combination of multiple women's.

Yet this is the only placebo-controlled study involving humans and placenta consumption (though one is in the works as we write this). Another pair of human studies on placenta consumption and milk production, published in 1918, had no control groups. All other studies supposedly supporting placentophagy benefits are either animal studies (usually rats, which tells us little about humans) or postpartum depression studies finding low levels of iron or certain hormones in depressed mothers (which doesn't mean that supplements, much less a placenta, would improve mood). The placenta is full of hormones, iron, and protein, but we don't know if the body can absorb these nutrients, especially if cooked or dried out.

Picking a Pediatrician

Few specialties allow for appointments unrelated to a current acute medical need when prospective clients might check out whether a provider would fit their needs, but pediatricians are an exception. Most pediatric offices have time set aside in the schedule each week for new potential clients to schedule an interview, lasting anywhere from 10 to 30 minutes. It's not a lot of time, but it's enough to get a sense of the practice and to ask questions about that provider's values, beliefs, and practices. To make the most of it, prepare questions ahead of time that will let you discover any deal breakers and help you get a sense of what you might expect if you choose that provider.

Research has found that doctors' personal experience, beliefs, and the extent to which they keep up with current medical literature and guidelines all influence the care they provide. For example, a 2010 study out of Canada asked 572 family doctors, urologists, obstetricians, pediatricians, and family-medicine residents what they use to make their decisions regarding circumcision. Just over three-quarters of them (77%) said they base their circumcision decisions on medical evidence. However, the survey also asked the men about their circumcision status and about their attitude toward circumcision: 68% of the 125 circumcised males supported circumcision, and 69% of the 106 uncircumcised males opposed circumcision. This is a fairly small group (and nearly half the original 1,009 physicians contacted didn't answer the survey), but clearly, male doctors' own circumcision status may influence their decisions—and recommendations—even if they believe they are basing those decisions only on the medical evidence.

We aren't advocating that you ask a prospective male doctor about his circumcision status—that might get a little awkward—but you can craft questions that will provide insight into that doctor's beliefs and knowledge on issues that matter to you. Start with any of the dozens of online lists of questions to ask pediatricians, and then incorporate into that the recommended questions on our website that appeal to you. It's not necessary to ask all these questions, and you may not have time anyway, so rank them and ask the most important ones first.

Circumcision is actually a good example, because decreasing rates of circumcision in the United States mean that some older doctors may be less knowledgeable about appropriate care for an uncircumcised penis. Further, one study found that 1 in 5 doctors (family doctors, internists, pediatricians, and ob-gyns) did not feel they understood the risks and benefits of newborn male circumcision well enough to advise parents. If your son is uncircumcised or you don't plan to circumcise a son you're expecting, you may want to ask a prospective pediatrician what percentage of his male patients are uncircumcised and what his familiarity is with the care of an uncircumcised penis.

Vaccines are another big issue to ask about. Just a few years after the chickenpox vaccine was added to the CDC recommended schedule, fewer than half of surveyed pediatricians in Washington State were recommending universal chickenpox vaccination, and their willingness to follow the recommendations appeared "influenced by personal experience, perceptions about the potential seriousness of varicella, and beliefs about the societal and medical cost-effectiveness of varicella vaccine." And then there are the vaccine policies of different practices, ranging from accommodating delayed vaccine administration to requiring children follow the recommended CDC schedule.

One area where pediatricians may particularly differ from one another in beliefs and practices is breastfeeding, a topic with documented deficits among many pediatricians. A survey in 2004 found that pediatricians were less likely then, compared to a decade earlier, to believe that the benefits of breastfeeding outweighed the difficulties or inconvenience. There were also fewer pediatricians in 2004 who believed almost all mothers could succeed in breastfeeding, and more who reported reasons they might recommend against breastfeeding. Similar to the findings with the circumcision data, however, pediatricians who had personal experience with breastfeeding were more than twice as likely to recommend supportive policies than those without those experiences. Even if a pediatrician is clearly very supportive of breastfeeding, he may lack sufficient knowledge to advise breastfeeding moms, or doctors and mothers may have different ideas about what "support" means and how long breastfeeding should extend.

Generally speaking, doctors are more likely to be in the loop about the most current research and changes to recommendations for various topics if they're involved with their professional association, usually the AAP for pediatricians or the American Academy of Family Physicians for family doctors. A Fellow of the American Academy of Pediatrics (FAAP) means the pediatrician passed a pediatric exam and maintains certification with ongoing continuing education. Being "board-certified" means that after medical school, a physician completed a residency of 3 to 5 years in a specialty (such as pediatrics) and then passed an exam in that specialty. ("Board-eligible" means they did the residency but haven't taken or haven't passed that exam.)

Finally, there are a variety of questions you can ask that will give you a more holistic feel for how providers think about problems and about healthcare in general, such as whether becoming a parent influenced the way they practice as doctors, or how they respond to parents who opt not to follow official recommendations. Be sure to include questions that might relate to any specific circumstances in your family. If your family has a substantial mental health history, or if you have a child with a developmental disorder or other special needs, be sure to ask about the pediatrician's experiences with that area. See the website TheInformedParentBook.com for a detailed list of questions to consider.

Labor Interventions: From Semen and Primrose Oil to Safety Considerations

Even though there appears to be agreement that interventions for and during labor should be applied only on a need-to basis, rather than routinely, according to one 2014 literature review, interventions such as labor induction and augmentation and episiotomy are on the increase worldwide. This pattern varies from country to country, however; for example, episiotomy rates in the United States, while still pretty high, are not as high as they were in the later 20th century.

What are the reasons for these interventions, and how compelling must the rationale be for their use relative to the discomfort and pain that many of them involve? In addition, how much do these interventions lead to other interventions or complications, as it is widely thought that they do? We have divided this section into three parts that track the progress of labor and delivery, beginning with interventions to induce labor, moving to discussing interventions intended to augment or otherwise facilitate the labor itself, and finally interventions for pain during labor.

Induction

First of all, it's important to understand the specific conditions that would require a labor induction in the first place. As a 2009 review in the obstetrics journal *BJOG* noted, inductions are ever increasing, so does that mean that the reasons for them are becoming more frequent too? The review authors identified several indications (in med-speak, "reasons for doing it") for induction in their review of 34 papers, most of them randomized trials. These indications included post-term gestation (longer than 41 weeks), intrauterine growth retardation, premature rupture of membrane, twin pregnancy, and maternal diabetes requiring insulin.

Based on their findings, induction even for what are considered to be established medical reasons can be a mixed bag. Doing it for intrauterine growth retardation, for example, reduces the risk of fetal death in utero but increases the risk of neonatal death and cesarean birth. Induction is definitively necessary for premature rupture of membranes at term or near term if fetal lungs are mature and recommended if gestation has passed the 41-week mark. But they say that evidence is insufficient to support induction for twin pregnancy, maternal diabetes requiring insulin, too little amniotic fluid, or maternal cardiac disease.

Once the decision to induce is made, the next question is how to go about it. No randomized controlled trials exist to support hypnosis as a way to induce labor, and the authors of an attempted Cochrane Review (they ended up having nothing to review) urge caution in trying hypnosis for fear that it might delay effective methods. Acupuncture has received more attention, and a Cochrane Review of this intervention for cervical ripening and labor induction found some evidence, in 14 trials involving 2,220 women, that acupuncture might affect cervical ripening. But labor in the acupuncture group was longer than in the group receiving standard induction. Otherwise, evidence supporting acupuncture as an intervention was limited.

The Internet abounds with suggestions and advice about inducing labor at home or "getting things moving" for the anxious mother-to-be. And an intervention involving tea, sex, or application of a little oil to the cervix does sound considerably more appealing than, say, a flood of Pitocin. But how effective are these various at-home solutions to the "get this baby out of here" problem? The verdict from Cochrane Reviews for castor oil and primrose oil is not at all, and there are hints that they might even increase the incidence of complications. Homeopathy gets no traction, although Cochrane Review authors give a nod to placebo effects by observing that "some women have found these remedies helpful." Blue cohosh, which is another "inducer" popular on the web, gets a strong negative and a warning against it. Case studies have associated it with fetal or infant stroke, heart attack, and neonatal heart failure, and it can cause abortion or miscarriage. Other than these reports and some in vitro data, blue cohosh remains a question mark, with some suggestion that it can have some very serious, if rare, adverse effects. The only reports of its effectiveness are anecdotal. On the plus side, breast stimulation—which will promote some oxytocin release—gets a small thumbs-up as a labor inducer, but raspberry leaf (as tea or pill is unclear) gets mixed reviews as well.

Sometimes, mechanical (as opposed to chemical) methods can be a way to get the uterus and its friend, the cervix, to cooperate. These methods can include stripping the membranes, in which the practitioner can use a finger to separate the cervix from the amniotic sac, which is thought to stimulate release of chemicals called prostaglandins that promote labor. The results of a Cochrane Review aren't promising for most of these; compared to no treatment, with cesarean birth and vaginal delivery within 24 hours as the outcome, mechanical stimulation was no different from doing nothing or having some actual prostaglandin E2 (or a synthetic) inserted into the cervix. However, using the mechanical approach was associated with a reduced risk of unwanted fetal heart rate elevation, and compared to oxytocin induction, mechanical stimulation was associated with a reduced risk of having a cesarean birth (based on 5 studies involving 398 women).

As with any medical intervention, a risk–benefit calculus goes into the induction decision. What are the risks associated with induction? Among the concerns is that a too-early induction can lead to prolonged labor and the need for cesarean delivery. A 2014 review and meta-analysis published in the *Canadian Medical Association Journal* included data from 157 randomized controlled trials, which has to make this one of the most studied questions in obstetrics. The population pool from these trials was 13,085 women. When the authors compared "watch-and-wait" (or "expectant management") with labor induction (with a variety of possible interventions), they found an overall decreased risk of cesarean delivery when labor was induced, a significant effect for full-term and post-term pregnancies. They looked at possible confounders, such as dilation progress and why induction was performed and still got the same result. In addition, induction was associated with a decrease of 50% for the risk of fetal death and a 14% decrease in risk for admission to NICU. Induction was not associated with an increased risk of maternal death.

Yet another systematic review and meta-analysis addressing the same question was published in *BJOG* in 2014. These authors reviewed 37 studies, 27 involving women with uncomplicated pregnancies. In their meta-analysis, and in agreement with the above study, they found that induction versus expectant management in women with intact membranes was associated with a reduced risk (17%) of having a cesarean birth. A 2012 Cochrane Review reached a similar conclusion and also suggested that induced labor versus expectant management was associated with fewer perinatal deaths and a lower incidence of meconium aspiration in pregnancies that were post-term. Adding to this stack of results pointing in the same direction is a 2014 paper published in *AJOGB* (*American Journal of Obstetrics and Gynecology*) examining outcomes for mother and baby with elective induction at term in low-risk pregnancies. This study involved 19 hospitals and two other health-care facilities and retrospectively examined data for 131,243 deliveries. Of these, a total of 13,242 involved elective induction, and the authors compared cesarean delivery outcomes between elective induction and expectant management at term. They found that from 37 to 40 weeks, induction was associated with a reduced risk of cesarean delivery and that this risk reduction steepened with each passing week up to 40 weeks. In addition, elective induction was associated with a reduced rate of maternal infection and lower rates of neonatal respiratory problems. According to their analysis, these reduced risks were unrelated to whether a woman had given birth before or not and the status of her cervix.

Augmentation

Induction refers to getting labor started. Tactics related to getting labor moving along or moving faster are referred to as augmentation. These interventions can be mechanical (amniotomy, or rupture of the membranes) or chemical (oxytocin, misoprostol), and special situations can apply. For example, epidural anesthesia has been associated with poky labor (known as labor dystocia) and increased surgical interventions, and oxytocin is commonly applied to remedy this issue—an example of "snowballing interventions" that worry some pregnant women. But how effective is this oxytocin augmentation?

A 2013 Cochrane Review that included only two studies with 319 women in total found no difference in outcomes associated with instrument-related interventions during the birth (forceps, vacuum, cesarean delivery) and being administered oxytocin or a placebo plus epidural analgesia and having oxytocin versus placebo with epidural analgesia. The use of oxytocin or placebo also didn't affect Apgar scores or NICU admissions or maternal hemorrhage risk postpartum. However, this group of women going into spontaneous labor was pretty small, and as noted, the review included only two studies. Another Cochrane Review from 2013 comparing high and low doses of oxytocin for delayed labor (epidural not required) found that while higher doses sped up the labor and were linked to a reduced risk of cesarean delivery, the differences from low doses weren't compelling enough to lead to recommendations for regular use of higher oxytocin doses.

Another tactic for augmenting labor is the mechanical approach of amniotomy, known more casually as "breaking the waters." In Emily's case, with her third son, this meant being handled like a football by her OB, who literally climbed up on the delivery table with the little grappling hook—called the OmniHook—clinicians use for this process in her mighty struggle to rupture Emily's amniotic membranes. But why rupture membranes, and how effective is it as a tactic? Let's look at a Cochrane Review from 2013 that included 15 randomized controlled trials involving a total of 5,583 women in spontaneous (that is, not induced) labor. Amniotomy appears to have done absolutely nothing for how long the first stage of labor (before the transition) lasted, risk for cesarean delivery, Apgar score, or maternal satisfaction. The trials were not uniform in terms of the status of the cervix when the amniotomy was performed. The authors recommend that their review be "made available to women offered an amniotomy," but given the conditions under which that usually happens, we suggest that discussing it with one's practitioner beforehand, as with all other potential interventions, might be more rational.

What happens when chemical and manual interventions are combined, when oxytocin and the OmniHook both come into play? A 2013 Cochrane Review looked at the combination of the two as a prevention or treatment for delayed labor. The authors broke their evaluation into the therapies used as prevention versus their use as treatment. The 14 trials they included involved 8,033 women, and the authors found a reduction in the risk of cesarean delivery with the combined augmentation in women experiencing slow labor. They caution, however, that this finding for women in the treatment group is questionable because "no effect at all" remains among the possible interpretations of the statistical results. For the women randomized to prevention of slow labor, however, the risk for cesarean delivery was reduced without any caveat, and labors were shorter by an hour and a half compared to women not receiving the combination preventive measures. The authors describe the prevention findings as "modest." So no fireworks, but some modest level of presumably desired effects.

One last intervention to mention during labor before we move onto pain is the episiotomy, the intervention intended to enlarge the vaginal opening, ostensibly to avoid perineal tears as the head pushes through. This surgical procedure became common practice during deliveries in the United States, applied in 30% to 35% of vaginal births by the turn of the 21st century. Oddly enough, according to a pretty definitive 2005 systematic review in the *Journal of the American Medical Association* (*JAMA*), episiotomy came into common practice without much of an evidence base. The *JAMA* authors note in their review of 26 studies that episiotomies generally tend to make things worse: they make tears worse, lengthen the healing process, and cause more pain. There was no evidence that their routine use was beneficial, and they were associated with pain when women began having intercourse again.

Pain

Speaking of pain, if there's anything people think of when they think of childbirth—beyond holding a baby at the end of it—it's pain. And one big question around pain management interventions in childbirth is, how safe are they?

Of all the questions obstetrics researchers address, this one might have the most abundant evidence base. It's so abundant, in fact, that Cochrane offers a review of the 18 systematic reviews on the subject, covering almost 300 trials that used either placebo or routine care as the comparison against the pain intervention. These authors helpfully broke the findings down into "what works," "what may work," and "insufficient evidence." In the first category, epidurals work, and combined spinal epidural—in which a local anesthetic is delivered that gives immediate pain relief and an ongoing epidural block is simultaneously administered through a catheter to give long-term relief—works faster. Inhaled nitrous oxide was associated with nausea, vomiting, and dizziness, and sedatives helped some with pain but not as much as opioids.

The pain relief from epidurals was effective in this huge analysis, but epidurals were associated with more instrumental births (forceps or vacuum) and with more cesarean deliveries as a result of fetal distress. In addition, epidurals were linked with maternal low blood pressure, acute walking difficulty, and inability to urinate, all of which are typically temporary. The combined spinal epidural was less associated with urinary retention than the traditional epidural but was associated with more itching, possibly because of the local anesthetic.

These authors found limited studies for "what may work." Local nerve blocks fell into this category, but they were associated with some discomfiting maternal side effects such as tingling and sweating and with a greater incidence of low fetal heart rates. Also in this category were immersion in water and various relaxation and massage techniques, but generally only with one trial to support the finding. Acupuncture seemed to be associated with fewer interventions and cesarean births. Given the contribution of anxiety to pain, it's not surprising that techniques targeting distraction and relaxation might be useful. Water immersion may be okay if membranes are intact, but the risks of giving birth in water include exposure to waterborne pathogens that at least in one 2014 case proved fatal to the newborn.

Among the interventions falling into the "insufficient evidence" column was "water injection," along with aromatherapy and biofeedback. Sterile water injection has recently become common enough for a 2012 Cochrane Review to evaluate its effects. These authors included seven randomized controlled trials in their review, looking at the outcome measure of 50% pain relief and maternal and neonatal health measures. In the data for the 766 women in these studies, the authors found no compelling evidence for water injection's benefit for pain or any other outcomes.

Baby's Arrival: Cesarean and Vaginal Births

Today, about 1 in 3 babies is delivered by cesarean section in the United States, but the numbers were not always so high. The serious climb began around 1996, when first-time birth ("primary") cesarean rates hovered around 15% and about 1 in 5 pregnant woman overall had one. Today, just under a quarter of first-time deliveries and about a third of all deliveries are cesarean births. But these national averages vary across different regions and even hospital by hospital, ranging from 7% to 70%. Even for low-risk women, the rate from one hospital to the next can vary by dozens of percentage points, partly due to the culture of the hospital and partly due to other factors, such as the population the hospital serves.

> About 1 in 3 babies is delivered by cesarean section.

The reasons for this increase are numerous: a study of more than 32,000 pregnant women at the Yale–New Haven teaching hospital in Connecticut identified that more than half the increase came from a jump in first-time cesarean births, which grew out of an increase in six indications, many of which should not (as far as the evidence suggests) have been automatic cesarean deliveries unless alternative treatments had been tried.

When the researchers broke down how much each of these reasons contributed to the overall increase, they found the following:

- 32% arose from a "nonreassuring" fetal status, based primarily on heart rate
- 18% came from stalled labor, usually a halt to cervical dilation
- 16% came from multiples (twins, triplets, etc.)
- 10% came from preeclampsia
- 10% came from a suspected big baby
- 8% came from mothers' requests
- 5% came from other conditions in the mother or fetus
- 1% came from other obstetric conditions

Several of these, such as multiples and suspected big babies, have little to no data to support an automatic cesarean delivery. No significant changes occurred in cesarean birth rates resulting from a baby's position (not having the head down), a halt in the baby's descent through the birth canal, or other conditions in the mother or fetus, such as placenta previa (where the placenta is partly or completely blocking the uterus) or cord prolapse, when the umbilical cord gets ahead of the baby and exits the vagina before the baby's head does.

What are the differences in risk between cesarean and vaginal birth? The absolute risks of complications are very low for both types of births, but because of a slightly higher risk of complications or poorer outcomes with cesarean birth along with climbing rates of the procedure, more hospitals and providers are making an effort to decrease the rates. The data support such an effort. Studies done in Canada and France, which won't translate perfectly to the United States, each showed that severe complications and death were about 3 times greater for cesarean births than for vaginal births of single babies. In real numbers, the severe complications rates were 0.9%

for vaginal delivery and 2.7% for cesarean delivery. Thus, for every 1,000 cesarean births, 18 additional complications of some kind occurred beyond what might be expected for vaginal births, though these differences do not account for planned versus emergency cesarean deliveries since the latter is already more prone to complications. Complications included uterine rupture (literally a rip in the uterus, a serious medical emergency), kidney failure, heart attack, shock, anesthesia complications, hemorrhage that required a transfusion or hysterectomy, a major blood clot, a major infection, or a major wound. The rate of each complication varies: for every 2,000 cesarean births, there are 3 extra maternal heart attacks, 5 anesthesia-related complications, and 8 major infections (some of these may be due to preexisting conditions). In the Canadian study, the death rate for vaginal and cesarean births was about the same, but in the French study, the maternal death rate was just under 3 times higher for cesarean births, which translates to about 133 deaths out of 1 million births, compared to 36 deaths out of 1 million vaginal births.

These numbers all refer to single-baby births. With twins, a Cochrane Review found an overall severe complications rate of 8.6% for vaginal birth and 9.2% for cesarean birth, so the differences with multiples is far less significant.

What about longer-term risks for either birth method? There is no difference in postpartum depression between mothers who have cesarean deliveries and those who have vaginal deliveries. There is also no difference in urinary incontinence 2 years after birth. (It's a little higher initially with vaginal births, but by 2 years, there is no difference. The good news is that there's good evidence that pelvic floor muscle training reduces this risk.)

Finally, the risk of respiratory problems in the baby is less than 1% in vaginal deliveries and somewhere between 1% and 4% in planned cesarean birth. (The risks are higher—depending on the situation—for cesarean deliveries that are initiated after labor begins, but this is often due to the reason indicating the procedure.) A small amount of preliminary evidence indicates that corticosteroids before a cesarean birth may decrease a baby's risk of admission to the NICU for breathing difficulties.

Other risks associated with cesarean deliveries don't have anything to do with your first birth, but they do come into play with future pregnancies, such as a higher risk of placental abnormalities and complications (see

TheInformedParentBook.com for our discussion of vaginal birth after cesarean, also known as VBAC). There's no evidence that cesarean deliveries increase future risk of ectopic pregnancy, and although a meta-analysis of studies suggested a very small increased risk for miscarriage or stillbirth, many of the included studies were poor quality, and most did not account for other factors that could be related to needing a cesarean delivery while independently contributing to miscarriage or stillbirth risk.

If giving birth by cesarean affects fertility, the effect is quite small. One analysis of 18 studies found a 9% lower rate of subsequent pregnancies and an 11% lower rate of subsequent births than among women who had vaginal births, but when the authors looked at the studies that accounted for women's age or adjusted for bias, that tiny difference was reduced further. Similarly, a number of investigations have found a higher risk of obesity in children born by cesarean delivery, but these usually didn't take into account other factors (especially related to the mother's health or the reason for the cesarean delivery) to support the idea that the obesity risk was actually related to cesarean birth.

The two most common reasons for cesarean deliveries are a stop in labor, which accounts for about a third, and a concern about the baby's heart rate in almost a quarter, followed by the baby's position (such as breech) and multiples.

Slowed/Stopped First-Stage Labor. Although stalling accounts for the highest proportion of cesarean deliveries, the most recent evidence suggests that labor moves more slowly than doctors have been taught to expect. While there still is no precise definition for how quickly or slowly the first stage should go, a study in 2010 of more than 62,000 women who gave birth to single, healthy babies found that cervical dilation rates were anywhere from 0.5 to 0.7 centimeters per hour in first-time moms and 0.5 to 1.3 centimeters per hour in moms who had already given birth once before. On average, it takes first-time moms about 6 hours (from 4 centimeters) and other moms 3 to 4 hours (from 5 centimeters) to fully dilate to 10 centimeters—but there's little reason to suggest someone's labor has stalled before she reaches 6 centimeters. If labor does stall and a woman receives oxytocin (Pitocin) to move things along (augmentation), it's fine if things move along slowly (as long as they're moving). One study found that getting oxytocin for 8 hours instead of 4 cut the rate of cesarean deliveries for first-time moms in half, with little risk to babies. So what actually qualifies as stalling out? At least 6 centimeters dilation, water broken, plus at least 4 hours of "adequate" contractions or 6 hours of "inadequate" contractions with no change in the cervix.

Long Second-Stage Labor. Again, this isn't clearly defined, and problems with babies (such as infection, NICU admission, and Apgar score under 4) haven't generally been linked to a lengthy second-stage labor, even when it surpassed 5 hours or pushing exceeded 3 hours. However, the risk of maternal infection, third- and fourth-degree perineal tears, and postpartum hemorrhage does increase with longer labors. The best evidence currently is that outcomes remain good for at least 3 hours of pushing in first-time moms and 2 hours in other moms. After that, it depends on the circumstances. If labor is dragging on too long, does that mean a cesarean delivery is essential? Well, that depends on your care provider's training. Use of forceps carries a slightly lower risk of hemorrhage than vacuum delivery or cesarean delivery, and fewer than 3% of women need a cesarean if a delivery using forceps or vacuum is attempted—as long as the provider has been trained to do these, because the procedures are taught less often now.

Fetal Heart Rate. Without getting into the weeds on this one, there is evidence that stimulation to the fetal scalp, position change for the mother, and injection of saline into the uterus (amnioinfusion) may help with heart rate irregularities. The biggest challenge here is that providers just don't have enough good data to guide them on the best way to respond to certain variations in heart rate, especially with all the factors that can influence it. Variation can result from fetal position, maternal blood pressure levels or fever, infection, umbilical cord location, mother's position, mother's heart rate, fetal sleep cycles, maternal medications, natural variations, and other issues, some of which could be serious problems and some of which are not.

Induction. Though we cover this on page 66, there are two important points here: an induction at 41 weeks actually reduces the likelihood of a cesarean birth and problems for a baby, and any induction (after accounting for the reasons for one) does not increase the risk of a cesarean delivery.

Breech Position. When a baby's still butt down, which occurs in 3% to 4% of pregnancies, many providers or hospitals will insist on a cesarean delivery (about 85% of women with a fetus in breech position deliver in this way), but there's an alternative to try first: a review of 11 studies found an external cephalic version—a procedure in which a care provider manipulates the baby through a woman's abdomen to a head-down position—resulted in a cesarean delivery rate of just 21%. Even after a successful turn, women were twice as likely to need a cesarean delivery for fetal distress or another difficulty with the baby's exit, but for every 3 women who received an external cephalic version, 1 woman delivered vaginally. In a different Cochrane Review, an external cephalic version cut the risk of breech birth in half and reduced cesarean births by a third. A different analysis assessed the risks of this procedure based on 84 studies involving almost 13,000 women and found 6% had complications (most commonly a change in the baby's heart rate) and 0.2% had serious complications.

Other Reasons. Unless a baby is at least 11 pounds without maternal gestational diabetes or at least 9 pounds, 14 ounces with maternal gestational diabetes, evidence supporting cesarean delivery for size is poor. Ultrasound is notoriously lousy at estimating fetal weight, and the evidence is pretty clear that there have likely been cesarean births for a "big baby" who wasn't that big and actually increased risks and didn't benefit the baby (or mom). For twins, if the first twin is head down, a cesarean birth doesn't lead to better outcomes, even if the second twin isn't head down. Herpes was once considered an indication for cesarean delivery, but taking the viral suppression drug acyclovir starting about a month before the due date can allow for vaginal delivery unless the infection is active. Doulas appear to be cesarean delivery preventives—a Cochrane Review of 12 trials and more than 15,000 women found that this support during labor increases maternal satisfaction and reduces cesarean delivery rates.

Circumcision

Until 1999, the AAP took a pretty neutral position on the cutting off of some or all of the foreskin covering the penis. They stated then that "potential medical benefits" exist for circumcising, but "these data are not sufficient to recommend routine neonatal circumcision." Since then, a great deal more research has been published, especially related to sexually transmitted infections (STIs) and from randomized trials in some African countries. So the AAP updated its recommendations in 2012 to suggest that the benefits of the procedure outweigh the risks (but not enough to recommend it routinely), reigniting the firestorm over the procedure. The two biggest clash points typically involve those whose religious beliefs require circumcision, as in Judaism, and those who actively, vocally oppose circumcision, often calling themselves "intactivists," who believe it is unethical to cut off a healthy foreskin without a child's consent. These camps represent the extremes, but they often define the debate in the public sphere. Most parents, of course, don't discuss their decisions publicly (for which their sons will likely be grateful later, since the Internet is forever), and those typically less vocal include those who support circumcision for its potential health benefits and those who oppose its routine use for its risks and drawbacks.

In the AAP's 2012 statement, the authors still fell short of recommending the procedure for all male babies, but they did come out more strongly in favor of certain specific health benefits, such as prevention of urinary tract infections, STIs, and penile cancer, noting that the "preventive health benefits of elective circumcision of male newborns outweigh the risks of the procedure." More simply, the consensus of research can be summed up thusly: the benefits of circumcision exist but are small—too small to recommend the procedure routinely—and the risks are far smaller.

Understanding the Risk–Benefit Analysis

Consider the three primary benefits that circumcision confers: lower risk of urinary tract infections during the first year, reduced risk of penile cancer, and reduced risk of HIV, human papillomavirus (HPV), and several other STIs during heterosexual sex. The risks of circumcision are most commonly bleeding, infection, or the wrong amount of tissue snipped off, occurring in about 1 of every 500 newborn boys (0.2%). Other studies have found higher rates, up to 2% to 3%, but these higher rates were also primarily minor bleeding. The AAP report even offered a comparison of a similar surgery: complications involving severe bleeding from tonsillectomies occur about 1.9% of the time in kids age 4 and under. Their statement also notes that, with circumcisions, "the majority of severe or even catastrophic injuries are so infrequent as to be reported as case reports."

These case reports do describe some horrific complications—glans or penile partial or complete amputation, transmission of herpes simplex, antibiotic-resistant bacterial infections, insufficient blood to the glans, tear in the urethra, and death. However, the case reports number dozens out of millions and millions of circumcisions performed, and the majority relate to ritualistic or traditional circumcisions rather than medical ones performed by health-care professionals. For example, the herpes transmissions occurred during traditional Jewish circumcision ceremonies in which the mohel performed *metzitzah*, or oral suction of the circumcised penis, during the procedure, an ancient practice that is rare today except in ultra-Orthodox communities. Two deaths recently occurred in New York City as a result of this practice by a rabbi who transmitted herpes to the infants. That risk does not exist for a child circumcised in sterile hospital conditions.

What Are the Benefits?

The risks in infancy are pretty low (more on post-infancy circumcision risks on page 82), but how beneficial are the benefits?

Let's start with the risk of penile cancer. The AAP committee notes that circumcision can reduce the risks of developing this cancer. The American Cancer Society estimates that 1,570 new cases will be diagnosed in 2012, leading to 310 deaths. This type of cancer is so rare in North America and Europe that fewer than 1 man in 100,000 will get it. Even among men with cancer, fewer than 1% have penile cancer. The risk reduction circumcision offers for this type of cancer was probably included because it's more common (up to 10% of male cancers) in Asia, Africa, and South America. But for North Americans and Europeans, the risk is not high in the first place. The current evidence from two studies suggests that somewhere between 909 and 322,000 boys would need to be circumcised to prevent one case of the cancer, though the study with the larger number was only of fair quality. The huge range results from the initial number of participants in the studies, the statistical methods, and where the study was done.

Then there are the benefits associated with a reduced risk for HIV and several other STIs. Circumcision reduces the odds of contracting HIV during male–female sex by 40% to 60%, based on dozens of studies done in African populations. When the CDC calculated that figure using HIV transmission rates during heterosexual sex in the United States, they came up with a 15.7% reduction. That means if 100 men were going to contract HIV, 15 fewer would get it if they were all circumcised. It's unclear, however, whether the African findings can be generalized to the US population, and a condom is far more effective. There's not much evidence that circumcision reduces HIV transmission during male–male sex. On the other side of the coin, one study found that circumcision can make it a little easier for women to contract HIV from a man.

Circumcised men are 30% to 40% less likely to get any type of HPV, including the relatively harmless strains and the ones that can raise the risk of cancer of the mouth, throat, penis, and anus, and can lead to cervical cancer in women. Some evidence suggests that circumcision reduces the risk of contracting herpes (HSV-2) by 28% to 34%, but these data come from just two studies in Africa. A tiny amount of evidence suggests protection against syphilis, but it's weak. There's no evidence that circumcision decreases the risk of contracting gonorrhea or chlamydia.

Plenty of evidence indicates that uncircumcised boys get more urinary tract infections than circumcised boys, in part because bacteria can thrive in that moist area under the foreskin. Estimates of UTIs vary from 1% to 2.5% among uncircumcised boys. (One older analysis finds a rate of 2.4% among circumcised boys and 20% among uncircumcised boys, but this strays considerably from the bulk of other research.) The AAP estimated 7 to 14 out of every 1,000 uncircumcised boys will develop a UTI before their first birthday, compared to 1 to 2 out of 1,000 circumcised boys. One meta-analysis of 12 studies calculated that it would require 111 circumcisions to prevent a single UTI.

While those numbers are small, 10% to 30% of UTIs involving a fever cause kidney scarring, and UTI complications can be severe. That same study estimated 11 boys with recurrent UTIs would need to be circumcised to prevent an additional UTI, and among those with vesicoureteral reflux (a bladder disorder in which urine can flow back up into the kidneys), 4 would need to be circumcised to prevent 1 UTI. Those authors suggested the preventive benefits of circumcision were mostly relevant for boys already at higher risk for an infection, such as those with kidney conditions or a history of UTIs.

But that suggestion does not consider risk across a life span. A different meta-analysis published after the AAP statement looked at 22 studies involving more than 110,000 uncut males and nearly 300,000 cut males and found lifetime risk of UTIs to be almost 4 times greater in uncut males. Broken down by age, the risk of UTIs was 10 times greater in infants, nearly 7 times greater in children ages 1 to 16, and about 3.5 times greater in those older than 16. While infancy is the highest-risk period for UTIs, the risk doesn't drop to zero after a child's first birthday, and problems become more likely again in old age. That analysis estimated that a third of all uncircumcised males would experience a UTI in their lifetime, compared to 9% of circumcised males. Every 4 to 5 boys circumcised, they found, would prevent 1 lifetime UTI.

Another concern for uncircumcised males is balanitis, a swelling or inflammation of the foreskin or penis. Foreskin infections affect up to 10% of uncircumcised males across a lifetime, estimated one analysis. The risk of balanitis is 3 times greater in uncut males than cut males. The same analysis estimated that 0.6% of uncircumcised males would experience a kidney infection at some point in their lives, a risk 10 times greater than among circumcised males.

So these benefits of being circumcised—a lower risk of UTIs, foreskin infections, and some STIs—then become the risks of *not* being circumcised. A UTI is usually treatable, although some cases can be very serious, and untreated UTIs can damage the kidneys. The frequency of foreskin infections generally fades as boys become school-age, when the foreskin retracts more and they can take better hygienic care of their penis. HIV still carries life-threatening danger, and the treatment is currently lifelong, costly, and variably effective. Of course, there are more prominent risk factors for HIV infection, particularly unprotected sex, regardless of circumcision status.

Why the Controversy?

So if there are benefits to circumcision, including avoiding infections that uncircumcised boys may experience, and the risks are extremely minute, why is the question such a contentious one? The answer is that some individuals perceive male circumcision to be a human rights issue, pitting "bodily mutilation" against "bodily integrity." That perspective is not invalid, but it's a moral and ethical perspective, not a scientific argument (and this book focuses on scientific evidence, not competing ethical positions). Some with this belief, however, will attempt to claim science "supports" not circumcising. It doesn't. It's true the evidence does not support routine circumcision for all male infants. But the evidence also does not support *not* circumcising without an urgent medical indication.

For example, one argument against circumcision suggests that the research shows that circumcision damages penile sensitivity and decreases sexual satisfaction. However, no reliable evidence supports this contention, and exploring this area is problematic anyway. Most studies looking at sexual pleasure come from African countries and involve men who were circumcised as adults in randomized trials looking at STI transmission and then asked about sexual satisfaction. Any changes in sensitivity after circumcision as adults may differ from how losing a foreskin at 1 or 2 weeks old may later affect sensitivity. One study commonly cited by anti-circumcision advocates tested "fine-touch pressure thresholds" among 91 circumcised and 68 uncircumcised men and found the glans of a circumcised penis to be less sensitive than that of an intact penis. But this single study doesn't really tell us anything about sexual satisfaction, which depends on far more than a lab-tested sensitivity analysis. (Other researchers also challenged this study's statistical methods.)

Two other difficulties with studying sexual satisfaction are that men circumcised as adults usually have the procedure for medical reasons that might also influence their sex lives, and cultural and social influences may affect how someone perceives his sex life. A Danish study by a well-known anti-circumcision researcher found a lower level of sexual satisfaction among circumcised Danish men. But very, very few Danish men are circumcised, and the cultural bias there is against circumcision, a fact that cannot be separated from their perceptions. Similarly, circumcision is valued in many African countries for reducing the risk of HIV, so that may affect how men there report on their sexual satisfaction.

Other arguments made against circumcision are that it causes infant behavior changes or that the trauma of the procedure irreparably harms infant brains, but no evidence supports these claims, and birth is arguably far more traumatic for an infant who is circumcised in his first few days of life.

For parents who want to leave the question of circumcision up to their sons, what are the risks of waiting? We know the highest risk period for UTIs is in the first year and that complication rates, pain, and recovery time from the procedure all increase as boys grow older. A study of more than 1.4 million males found that 0.5% experienced complications, but this proportion varied greatly by age. Compared to boys circumcised before their first birthday, adverse events were 20 times greater among boys ages 1 to 9 years and 10 times greater among those older than 10 (though, keep in mind the overall rates were still very low, and some of the complications may have been related to whatever medical situation might have led to circumcision).

It's not hard to find anecdotes online of men who felt betrayed when they discovered that they had been circumcised. Those stories are anecdata that have not been adequately verified or quantified, and not much research has explored how many men regret being circumcised as infants. However, it is unlikely to be vast numbers, or circumcision rates would have plummeted. Rates have decreased, from somewhere around three-quarters of all boys in the 1960s to 55% to 59% in 2010, but they haven't plummeted. Ultimately, the evidence does not conclusively support circumcising any more than it conclusively supports not circumcising.

What We Did: Neither of us will divulge publicly what our sons' penises look like. However, we can say that among our five boys combined, they vary in appearance.

Diapers: Cloth vs. Disposable

Most families in the United States—about 95%—use disposable diapers, so for the vast majority of parents, this question has been answered. Many parents who raise it do so because of a perception that cloth diapers might be more environmentally friendly than disposable ones; however, an incredibly detailed UK analysis of the two options for "nappies" called it a virtual tie based on what's required to make them, use them, and clean or dispose of them. The AAP, uncharacteristically, has no stance on this question, although the literature on diapers is relatively substantial (for example, there are more than 400 hits in PubMed). The EPA sees disposable diapers as nonhazardous and just a part of municipal solid waste in the landfill, and compostable diapers might be the wave of the municipal solid waste future, because, according to one 2013 analysis, they could be transformable into "high-quality compost." This possibility could ultimately give the environmental edge to disposables. Because disposables might be better at preventing diaper rash and yeast infections, parents who do choose cloth should be mindful of the need for frequent changes. One 2005 study in the journal *Pediatrics* found that the dyes in diapers might trigger rashes in some children, but a later paper refuted that assertion, saying that numerous allergen tests showed no evidence of skin irritation or sensitization. Day care centers generally require disposables. In short, neither beats the other in the big picture.

Breastfeeding and Formula Feeding

When it comes to charged topics in the "mommy wars," the way parents feed their children always throws them onto the front lines. The issue also becomes political very quickly since social policies play a role in the choices women have (or don't have) in the first place, and little good ever comes of mixing politics with parenting choices. The reality is that not all women have the same choices when it comes to whether they will breastfeed and/or formula-feed. Some women physically cannot breastfeed or cannot do so exclusively while financial constraints, work obligations, medical conditions, family situations, personal history, mental health concerns, and other factors can affect the risk–benefit assessment of feeding options for others.

While the evidence shows a range of better outcomes for breastfed children, breastfeeding mothers in the United States are more likely than other mothers to have higher incomes, more education, healthier lifestyles (including lower smoking and drinking rates), better nutrition, and better access to healthcare and quality schools. The trick is figuring out what the benefits are when all other things are equal.

Breast milk is pretty amazing stuff. "Liquid gold" might be a stretch considering all the environmental pollutants it can contain, from pesticides to plastics compounds to pharmaceuticals, but milk production is responsive to an infant's needs. One study found more white blood cells—immune cells—in the milk of mothers whose children had active infections than in the milk of mothers of healthy infants. Animal studies have also found that breast milk composition will change according to an infant's nutrient needs.

That doesn't mean breast milk is perfect, however. Exclusively breastfed babies do not get enough vitamin K to remove the risk of vitamin K deficiency bleeding—hence the need for a vitamin K shot at birth, discussed on page 124—and breastfed babies may frequently need iron and vitamin D supplements (the latter because babies get less direct sunlight these days).

These aren't issues for formula-fed babies because formula is some pretty remarkable stuff too, and it's usually fortified with vitamin K, vitamin D, and iron. Thousands of babies died from food-borne infections or malnutrition before infant formula arrived on the scene, so the importance of having a safe, nutritious option aside from breast milk that meets infants' needs cannot be overstated.

One of the biggest fallacies in this mother of all mommy battles is the idea that you must only breastfeed *or* formula-feed, as though they are mutually exclusive options. A related fallacy is that supplementing with formula is some sort of failure or concession. Yet in the countries often held up as models of widespread breastfeeding, it's rarely all or nothing. In Norway, for example, where women have lengthy paid maternity leaves, strong postpartum breastfeeding support, and laws against formula advertising and marketing, up to 99% of women breastfeed. Yet a closer look at their stats reveals something that might surprise the most strident "lactivist." One study of nearly 30,000 Norwegian mothers found that 97% were breastfeeding when their babies were 1 month old, 91% at 3 months, and 80% at 6 months. But guess what? Only 85% were *exclusively* breastfeeding their 1-month-old infants. That dropped to 71% at 3 months, then 44% at 4 months, 17% at 5 months, and 2% at 6 months. By contrast, nearly 80% of US infants have ever received breast milk, 40% are exclusively breastfeeding at 3 months old, and 19% are exclusively breastfeeding at 6 months old.

There's no doubt that breast milk offers various health benefits that formula can't offer, and most are dose-dependent: the more breast milk your child gets, the more benefit your child reaps. The majority of these clinical benefits include lower risks for certain health conditions in infancy and early childhood. As children grow past the preschool years, the health benefits of having been breastfed over formula-fed gradually recede into clinical insignificance because other genetic and environmental factors begin playing a bigger role. By the time kids are teens, having been breastfed plays almost no role in their current health.

But for an individual woman, those health benefits (which we'll get to shortly) may or may not outweigh other considerations or possible harms of breastfeeding. There is little to no research on this issue, but anecdotes abound of women who had the physical ability to breastfeed but doing so incurred significant burdens, financial stress (for example, lost wages), or psychological harm due to a history of sexual abuse or other mental health concerns. Breast-feeding is associated with a lower risk of postpartum depression, but the reasons are complex and a bit of a chicken-and-egg dilemma. Some research links the reduced risk to prolactin and oxytocin's effects on women's moods, but postpartum depression can also precede the decision to stop breastfeeding. And if "choosing" to breastfeed leads to postpartum depression, as it can for some women, then is the benefit of a child's lower risk of ear infection worth the increased risk of having social or emotional difficulties because mom is mentally unwell? But before delving into the morass of social, emotional, and cognitive outcomes, we'll cover the health benefits, which are far better established in the evidence base.

Health Benefits of Breastfeeding

At the risk of overwhelming you with (rounded) numbers, this list provides an overview from multiple studies and reviews, all stated in relative risk, which means the absolute reduction in cases will depend on how common the condition is in the first case:

- Babies exclusively breastfed for at least 4 months have about a 70% reduced risk of being hospitalized for lower respiratory tract infections, and the severity of respiratory syncytial virus infections drops by almost 75%. Two more months of exclusive breastfeeding cuts pneumonia risk by 4 times.
- Infants getting any breastfeeding have a quarter lower risk of ear infections, or half the risk if breastfed exclusively for 3 months. Adding 3 more exclusive months cuts the risk of colds and ear and throat infections in half.
- Infants getting any breast milk are half as likely as those getting none to have gastrointestinal tract infections, a benefit that lasts up to 2 months after they stop breastfeeding.
- Babies exclusively breastfed for 3 to 4 months appear slightly less likely to develop asthma, eczema, and allergic dermatitis, particularly if family history already predisposes them to allergy risk, but the evidence surrounding allergy risk and breastfeeding is complicated and in flux due to confounders.

- Breastfed babies have about a 30% lower risk of inflammatory bowel disease, which affects approximately 1 in 5 children across childhood.
- Limited evidence suggests babies exclusively breastfed for at least 3 months may have up to a 30% lower risk of type 1 diabetes and up to a 40% lower risk of type 2 (perhaps due to lower obesity risk).
- Evidence on cardiovascular health benefits is inconclusive.
- Although breastfed babies have a 10% to 15% lower risk of acute myeloid leukemia and a 12% to 20% lower risk of acute lymphocytic leukemia (both rare in childhood), it's not clear whether the lower risk actually results from the breastfeeding or other factors.
- One ongoing long-term study of more than 1,200 children found that children breastfed at least 9 months had a lower risk of ear, throat, and sinus infections at age 6 than those breastfed fewer than 3 months.
- As we discuss in Chapter 6, breastfeeding cuts the risk of sudden infant death syndrome (SIDS) in half. It does appear that breast milk actually causes this reduced risk through two proposed mechanisms: (1) the influence of breast milk's immune properties reduces infection risk, which reduces risk periods when a baby may be more susceptible to SIDS, and (2) breastfed infants don't sleep as deeply as formula-fed ones, so they arouse more easily.

The powers of breast milk are most evident among very preterm and underweight newborns. The earlier a baby is born, the bigger an impact breast milk can have on that child's chances of survival and avoiding infection. The evidence is so clear in this area that donor breast milk is recommended over formula when a mother cannot provide her own breast milk. Preemies who receive breast milk are considerably less likely to develop infection or necrotizing enterocolitis (NEC), a serious condition in which the intestinal tissue dies off. NEC is one of the biggest risks preemies and low-birth-weight newborns face, because an estimated quarter of infants who develop it will die. A 2014 Cochrane Review found that NEC was more than twice as likely in preemies or low-birth-weight infants receiving formula instead of donor milk, though the formula-fed ones gained more weight in the hospital.

Preemies fed breast milk are also less likely to be readmitted to the hospital during their first year of life, and they have better long-term growth with a lower risk of neurodevelopmental disability, though the children who do experience growth and neurodevelopmental problems are those who developed NEC. Other benefits include a reduced risk of severe retinopathy of prematurity (an eye condition in premature infants that may lead to blindness) and, in adolescence, lower blood pressure, better cholesterol levels, and better insulin metabolism.

The most immediate health benefit for mothers who breastfeed is a lower risk of postpartum blood loss and faster contraction of the uterus. The idea that breastfeeding helps moms lose weight is problematic. The research on this is all over the map, most likely because it depends on so many other factors in women's lifestyles, genetics, and environments. Some women lose weight quickly while breastfeeding. Others gain. Others remain stable. Even one of the largest, strongest studies showing greater weight loss in breastfeeding moms found a difference of only 3 pounds. Another possible benefit that's dependent on women's current health is diabetes risk: mothers without a history of gestational diabetes have a modest 4% to 12% lower risk of type 2 diabetes for each year of breastfeeding, but no effect has been found for women who had gestational diabetes.

The risk of rheumatoid arthritis appears to drop by 20% to 50% among women who breastfeed, based on three studies, and the risk of hypertension, high cholesterol levels, and heart disease also drops slightly, but it's a less than 10% risk reduction and is based on scant evidence. Stronger evidence supports the reduced risk for breast cancer (mostly before menopause) and ovarian cancer, a nearly 30% drop in risk for those who breastfeed longer than a year. A handful of studies have reported risks "per year of breastfeeding," but none of these calculate the benefits beyond 24 months of breastfeeding, so there's no way to know if the benefit keeps increasing or tapers off.

Social, Emotional, and Cognitive Development

Here the evidence base gets very messy. It's nearly impossible to separate the decision to breastfeed from the effects of breastfeeding: a mother who chooses to breastfeed and/or does so will differ from those who never choose to (or are unable to do so) in ways that may not ever fully be understood. One six-year ongoing long-term study of more than 1,400 mom–child pairs found lower odds of emotional, behavioral, and social difficulties among breastfed children, but this finding vanished after adjustment for other factors that could influence emotional and social development. Another study of siblings in which one was breastfed and one was formula-fed (thereby controlling for many—though not all—other environmental factors) found no evidence that breastfed children had better behavior, reading or vocabulary comprehension, math ability, or memory.

Some evidence suggests greater white matter development and a higher IQ in preemies who were breastfed, but this evidence is limited to preterm and low-birth-weight babies, and the white matter study found no effect in girls. Other studies purporting to find stronger cognitive development in near- or full-term babies who were breastfed don't account for enough other factors that can influence IQ and cognitive outcomes, especially parent education, parent IQ, home environment, and socioeconomic status. A review that covered about 400 studies found no evidence that breastfeeding enhances cognitive performance.

The largest randomized controlled trial ever conducted related to breastfeeding, involving more than 17,000 pairs of mothers and children in Belarus, "found no evidence of risks or benefits of prolonged and exclusive breastfeeding for child and maternal behavior." Though a trial cannot ethically randomize infants to be breastfed versus formula-fed, this trial tested an intervention to promote breastfeeding, so it's as close as we can get to a true experiment on the effects of breastfeeding. The same trial also looked at cognitive outcomes and found contradictory results. There were no differences reaching statistical significance on overall IQ and related measures, but the breastfed babies did have stronger vocabulary skills and an average 7.5 points higher verbal IQ as tested by their pediatricians (who were aware of the study). Yet teacher ratings of more than 10,000 children's academic performances in reading, writing, math, and other subjects showed no differences between the breastfed and formula-fed babies. The authors suggest "some constituent of breast milk" or else "the physical and social interactions inherent in breastfeeding" might strengthen cognitive development, but the modest findings and weaknesses in the study make it tough to draw the conclusion that breastfeeding "caused" the higher verbal IQ scores. If it did, and if the reason is due to "the physical and social interactions inherent in breastfeeding," then these interactions would be something formula-feeding mothers could achieve through increased skin-to-skin contact and close interaction with their children.

Obesity Risk, Self-Regulation, and Bottle-Feeding

The evidence on breastfeeding as obesity prevention in children is also muddled, partly because so many factors can affect a child's obesity risk. Together, the evidence shows a range of 15% to 30% lower risk of obesity among babies who did any breastfeeding, though, again, tons of interacting factors in these studies make it hard to know how much is related to the breastfeeding (or breast milk) itself. One study of almost 500 pairs of siblings (one breastfed and one not) found that breastfed siblings had lower weight in adolescence than their formula-fed siblings, a difference that equated to being about 13 pounds lighter at age 14. But the study adjusted only for mother's employment status and the pregnancy weeks when the siblings were born, and other factors might affect why one child was breastfed and another was not. Another long-term study of more than 35,000 women found no link between their lifetime obesity risk and whether they were breastfed. Dozens of other studies are similarly contradictory.

Even a systematic review's finding that each month of breastfeeding reduced the risk of being overweight by 4% was deeply flawed by the many differences among the studies and too few adjustments for other factors.

But more recently, one mechanism has clarified how breastfeeding might reduce the risk of obesity, and understanding it can be useful to formula-feeding parents as well: bottle-feeding has the potential to interfere with regulating food intake. Researchers compared how many of 1,200 kids emptied a bottle or a cup of milk in late infancy; some had been exclusively breastfed, some exclusively bottle-fed, and the rest were both breastfed and bottle-fed in early infancy. While only 27% of exclusively breastfed kids polished off the milk, 54% of mixed-fed kids and 68% of exclusively bottle-fed kids downed the whole cup. Children who fed from a bottle at least two-thirds of the time were twice as likely to empty their cup than those fed from a bottle less than a third of the time—regardless of whether their bottle contained formula or breast milk. It was the bottle-feeding and its frequency, not what was in the bottle, that made the difference.

The authors suggested several possible reasons for their findings. Babies feeding at the breast decide when to start and stop sucking, thereby controlling what they get. They can also more easily express that they want a small amount of milk, maybe just a sip, by pulling on mom's shirt as opposed to having to get truly hungry and signal their hunger with a cry or to wait until someone makes a bottle. Breastfeeding moms may be less likely to encourage a baby to keep feeding at the breast whereas bottle-fed babies may be encouraged to empty a bottle, regardless of whether it's formula (that stuff is expensive!) or breast milk (that precious time pumping!). During suckling itself, infants also control milk flow by adjusting their suck and sometimes sucking non-nutritively (sucking without actually taking in milk). Finally, breast milk varies throughout a feeding, with the fattier hind milk coming at the end and signaling that the feeding will end soon, which may enhance self-regulation.

Other studies have yielded similar results, all pointing to breastfeeding as helpful in infant ability to self-regulate, but these results don't mean that bottle-fed babies don't or can't learn to self-regulate, and we don't know if any of these effects last past childhood. A child who was bottle-fed but whose mother doesn't insist that the dinner plate is cleared off each night can still learn healthy eating habits.

Who Shouldn't Breastfeed

Not all women and/or infants can or should breastfeed, as we note in "Breastfeeding Blues" on page 134. Women with HIV in the developed world can transmit the virus through breast milk, which is a significant risk when clean water is available for formula. Women with active tuberculosis or herpes lesions on their breasts and mothers with an active shingles infection should not breastfeed as long as those infections are contagious. Infants with certain metabolic disorders cannot breastfeed or may require special modified formulas, and infants with human milk allergies obviously cannot breastfeed or receive donor milk.

When Baby Feeding Gets Personal

Although other parenting debates might share the intensity of the "boob versus bottle" minefield, few reach so deeply into women's psyches as this one, though this area has unfortunately been little studied. A single article in an Australian breastfeeding journal in 2014 suggested that the experience of breastfeeding for a small minority of women can "evoke existential vulnerability" and involve "shameful feelings, such as dislike of breastfeeding, aversion to the milk-producing body, and anger towards the child." Clearly, that situation isn't good, but many women, including those discussed in that paper, feel external and internal pressures to keep breastfeeding anyway, despite the potential negative consequences for the mother–child relationship and the child's long-term emotional health. Various studies have investigated postpartum depression and breastfeeding, but almost none have explored the possibility that breastfeeding might cause depression and anxiety in some women, especially in those who struggle with breastfeeding. A few explore the feelings of women beginning to formula-feed and finding a lack of support or even disapproval.

In one review of 23 studies, mothers "who bottle-fed their babies experienced negative emotions such as guilt, anger, worry, uncertainty, and a sense of failure." They also received little information about bottle-feeding, did not feel empowered to make decisions, and frequently made mistakes in bottle preparation. Another study surveyed more than 500 British mothers in 2004 and found a third felt both "guilt" and a "sense of failure about not breastfeeding" when they first fed their baby formula. Although 88% felt relieved that their baby was being fed, almost half were "uncertain they were doing the right thing." A quarter worried what a midwife or healthcare provider might say to them, and 1 in 5 worried about the effects of formula on her baby's health. Half of all women in that survey agreed that "women are put under pressure to breastfeed," and 44% agreed "women who don't breastfeed are made to feel guilty about it." Perhaps contributing to that pressure was the 4 in 10 moms who agreed that "breastfeeding is natural and all mothers can do it."

The refreshing exception to the complete neglect in this area was a 2014 paper that, strikingly, explored the shame that *both* breastfeeding *and* formula-feeding mothers felt. The authors conducted intensive interviews with 63 mostly white English mothers, about half of whom breastfed exclusively and the rest either formula-fed exclusively or used both breast milk and formula. Three themes about the shame women experienced emerged from these interviews: "exposure of women's bodies and infant feeding methods," "undermining and insufficient support," and "perceptions of inadequate mothering." Breastfeeding moms felt pressure to hide their breasts in public, but formula-feeding moms felt pressure to hide their bottles. Self-doubt and anxiety were common among formula-feeders, who experienced betrayal, disapproval, and the implication that they were "bad" or "second best" mothers "depriving" their children of the "best." Meanwhile, breastfeeding mothers felt self-conscious and unsupported with mixed messages: they were expected to breastfeed, but not in public, where they were stared at or frowned upon.

Ultimately, the moms were damned if they did and damned if they didn't. Perhaps one step to changing this reality might be more research that helps everyone realize that both breastfeeders and formula-feeders experience social pressure, judgment, and shame, and little good will come of arguing over who has it worse.

What We Did: Tara exclusively breastfed her first son (except the first night home from the hospital, when he received a couple of ounces of formula), until he was 5 months old. Tara experienced partial secondary lactation failure with her second child due partly to disorganized suckling in a child born a couple of weeks early. Her second son, who initially did not gain adequate weight, subsequently received about 60% formula and 40% breast milk until he started on solids at around 7 months old. She also had a kick-ass lactation consultant for her second son. Emily breastfed her first two for varying periods under one year, with formula introduced for both within the first 6 months. Her second son had a tongue-tie that required clipping before breastfeeding worked for him, and her third son was unable to breastfeed, despite the support of a midwife and two lactation consultants, or even to use most bottles, probably because of a developmental condition. He also could not tolerate regular formula, so she pumped for him and fed him a specialized formula.

Vaccine Schedules: One Has an Evidence Base

Tara remembers cradling her 2-month-old son at his first well-child visit with vaccines, trying to push aside her dread. Three shots and an oral vaccine—a total of 8 immunizations—seemed like a lot for a boy who weighed 11 pounds, 5 ounces and was not yet 2 feet long. Decisions surrounding vaccination can be fraught for the most confident parents, and the misinformation in this area might exceed all others—and with some of the highest stakes.

Some parents never question vaccines, feeling secure in the CDC's or their doctor's recommendation, while others don't trust vaccines, ever, no matter what. But most fall between these extremes. Most parents recognize that vaccines work and want to protect their children from disease, but many are concerned about other effects of vaccines besides protective ones. Because this subject could fill several tomes, we've organized it so you can skim for the specific information you want. Then an appendix on our website, The InformedParentBook.com, lists each childhood vaccine with vital information on each one, including a description of the disease, the vaccine's effectiveness, risks from the vaccine, possible complications from the disease, and special considerations (if any) for that particular vaccine or disease.

The Difficulty of Doing Your Own Research

Most people start their research these days with Google. But googling can lead to frustration and confusion as you click through government sites touting the safety and effectiveness of vaccines and through homegrown, only slightly less polished sites that throw up graphs and dozens of links about how toxic vaccines could be. Images of red-pocked children on government sites compete against heartbreaking anecdotes from parents who feel their children suffered permanent damage from an immunization. Both sides cite peer-reviewed studies and quote medical doctors.

Separating the myths, misconceptions, and half-truths from the facts and bona fide science can be tough. Even PubMed, probably the largest database of peer-reviewed medical studies, is not always helpful. Plenty of junk science gets published in peer-reviewed journals, and properly interpreting abstracts or full studies often requires extensive training.

Just as challenging as finding the information you want is avoiding some of the common thinking errors that lead people to misinterpret the information they find. We cover these in more detail in the section on cognitive traps on page 305, but this section more than any other merits some reminders.

Common Problems in Evaluating Vaccine Studies

Confirmation Bias. Chances are, before you even bought this book, you had some kind of opinion about vaccines, which may make it more difficult to consider information here if something contradicts your beliefs. It's not always something you can easily guard against, but awareness can't hurt.

Confusing Correlation and Causation. Just because two things happen in close proximity does not mean that one caused the other. The most common anecdote illustrating this error is the child who has signs of autism after a vaccine. Parents state their child was fine until receiving the MMR (measles, mumps, rubella) vaccine or another set of shots. Then the child suddenly shuts down within weeks after immunizations. But there are three reasons to check that assumption. First, most children receive the MMR vaccine at 12 months of age, about the same time many detectable signs or symptoms of autism become apparent. Second, parents may be more attentive to these indications of autism after a child's shots because of their fears—even if they missed earlier signs and symptoms. Third, parents might unwittingly assume that coincidences cannot occur: if a person's child got hit by a car the day after he was vaccinated, almost no one would blame the vaccine. But the same possibility of coincidence holds true with other conditions that might happen to occur around the same time a child receives a vaccine. Although we used the example of autism here, the same potential to mistake correlation for causation exists for any apparent "reaction" after vaccines. Every once in a while, a condition *is* due to the vaccine, especially if it's a known risk. Most of the time, it really is a coincidence.

Dosage Matters. Substances like formaldehyde and aluminum may raise concerns until we remember the first rule of toxicology: the dose makes the poison. Every substance on earth—even oxygen and water—can be toxic in the right dose or by a specific exposure route. A child can swim in water for hours without the skin exposure causing harm, but obviously inhaling water can be deadly. Even drinking excessive water can be deadly in rare circumstances. Conversely, many toxic-sounding substances are harmless in low enough doses.

Dunning–Kruger Effect. Our occasional inability to accurately estimate how much we know and how much others know can especially hamper our assessment of the evidence here. An unskilled person often tends to overestimate her skill or knowledge, especially when she has just learned new information about it. For example, a person who reads about a medical condition ahead of a doctor's appointment may arrive at his doctor's office believing he knows as much as his care provider about that condition—but lacks the training, knowledge, and experience of his doctor. Consider everything you know about your child. If someone read a little about your child—say, all his school files—that person might think she had a complete picture of your child's abilities. But you obviously know much, much more.

Misinterpreting the Science. Science is a process, not a body of knowledge, and it's essential to understand how the scientific method works and what it is and isn't capable of doing. Some people want "science" to do things it can't, like prove something is "safe," which is impossible given the constraints of the scientific method. Even those well versed in the scientific method may lack the statistical knowledge or precise terminology to adequately assess a study's findings.

Neglecting a Source's Limitations. Not all sources are created equal, and all have drawbacks. The information in vaccine product inserts and the incidents in the Vaccine Adverse Event Reporting System (VAERS), a database of adverse events (and possible side effects) that occurred to people after being vaccinated, cannot all be taken at face value.

Vaccine product inserts list every ingredient in that vaccine (including trace amounts that may or may not actually be present) as well as every remotely possible thing that might possibly one day potentially happen after getting vaccinated—maybe. These frightening lists do not necessarily mean that those things will happen, or even have happened, because of a vaccine. They are written for legal reasons, not scientific ones. If a person were hit by a bus 5 minutes after getting vaccinated, then that very well might be listed in a vaccine insert just for liability reasons.

VAERS has similar limitations. This government reporting system allows people to report any possible illness or event that occurred after a person received a vaccination so that researchers can periodically comb it for possible vaccine reactions previously missed. *Any* report an individual submits appears in the system, regardless of how truthful it is (or isn't) and whether it had anything to do with a vaccine. (Even car accidents are listed in VAERS.) A single event, such as a child's fever, reported by more than one person (such as the child's parent and the child's doctor) also shows up as two separate entries, which can inflate the numbers. VAERS reports are helpful to researchers but rarely mean anything to individual consumers. (To make a point, one scientist actually submitted a VAERS report claiming he turned into the Incredible Hulk after being vaccinated. That report remains in the system today.) Furthermore, VAERS contains only reports of adverse events, not a record of all the children who received vaccines and nothing happened. Therefore, VAERS does not track information in a way that could show what the risk of a particular occurrence was even if it was related to the vaccine.

Mistaking Personal Experience for Universal Fact. The power of the anecdote is hard to deny. Anecdotes are compelling, personal stories. But they are unreliable and, like any story, easily spun. Furthermore, something that happened to you may not be common or apply to others. And something that didn't happen to you may actually be common among others.

What Was It Like Before Vaccines?

There was a time when whatever risks might be associated with vaccines couldn't compete with public fears of rampaging diseases such as polio. It wasn't hard for most parents to decide whether to inoculate their children against polio in 1955: although 1 in 2.4 million children inoculated with the oral polio vaccine could develop paralytic polio, the chances they would catch the disease itself—potentially causing paralysis or death—were much higher, and the evidence was all around them. Local newspapers even published the number of polio victims each day.

Polio no longer occurs in the United States, and several other diseases have all but vanished. In Massachusetts in the 1880s and 1890s, for example, 10% of all deaths were from diphtheria. Yet only seven cases of this bacterial respiratory disease were reported to the CDC from 1998 to 2004. Certainly, improvements in sanitation and hygiene have also contributed to a drop in disease rates generally, but most diseases we vaccinate against in the United States are not diseases of sanitation. Furthermore, fewer people died from various diseases as medical care improved, but the actual number of disease cases did not drop until vaccines for each one were introduced—and surviving doesn't mean those people didn't suffer or experience long-term disabilities.

Vaccines have become victims of their own success: they have so effectively reduced infection rates that fewer people today are familiar with most of the diseases for which vaccines exist, making it

> Vaccines have become victims of their own success.

harder to see the upside of vaccines. They might hear about these diseases in other countries, but they don't see them up close. They might also attribute the diseases in other countries more to poor sanitation and poor medical care instead of the absence of vaccines. (It's usually all three.) Returning outbreaks—such as the measles outbreak starting at Disneyland in winter of 2014 to 2015—have put the spotlight on vaccines again.

Whooping cough, the common name for pertussis, is one of the few vaccine-preventable diseases that is still endemic (regularly circulating) in the United States today, though the vaccine has dramatically reduced its incidence. Before the pertussis vaccine, between 150,000 and 260,000 cases were reported annually, with up to 9,000 pertussis-related deaths and thousands left with brain damage, seizures, and intellectual disability. Cases are far lower now—just under 17,000 pertussis cases occurred in 2009—but numbers have begun climbing again. The main factors driving the increase have to do with improved laboratory tests for identifying and diagnosing the illness and a change in vaccines. An older pertussis vaccine was very effective but could cause frightening, albeit not life-threatening, reactions, such as seizure from a high fever. A new vaccine replaced it in the 1990s and was also very effective— at first. But the antibodies it triggers fade after several years, so researchers are now working on improving the current vaccine. In the meantime, even the higher current numbers are still well under pre-vaccine historic rates.

Why Vaccines Frighten People

Despite vaccines' success in reducing so much disease, several factors contribute to parents' anxiety about them. First, it's counterintuitive to give an injection to an otherwise healthy person. We tend to associate needles (which are scary in and of themselves) with illness, so when there is no disease, it's harder to justify to ourselves why we should give someone a shot. Plus, needles hurt and our kids cry. Furthermore, most people don't know what's in vaccines. Simply the list of virus and bacteria bits, preservatives, and other additives can scare off some. And then, without seeing the disease as often, it's understandable that some people would transfer fear from the diseases to possible side effects of the vaccines, no matter how rare or unlikely those side effects may be.

But the three factors that have probably played the biggest role in people's fear of vaccines are the media, the actual history of some vaccines, and the mountains of misinformation propagated by a small group of anti-vaccine advocates. It's easy to become preoccupied with concerns about vaccine side effects—real, imagined, or exaggerated—when they regularly appear in the news or online even if the sources can be unreliable. Sometimes poorly done media coverage of real vaccine research or of anti-vaccine advocates plants fear. When Minnesota congresswoman Michele Bachmann said that the HPV vaccine could lead to "mental retardation," the media covered it extensively. Most coverage correctly debunked the statement, but like negative campaign ads, the negative often sticks around longer than the facts, even if subconsciously. Even before Bachmann's statement, media reports about the relatively new HPV vaccine could be contradictory, incomplete, and controversial, causing some to skip the shots for fear of blood clots or other serious complications. (There was initially an increase in reported blood clots in girls receiving the HPV vaccine, but these associations later vanished when researchers found that more than 90% of the girls had an underlying condition, such as obesity or taking birth control pills, that predisposed them to blood clots. No link exists between the HPV vaccine and blood clots or any other serious condition.)

Sometimes, the media manufactures vaccine controversies: the media jumped the gun on a discredited and eventually retracted 1998 study headed by Andrew Wakefield linking the MMR vaccine to autism. Wakefield's paper was only a case series (not a randomized trial) of a dozen children and was later found to contain fraudulent data. The concern about an autism link quickly ceased to be a controversy among scientists following further studies, but the media was slower to report the studies that contradicted Wakefield's findings. It wasn't until 2010 that the *Lancet*, where the study first appeared, formally retracted the article, yet the myth of a vaccine–autism link lives on in the minds of many parents and on dozens of websites.

While the media has (mostly) grown wiser in the past decade, especially as some disease rates have begun climbing again, the anti-vaccine movement is alive and kicking, and anti-vaccine advocates have been very sophisticated at disguising misinformation as middle-of-the-road or "reasonable" and "scientific" information. The most influential organization is the National Vaccine Information Center, which claims not to be anti-vaccine but acts the part in every way. Just as nefarious, however, are sites that profit from inaccurate fearmongering about vaccines by selling supplements, books, DVDs, and other products. Many well-meaning people are part of the anti-vaccine camp as well, having fallen prey to some of the same cognitive traps we discussed previously in assessing the misinformation spread by the anti-vaccine profiteers. The advent of social media has made it more difficult than ever to help parents distinguish between accurate and inaccurate data.

But real issues in the history of vaccines may initially explain some people's hesitation. Consider the following:

- In the infamous "Cutter incident" of 1955, California-based Cutter Laboratories improperly stored their polio vaccine and administered doses containing not-completely-killed poliovirus. After 11 children died and hundreds were paralyzed, health officials passed a series of requirements to improve vaccine safety.
- During the 1976–1977 national swine flu vaccination campaign, several hundred cases of Guillain-Barré syndrome, an autoimmune disease in which the body mistakenly attacks part of the nervous system, were attributed to the flu vaccine—and the swine flu itself never arrived.
- In 1999, the first rotavirus vaccine, RotaShield, manufactured by Wyeth, was withdrawn when it was shown to cause a rare intestinal problem called intussusception, which caused severe diarrhea and could be fatal, in approximately 1 out of every 10,000 children. No children died, and the vaccine was pulled from use, but authorities conceded that future vaccines needed to be tested in larger groups of children to identify the risk of similar events sooner.
- Even as recently as the 2009–2010 flu season, the H1N1 flu vaccine manufactured by GlaxoSmithKline and used in Europe (but not in the United States) was linked to an increase in narcolepsy cases among children, which researchers are still investigating. (The vaccine's use was suspended when the problem came to light.)

Each of these events, however, led to the better monitoring that make today's vaccines safer than ever. In fact, improvements following earlier experiences are the reason that the link between intussusception and RotaShield was found and addressed so quickly. Vaccines are different from most other medications—the threshold for safety must be very high since healthy children receive them, and the tolerance for side effects very low unless the benefit is truly exceptional. For example, the smallpox vaccine—no longer given—could cause death in 1 out of every 1 million recipients, but when smallpox was still rampant, that risk was reasonable. Today it's not. Similarly, the live oral polio vaccine, discontinued in the United States in 2000, could cause paralysis in approximately 1 out of every 1 million doses. Today, with polio eliminated from the United States, that risk is unacceptable and the inactivated polio vaccine, which does not carry this risk, is used instead.

Because the government has made mistakes and vaccines can have side effects—sometimes very serious ones—many parents are left wondering how to determine what's greater: the risk of their child contracting the disease or the risk of their child experiencing serious side effects? How can we make a reasoned, informed decision when we feel we lack all the information necessary to tell us exactly what risks we're taking? We can never know or control all the variables associated with exposure to a vaccine-preventable disease. But the scientific evidence base on vaccine safety and effectiveness is extensive. The IOM has also issued more than two dozen safety reports addressing just about every concern a parent might have about vaccines, including a 2013 report that assessed the entire CDC childhood immunization schedule and found it to be the safest, most effective way to protect children from disease. There is no doubt that vaccines carry risks, but risks surround us every day of our lives. The question is whether the benefits outweigh the risks, and the evidence clearly shows they do. It's not possible to outline all the specific studies here, though we've both written extensively about them online. Instead, we offer an overview of what the evidence clearly shows overall for the most common questions parents have.

Q: **How does a vaccine work?**

A: In all types of vaccines, the components of the bacterial or viral disease—whether it's live or inactivated, the complete agent, or a piece of it—is called an antigen. The body sees antigens as intruders and gears up for battle, calling on B and T cells—two types of white blood cells that fight disease—to start attacking. B cells produce the antibodies.

One type of T cell directs B cells in stopping and starting antibody production while another type of T cell destroys cells that have taken up viruses, bacteria, or vaccine components. B and T cells make short work of vaccine components without causing significant symptoms; some immune cells then become a specialized standing army with a long memory, waiting for the next time that particular antigen, or its close cousin, intrudes again. If it does, the army destroys it before it has a chance to make the person sick.

Thus, by introducing a weakened or killed form or particle of a disease-causing agent or its "toxoids" (toxins with the harmful part removed), a vaccine tricks the immune system into entering battle mode and then producing memory cells that can recognize and swiftly trigger a defense against the real deal if and when it comes knocking—without the person ever knowing.

Q: **How are vaccines tested?**

A: Vaccines are extensively tested in four phases of clinical trials that last 15 to 20 years before the FDA assesses the product for approval. First, an ethics committee reviews evidence on a vaccine, including any from animal trials, and must approve a promising vaccine candidate before it can be tested in humans. Phase I, involving 10 to 50 people, tests whether an immune response occurs. Phase II, involving hundreds of people, tests the safety, level of immune response, and dosages in healthy adults or the population who would receive the vaccine. Phase III involves at least tens of thousands of people and focuses first on safety, followed by efficacy and immune response. The vaccines must not cause harmful reactions, but they do need to stimulate a protective immune response. A Phase III trial is also a randomized controlled trial involving a placebo or another vaccine whose safety profile is well understood. If the trial shows the test vaccine to be safe and effective, the FDA reviews the data to decide whether it should be licensed, what age groups should receive it, and how many doses are needed. Then the CDC's Advisory Committee on Immunization Practices (ACIP) decides whether to recommend the vaccine on the schedule. Phase IV refers to the ongoing surveillance of the vaccine in follow-up studies after licensure to look for extremely rare adverse events (the type that would only show up in millions of people) and to keep an eye on effectiveness. While efficacy refers to how well the vaccine works in clinical trials, effectiveness is how well it works in real life with a diverse population.

Q: **I've heard that vaccines contain antifreeze, formaldehyde, thimerosal (a mercury-containing preservative), and aluminum. Are these or any other ingredients toxic to my child?**

A: First, again recall that the dose makes the poison. Everything is toxic in some amount, and tiny enough trace amounts of almost anything will not harm us. Besides the antigens, vaccines contain a variety of other ingredients (additives or excipients) that serve one of three purposes:

- Carry the vaccine (such as water or a saline solution)
- Preserve or stabilize the vaccine
- Make the immune response stronger (the role of adjuvants)

Gelatin, monosodium glutamate (MSG), or a protein like albumin stabilizes some vaccines to ensure the components do not degrade over time or when exposed to humidity, heat, or light. (Someone with a severe allergic reaction to gelatin could suffer a serious reaction; fewer than 1 in 1 million people are thought to have this severe an allergy.)

Trace amounts of **egg protein** may remain in the vaccines that use eggs to grow viruses, such as flu or MMR vaccines. Current evidence suggests that those with egg allergies can receive these vaccines, but they should consult their allergist, especially if their allergy is severe.

Some vaccines contain **antibiotics**, such as neomycin, to prevent bacterial growth while the vaccine is made and stored.

Formaldehyde inactivates live viruses during vaccine production, and trace amounts remain in the final vaccine. However, our own bodies actually make far more formaldehyde that flows through our blood than what is contained in a vaccine. We also encounter much more formaldehyde every day from car exhaust and various household objects, such as fingernail polish, plywood, laminates, and even grocery bags. We breathe out formaldehyde, and we eat it in fruits and vegetables. The fact that the formaldehyde is in an injection, rather than something we consume, does not make it more harmful, especially since the most harmful exposure route for formaldehyde is inhalation.

Thimerosal, a preservative, was once in other childhood vaccines but is now in only the multidose flu vaccine and one multidose formulation of the meningitis vaccine for adolescents in the United States. Because multidose vials receive repeated needle insertions, the preservative prevents bacteria or fungi from being introduced into the vaccine. Few vaccine ingredients have been as intensely studied as thimerosal, and every valid scientific study has exonerated it of any connection with autism or any other adverse reaction. Yet the thimerosal issue keeps popping up because it contains the mercury atom, which immediately calls to mind the neurotoxic properties of mercury in fish or in the environment. The mercury in fish, however, is methylmercury, a neurotoxin that can accumulate in the body and affect child development. Thimerosal breaks down into only ethylmercury, a type little studied until vaccine safety concerns thrust it into the spotlight. The two types are as different as methanol (antifreeze) and ethanol (Chardonnay). Although massive amounts of ethylmercury can cause neurotoxicity and kidney damage, it's not nearly as dangerous as methylmercury, and the body metabolizes it quickly—within a week or two—rather than retains it. The small amounts in vaccines, past and present, are harmless.

Aluminum is another ingredient that concerns some parents. It's an adjuvant that enhances the immune response so that immunity is stronger and longer lasting. Several vaccines contain aluminum salts, but the amounts are far less than what babies already receive through their environment and even through breast milk and formula. Ingested aluminum gets absorbed and ends up in the same places injected aluminum might end up—until the body eventually excretes it. The only reaction associated with aluminum-containing vaccines is a greater likelihood of swelling, redness, and pain at the injection site than other shots—but that's because of the strong immune response, not the aluminum itself.

No **cells from human fetuses** are present in vaccines. The bacteria or viruses for some vaccines are grown in one of two human cell lines originally derived from fetuses that had been legally aborted for medical or personal reasons unrelated to vaccines. Every religious authority from the Pope to Imans has officially sanctioned the use of these vaccines. And finally, no vaccines contain antifreeze or its components.

Q: **Can too many vaccines at once overload my child's immune system; or, is my child's immune system too underdeveloped to handle vaccines?**

A: This concern rates high among parents, partly because children receive more shots today—up to 31 by age 6 if they receive all annual flu vaccines and no combination vaccines, plus 2 to 3 oral doses of rotavirus vaccine—than children did in the 1980s or earlier. Of course, we also protect against far more diseases than we did back then, and it's what's inside the shots that matters, specifically the number of antigens that activate the body's immune response (and are usually responsible for local reactions like redness and swelling). The immune system does not count the shots—it counts the antigens. The 3 vaccines (protecting against 7 diseases, excluding flu) in the 1980 CDC schedule contained more than 3,000 antigens in total. All 10 of today's vaccines (protecting against 14 diseases, including flu) combined have an antigen number in the low hundreds.

Additionally, a baby's immune system is better developed than you might expect at birth; by 14 weeks in the womb, B and T cells are already present, and a study in 2014 discovered that a newborn's T cells can release a previously unrecognized protein that attacks bacteria, mounting a stronger response than researchers previously thought possible. Multiple concurrent vaccines also won't "overwhelm" a child's immune system because vaccines simply can't hold a candle to what the body— even a tiny newborn's—fights daily. Moments after birth, babies encounter trillions of bacteria from the air, breast milk, or formula, everything they touch or that touches them—and many of these end up on and in their bodies: in their guts, mucus, lungs, blood, everywhere. Some bacteria are harmless, others are not. The multiple layers of the body's defense system fight off most of the harmful ones before they actually get inside the body, but many get through anyway. The infant's body must fight back, just as infants fight off the dozens of viruses they encounter their first year of life. The thousands of antigens in the trillions of bacteria the body is already battling puts into perspective those couple hundred vaccine antigens (spread across several years).

In fact, two immunologists at the University of California, San Diego, once calculated that an infant's body could theoretically handle 10,000 vaccines at once if they consisted of only the antigens they contained. (That calculation did not take into account the other ingredients, which might pose a problem at 10,000 shots, but not at 31.) Sound unbelievable? Yes, well, the human body is pretty remarkable—even at a few months old.

Q: **Can vaccines cause autism, multiple sclerosis, asthma, diabetes, or other chronic illnesses?**

A: More than two dozen studies have shown that there is no link between any vaccines and autism. Eight reports from the IOM, analyzing hundreds of studies, have conclusively determined there is no evidence to show that vaccines lead to asthma, multiple sclerosis, diabetes, SIDS, AIDS, cancer, inflammatory bowel syndrome, mad cow disease, deafness, or autoimmune disorders in children who receive vaccines, or congenital anomalies in children born to mothers who get vaccines. For more information on the specifics of this question, you can look up the IOM reports (online at Iom.edu) and/or check out the excellent book *Do Vaccines Cause That?!* by Martin G. Myers, MD, and Diego Pineda.

Q: **If vaccines are not 100% effective, why do we still vaccinate?**

A: First of all, nothing is 100% effective. No medicine on the planet cures a certain condition every time, just as car seats don't prevent all child deaths from car accidents. But some protection is better than none, and most vaccines offer somewhere between 80% and 99% protection.

And then there's herd immunity. When a high enough percentage of a community is vaccinated against a particular disease, the whole community—vaccinated or not—is protected. Herd immunity (or community immunity) was illustrated during a measles outbreak of 4,000 people in the Netherlands in 1999–2000. The measles vaccine is 90% to 95% effective with the first dose (higher with the second), and measles is extremely contagious. During the outbreak, unvaccinated individuals who lived in a community with a high vaccination rate were less likely to get measles than vaccinated individuals who lived in a relatively unvaccinated community.

Unvaccinated individuals erode herd immunity—unless they are the ones herd immunity is designed to protect: infants too young to be vaccinated, individuals with immune-compromised conditions (such as those undergoing chemotherapy), and individuals who cannot be vaccinated due to medical conditions. As herd immunity drops, everyone—even the vaccinated—are at higher risk for the disease because vaccines cannot offer 100% protection to everyone who receives them. Vaccines can fail in two ways: the immune system doesn't respond initially (called failed seroconversion, or primary vaccine failure) or the antibodies wane over time, called secondary vaccine failure. Herd immunity offers a second line of defense.

Need another example? Here's one from Larry Pickering, executive secretary of the ACIP: "When the conjugated pneumococcal vaccine was introduced into the childhood immunization schedule several years ago, we saw a dramatic decline in invasive pneumococcal disease in children. But we also saw a dramatic decline in disease in adults." In fact, they discovered in adults the same serotypes, or microorganisms, that were in the vaccine children received. "This conjugated vaccine not only prevents disease but it prevents the carriage. Nobody expected that," he said.

Q: **What are the risks and benefits of using a delayed or "alternative" schedule for vaccines instead of the CDC one?**

A: Although there is only one recommended CDC schedule, other "alternative" vaccination schedules have been publicized and seem to offer an attractive choice for parents to go more slowly with vaccines. It's hard to argue that a delayed or selective schedule would offer peace of mind to an uneasy parent, and some parents space out individual vaccines so they can watch for a reaction following each one. For a child with allergies, a known former reaction to a vaccine, or another known condition, that can be a reasonable choice, and it's usually still possible to adhere closely to the CDC recommended schedule while giving the shots individually. It simply means more doctors' visits over a month's time.

But there are significant drawbacks to delaying vaccines, spacing them out, or choosing to follow a different schedule than the CDC's. First, *no other US schedule besides the CDC's has actually been tested for safety and effectiveness.* Before being added to the schedule, every single vaccine has to be tested against all the others to be sure it doesn't create safety concerns or influence the effectiveness of other vaccines and that they likewise don't affect it. The most popular "alternative" schedules aren't alternative at all: they were invented by a celebrity pediatrician who has no training in immunology or vaccine research or development and who readily admits there is no evidence to support their use. That alone is concerning—after all, this book relies entirely on evidence, and there is none to support delayed or selective schedules—but a bigger issue is that there is evidence to show greater risks with such schedules. The most obvious risk is that children are unprotected from those diseases for a longer period of time, and the evidence-based CDC vaccine schedule targets protecting them when they are most vulnerable. If a parent is relying on herd immunity for protection during that time (social responsibility ethics aside), that may be an effective strategy— until an outbreak occurs, or unless others in the community have made a similar decision and herd immunity is too low.

But there are also more risks to getting the shots themselves following an alternative schedule. The MMR vaccine, recommended between 12 and 15 months, is twice as likely to cause a seizure from a fever if given between 16 and 23 months instead. A febrile seizure does not cause long-term harm, but it's frightening, and it completely undoes the peace of mind a parent may have been trying to achieve. The risk of febrile seizure goes from 1 in 3,000 to 1 in 1,500 when delayed in that time frame.

In addition, each extra visit to the doctor's office means being exposed to whatever germs walked in the door that day. Evidence has shown that some adverse events following vaccination were actually due to catching something in the waiting room, so each extra visit increases that risk even if your doctor has separate well-child and sick-child waiting rooms. And needle phobia? Extra visits may contribute to that as well, though the evidence isn't as solid. One study found an increase in children's cortisol levels (stress hormone), as expected, following a shot, but the increase was the same after one shot or two. Multiple shots at one time didn't make a difference, but the increase would occur with each subsequent visit. (Cortisol increases declined as children got older.) Finally, interestingly, a study in 2010 found that children who received their vaccines on time performed better on several cognitive tests than kids who didn't. The difference was slight and potentially due to other factors, such as parental income, but it certainly showed on-time vaccination did not cause cognitive problems.

Q: **Is there anyone who can't get vaccinated?**

A: Yes. Not everyone can receive all vaccines. In fact, that's one of the reasons it's so important for others around them to be vaccinated, to maintain herd immunity. Individuals with compromised immune systems, such as those undergoing chemotherapy, cannot receive live vaccines. Pregnant women cannot receive live vaccines, either, though there are a couple of non-live vaccines recommended for them. And a handful of medical conditions, such as severe allergies to vaccine ingredients, some autoimmune diseases, and some rare conditions, may mean that someone cannot get one or more vaccines. Although most individuals, even with various chronic conditions, can receive vaccines, parents can see what contraindications exist for different vaccines on the CDC website and can ask their doctors about specific conditions.

Q: **What's cocooning?**

A: While herd immunity works on the macro scale in a community, cocooning is the micro version in your own home. Let's say you have a child with leukemia who is undergoing chemotherapy and cannot receive the flu vaccine. When flu season rolls around, everyone else in the house can get the vaccine to provide a protective "cocoon" for the child who can't get the vaccine. The success of cocooning varies from one vaccine to the next depending on the particular vaccine's effectiveness and the disease's infectiousness. It was previously thought that cocooning was a good strategy for protecting infants against pertussis—babies can't get the vaccine until 2 months old, and the youngest babies are at the highest risk of death—but it turns out the current vaccine may not be an effective one for cocooning. Getting mom, dad, grandparents, and siblings vaccinated does slightly reduce a baby's risk of contracting pertussis, but the best protection is provided from a dose of Tdap (tetanus, diphtheria, pertussis vaccine for teens and adults) during pregnancy.

Q: **Can vaccines shed and make others sick?**

A: Viral shedding occurs when a person with a viral infection can "shed" the virus in bodily fluids or by touching a wound, potentially transmitting the virus to others. Some parents may have concerns that live vaccines can shed and make others around a recently vaccinated child sick. Inactivated vaccines cannot shed at all—the virus or bacterium cannot replicate or cause disease. Live vaccines have been severely weakened so that they don't cause disease, but they can replicate in the body. Children might receive four live vaccines: the MMR, flu nasal, chicken pox (varicella), and rotavirus. Of these, the MMR sheds only rarely from immune-compromised individuals. The rotavirus vaccine can shed in the stools of a vaccinated infant, which means good hygiene, such as hand washing after changing diapers, is preventive. Transmission can occur only with direct contact with the virus in the stool, so immune-compromised people should avoid changing diapers for at least a week after a child's rotavirus vaccination. One study looking at NICUs did not find any transmission of rotavirus from shedding. Shedding of the chicken pox virus can occur only if a child develops a breakthrough rash from the vaccine—which is very rare but possible—and someone has direct contact with the rash. There is no evidence that the nasal flu vaccine has led to flu transmission even among those with weakened immune systems, though it is theoretically possible.

Q: **Why does it seem that more vaccinated people than unvaccinated people get sick with a disease during outbreaks?**

A: Often during outbreaks of vaccine-preventable diseases in the United States, if the outbreak gets large enough, more vaccinated individuals than unvaccinated individuals may get sick. At first, this doesn't make sense. Doesn't that mean the vaccine didn't work? But vaccines are not 100% effective, and there are nearly always *far* more vaccinated than unvaccinated people. So let's do a little math: let's say 9,600 people in a community of 10,000 are vaccinated. A measles outbreak occurs. We'll say 200 unvaccinated people get sick and 1,000 vaccinated people get sick. That means 5 times as many people who were vaccinated got the measles than weren't vaccinated, right? But wait—1,000 out of 9,600 vaccinated people is 10%. And 200 out of 400 unvaccinated people is 50%. Just 1 out of every 10 vaccinated people got sick while half of those who were unvaccinated got sick. So in our hypothetical example, the risk for the unvaccinated was actually 5 times greater. It's important to consider not the numbers but the percentages: a small percentage of a very big number (i.e., the sick individuals among the vaccinated) will be larger than a large percentage of a very small number (sick individuals among the unvaccinated), but the odds still favor the vaccinated individuals.

Q: **Is natural immunity superior to immunity from a vaccine?**

A: For some vaccines, a natural infection leads to stronger immunity than the vaccine provides, or the immunity from an infection might last longer, especially if the body developed immune cells with especially long memories while fighting the infection. But for most diseases, immunity from a natural infection differs little from immunity from the vaccine. The difference in gaining that immunity, however, is huge: one comes from a vaccine, with some temporary discomfort and a low risk of serious side effects. A natural infection, well, that's the disease, the whole thing we're trying to avoid! The risk of brain swelling in 1 out of 1,000 measles cases, for example, is a far greater risk than the risk of a severe allergic reaction, which occurs in 1 out of 1 million MMR doses.

Q: **Why are vaccines needed if I'm breastfeeding?**

A: It's true that breast milk delivers antibodies to your baby. The problem is that of the 5 types of antibodies—immunoglobulins (Ig) A, M, G, E, and D—the ones the mother has for fighting off vaccine-preventable diseases, IgG, are transmitted only in tiny amounts in breast milk. Human milk is loaded with IgA, however, which helps with intestine-related immunity. The good news is that IgG can cross the placenta (they're the only ones that can) and fortify a fetus with mom's antibodies against specific bacteria and viral agents. The reason for recommending the pertussis vaccine in late pregnancy is to give newborns a small store of anti-pertussis antibodies until their first pertussis vaccines. But the maternal antibodies delivered by the placenta don't last forever. In fact, they start to decay almost from birth, dropping by half each month, and are usually gone by a child's first birthday. The antibodies from live vaccines, such as the MMR, are robust enough that they last awhile. This is great for disease protection for several months, but if a baby already has a decent store of mom's antibodies, the baby's immune system doesn't respond to the vaccine. That's why the MMR isn't given until 12 months old—after mom's transferred defenses are gone.

Q: **What are the most serious possible risks from vaccines?**

A: When something negative happens after a vaccination, it's called an adverse event. An adverse event can be *anything* that happens, from a seizure to a car accident. Some of these things—such as a seizure caused by a fever—might be related to the vaccine, so that could be considered a possible side effect. Others, such as a car accident, clearly aren't. The problem is figuring out which adverse events are side effects. Fortunately, hundreds of studies have helped researchers sort this out, and others are always ongoing to ensure any other adverse events related to a vaccine are quickly identified.

We discuss each of the mild, moderate, and severe risks for each vaccine in the online appendix at TheInformedParentBook.com, but a couple of reactions are worth noting here. A person with severe allergies to specific vaccine ingredients, such as gelatin or an antibiotic, could have a severe allergic reaction (anaphylaxis), and these reactions carry a low risk of death. An estimated 1 in 1 to 2 million people will experience an anaphylactic reaction. The MMR, chicken pox, influenza, hepatitis B, meningococcal, and tetanus-containing (Tdap and DTaP) vaccines have been linked to severe allergic reactions related to eggs or gelatin. How rare is such a reaction? One study using the Vaccine Safety Datalink found 5 cases of severe allergic reactions among 7,644,049 vaccine administrations—less than 1 dose per million. No one died.

Vaccines can also cause fevers, usually a mild or moderate reaction, and these can sometimes lead to a seizure. (Children are already more prone to febrile seizures in toddlerhood.) These febrile seizures, typically tied to the MMR, can be scary, but they do not result in long-term damage. There have been reports of children developing epilepsy or another seizure disorder after getting a vaccination. A remarkably thorough study in 2014 followed up with almost 1,000 children who had a seizure around the time of vaccination and investigated each case in which the child developed epilepsy or any other (mostly rare) seizure disorders either within 24 hours of an inactivated vaccine or 5 to 12 days after a live vaccine. The researchers found that genetic or other preexisting biological conditions were the underlying cause of the children's seizure disorders. Basically, the seizure disorder would eventually have shown itself, but the first seizure of those that would inevitably have come later might have been triggered by the vaccine instead of a different trigger later on.

A National Vaccine Injury Compensation Program (NVICP) provides payments for individuals who have suffered an adverse vaccine reaction for which the evidence supports causality (that is, there is reason to believe the vaccine could have caused the event). An NVICP payout, however, does not mean the vaccine definitely caused the apparent reaction, just that there is legally a sufficient burden of proof that it was plausible.

Q: **Why is the flu vaccine necessary? Can it give you the flu?**

A: The flu vaccine cannot give you the flu. Period. Can it give you a fever? Possibly. Can you feel a bit crummy in the week or so afterward? Sure. But it will not give you the flu. And feeling crummy with a fever is not the flu. Trust us. The flu is much worse.

The flu vaccine is problematic, though, for a couple of reasons. For one thing, right now, you have to get a new vaccination every year because researchers reformulate it based on what they predict will be that year's most common flu strains. In addition, it can be less effective if the eventual strains that do hit are ones they didn't include as targets in that year's vaccine. However, the flu vaccine is still one of the best ways to reduce your risk of getting the flu or, at the very least, having a less severe infection if you do get it.

The problem is, most people don't realize how bad influenza is. It's not just a really bad cold with a fever. The flu kills people—including healthy people. Every single year. Young children and the elderly are most at risk, but even teenagers and young adults have died from the flu, usually when it progresses to pneumonia or because of another underlying condition. But healthy teens die from it too. Anywhere from 3,000 to 49,000 people die each year from the flu, depending on how virulent the virus is and whether the predominant strain is included in the vaccine that year. The flu has been listed among the CDC's top 10 causes of death for several recent years.

So the flu vaccine is worth getting to protect yourself and those around you. A bonus is that researchers are finding other side benefits to the vaccine, such as a slightly reduced risk of cardiovascular disease and a slightly higher rate of healthy pregnancy outcomes among women who get the flu shot while pregnant (a flu shot is recommended for pregnant women, but not the nasal vaccine). Scientists don't completely understand all the reasons for these extra benefits, but they have been observed in a number of studies.

Bottom line: What should you do? A book cannot give you medical advice that is specific to your particular situation, so it would be irresponsible to say every single person reading this book should vaccinate their children. If your child has leukemia and is receiving chemotherapy, or if your child has a severe egg allergy, these are certainly considerations that might mean your child should not get certain vaccines. The big takeaway should be this: the benefits of vaccines far, far, far outweigh the risks. The scary-sounding adverse events that parents worry about either are not caused by vaccines or, in the handful that can be, occur in fewer than 1 in several million cases. So keep that risk–benefit ratio in mind, consider your child's individual circumstances, research your additional questions using reputable, reliable, science-based resources, and then talk to a doctor you trust about any concerns.

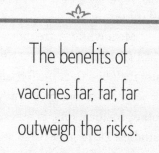

The benefits of vaccines far, far, far outweigh the risks.

Vaccines in Pregnancy

Two vaccines are recommended in pregnancy: the flu vaccine (if you'll be pregnant during flu season, which is true for nearly all pregnant women) and the Tdap, a combined tetanus-diphtheria-pertussis vaccine recommended specifically for the pertussis component. As we discussed earlier, pertussis rates have been climbing, and cocooning is not the most effective strategy for protecting newborns until they can get their pertussis vaccination. Since October 2012, the CDC has recommended pregnant women receive the Tdap in the third trimester of every pregnancy. First, having the shot reduces the likelihood that mothers will catch pertussis and pass it on to their infants (one study found babies were 4 times more likely to catch pertussis from their moms than from others). Second, the antibodies women develop in the 2 weeks after the shot cross the placenta and provide some protection to the fetus, protection that continues after birth. A small trial of 48 women found that babies of women who got the Tdap booster in pregnancy had 5 times as many antibodies against pertussis as infants whose mothers got the booster after giving birth. The third trimester is best so that the antibodies last as long as possible for the newborn.

What about safety? A study of more than 120,000 women found those who got the Tdap were no more likely to have preemies or underweight babies than those who didn't, and another study of more than 20,000 women looked for higher rates of stillbirth, mother or newborn death, preeclampsia, hemorrhage, fetal distress, uterine rupture, placenta previa, cesarean delivery, low birth weight, or newborn kidney failure—and found no evidence for any of these.

Meanwhile, a frequent concern about the influenza vaccine is that it "isn't tested" in pregnant women. While it's true that pregnant women were not included in clinical trials for flu vaccines, this is common for the majority of medications pregnant women take. Flu vaccine safety, like that of many other medications, is assessed after licensing through large observational studies. Dozens of these studies have investigated the flu vaccine in every trimester of pregnancy, and the consensus is that getting it in any trimester reduces the risk of influenza among pregnant women and leads to better outcomes—fewer preterm births, fewer underweight babies, and fewer miscarriages and fetal deaths.

In addition to lower flu rates, the lower risks of pregnancy problems may also be because women who get the flu vaccine likely have other healthy habits and receive better prenatal care. We reviewed more than a dozen other studies involving tens or hundreds of thousands of women: each one consistently found no increased risks to pregnant women or their fetuses from the flu shot but frequently identified better outcomes in association with the flu shot.

What if the only flu vaccine available is the multidose vial containing the preservative thimerosal? Again, despite looking for developmental, neurological, psychological, and other physical problems, researchers have found no evidence of harmful effects from thimerosal on mothers or on their developing fetuses.

What We Did: Tara vaccinated both of her children according to the CDC recommended schedule except for her first son's hepatitis B shot, which he received at his 2-month well-child visit. She got the flu shot during both pregnancies, including one with thimerosal in her second pregnancy. She got the Tdap during the third trimester of her second pregnancy even though she had gotten a Tdap the year before. Emily has vaccinated according to the schedule, delaying a shot only if her sons had a fever.

"I Want to Bank Your (Cord) Blood"

One person's trash is another's treasure, right? Until relatively recently, umbilical cord blood was among the discards of birth. But that was before we knew what treasures lay within, namely hematopoietic stem cells. These are the same stem cells found in bone marrow and have a pretty awesome super-power: imagine them as amorphous mounds of clay waiting to be shaped into whatever kind of blood or immune cell the body needs . . . with the abil-ity to clone themselves. These cells can mature into red or white blood cells and have been successfully used in thousands of transplants since 1988 to treat a variety of blood, immune, and metabolic conditions.

Although most of these conditions are quite rare, a growing industry sells "biological insurance" to parents who are able and willing to shell out about $2,000—and then another $100 to $300 a year—to store their child's cord blood in a private cord blood bank. Just in case.

The question is, just in case . . . of what, exactly? Just in case the child needs it later? Or a family member? Who can be treated with it? What spe-cific diseases or disorders can a cord blood transplant treat, and under what conditions? How likely is it that your child or a family member may need it? And how long is the frozen blood potentially useful? Is it really worth it to invest in private cord blood banking?

First, know that one alternative to private banking or discarding cord blood is to donate it to a public cord blood bank, which costs nothing and screens and stores the blood according to FDA guidelines. Donating your baby's cord blood to a public bank means you likely won't be able to retrieve it later, but if you have someone in your family with a known condition that cord blood may be able to treat, you can make a "directed donation," setting it aside at the public blood bank for that person's use. (Commercial blood banks will do this for free as well.)

Compared to bone marrow transplants, previously the only option for var-ious blood cancers or rare conditions requiring an infusion of healthy blood or immune cells, hematopoietic stem cells have a lower risk of blood-borne infection and rejection by the recipient's body of the donor cells. But there also aren't many cells in the 3 to 5 ounces of blood you can get from the cord, typically just enough for a child but not for an adult (unless combined with other cord blood donations, an increasing and, so far, mostly successful practice). Furthermore, engraftment—in which the transplanted cells grow and reproduce—fails more often with cord blood than with bone marrow and may also take longer, which means the immune system isn't up and running as quickly, and the window for possible infections is open longer.

So it would seem helpful to have cord blood stem cells available if your child ended up needing such a procedure, a possibility that private cord blood banking companies are, uh, banking on when they try to sell you their services, right? But here's the thing: a person's own cord blood can't help him if his condition is genetic—the cord blood contains the same DNA. And it's also unlikely to help him even if the condition isn't genetic, because with, say, leukemia, more of the same immune cells aren't going to fight the cancer as effectively as well-matched donor cells will (since those original immune cells failed to successfully fight it in the first place). In fact, one estimate puts the number of transplants in which a person used his own cord blood at fewer than two dozen, ever. His cord blood could help a sibling, however . . . in the 25% chance that the blood is a match for the sibling.

So banking your baby's cord blood is not actually as much of an insurance policy for your baby as it might be for others in your immediate family. Even then, hematopoietic stem cells can be used only currently to treat just five types of conditions: blood cancers, bone marrow failure, genetic blood disorders, immunodeficiencies, and genetic metabolic disorders. The likelihood that your child or an immediate family member will use that cord blood ranges from 1 in 1,000 to 1 in 200,000, but the most accepted approximation is about 1 in 2,700. (Cord blood companies put the lifetime odds of needing a stem cell transplant at about 1 in 217, but that's assuming "universal donor availability" and "broadening of use" of the blood, among other assumptions—and even then the stem cells could come from a public blood bank.)

But wait—what if science finds ways to cure diabetes or schizophrenia or neurological disease or cystic fibrosis? That what-if is basically what cord blood companies are selling. "Who knows what we'll be able to do with cord blood in 20 years?" Well, who knows what other treatments for those conditions we might come up with in that time besides stem cell use? Or maybe we'll discover other ways to harvest stem cells. Selling an insurance policy on that kind of what-if is like selling property on Mars when it's just as likely we'll colonize the moon first . . . and forget Mars was ever an option.

There are ongoing clinical trials for using cord blood cells to treat cerebral palsy, type 1 diabetes, several autoimmune disorders, and other conditions. But studying something doesn't guarantee the research will yield fruit. Private cord blood companies will also tell you that cord blood cells have already been used to treat deafness, lung injury, stroke, Parkinson's disease, cirrhosis of the liver, heart damage, rheumatoid arthritis, and a dozen or so other conditions . . . in rats. But if curing something in rats meant anything for humans, then we'd have cured cancer decades ago. Right now, cord blood can be used for those five conditions mentioned earlier, and that's it. And we don't know one way or another if it will ever be useful for anything else.

If you do decide to go with a private cord blood bank, be sure to research them carefully. An investigation by the *Wall Street Journal* found that a number of the small private cord blood banks are facing lawsuits for poor conditions or failure to store the cord blood adequately, and others have received poor inspections from the FDA.

What We Did: Emily banked her first son's blood at a commercial bank, 14 years ago. Tara did not bank either baby's blood at all.

CHAPTER 4

The Birth Day

How Important Are Apgar Scores?

This score, named after Virginia Apgar, who developed the screening tool in 1966, is often described as one of the first grades your baby will receive. The assessment comes at 1 minute and again at 5 minutes after birth and involves evaluation of breathing, heart rate, muscle tone, reflexes, and skin color. For each category, your child will receive a 0, 1, or 2, with 2 being the maximum and 10 being the best possible total Apgar score. For breathing, no breathing gets a 0 while lusty crying gets a 2. For heart rate, more than 100 beats a minute gets a 2, and no heartbeat gets a 0. Muscle tone ranges from 0 for loose and floppy to good movement, which gets a 2. Making a face—grimacing—is actually a good thing, and a good grimace after a stimulus like a little pinch gets a newborn a 2 whereas no facial reaction gets a 0. Finally, pink is the target skin color for the newborn and gets a 2, but blue, which suggests lack of oxygen to tissues, gets a 0.

A score of 7 or above is considered good, and there's no need to obsess about a perfect 10, because little blue feet or hands are common and normal and get baby a 1 for skin color. The 5-minute Apgar is intended as a reassessment and, when interventions have been performed based on a low first Apgar, to check for improvement.

What is the purpose of this score? It has one primary purpose, and the systems it incorporates hint at it: to indicate the immediate health status of the infant, particularly as it relates to breathing and oxygenation, and to determine if resuscitation measures are needed. According to a 2006 AAP opinion on Apgar scores, the 1-minute Apgar does not serve as any kind of predictor of long-term outcomes. A low 5-minute score—which, remember, can reflect the success level of interventions—can be a predictor of neonatal mortality, according to one study, and of cerebral palsy as well, according to another analysis. A low score on the 5-minute Apgar does not, however, show a strong correlation with future neurological conditions such as seizures, and even the association with cerebral palsy is not strong; 75% of people with cerebral palsy have a normal 5-minute Apgar score.

Finally, the Apgar score carries a subjective element—determination of skin color, intensity of grimace, evaluation of muscle tone. So even within those hard numbers and science, there is a great deal of human art and subjectivity. The influence of this factor becomes clear when you consider that studies have found that healthcare providers barely manage a 50% consistency rating in assigning Apgar scores for the same cases.

Baby Weight

The average weight of a newborn in the United States is 7.5 pounds, but anything between 5.5 pounds (2,500 grams) and 8.8 pounds (4,000 grams) is considered normal. About 5% of newborns fall outside this range, and falling either above or below is linked to a higher risk of various conditions, particularly falling below. Before we discuss these, it's important to know the two ways to classify weight outside the norm: absolute birth weight and weight-for-gestational age. It's easy to confuse "low birth weight" with "small for gestational age," for example.

- Low birth weight refers to a baby who weighs fewer than 5.5 pounds (2,500 grams), regardless of what week of pregnancy the baby is born. Very low birth weight (VLBW) is below 3.3 pounds (1,500 grams), and extremely low birth weight (ELBW) is below 2.2 pounds (1,000 grams).
- High birth weight, also called macrosomia, refers to babies who weigh more than 8 pounds, 13 ounces (4,000 grams) or 9 pounds,

15 ounces (4,500 grams), depending on the study, again independent of when the baby is born during the pregnancy.

- Small for gestational age (SGA) means a baby is smaller than would
be expected—below the 10th percentile—for the week she was born
(gestational age) during the pregnancy. It is possible for a baby to
have both a low birth weight and be small for gestational age, but
they are not the same thing. A baby born several weeks early, for
example, might have a low birth weight but not necessarily be smaller
than expected considering how early she was born. An SGA baby is
also referred to as being "underweight" in this book.

- Large for gestational age (LGA), as you might guess, means the baby
is bigger than would be expected—above the 90th percentile—for
his gestational age. Weighing 8 pounds at birth would not be considered high birth weight, but it could be considered large for gestational age if the child was born at 32 weeks.

But what does all this actually mean? Birth weight acts as an intermedi-
ary, or a proxy, when it comes to risk. It's a biomarker, a characteristic that is
used to estimate risk of presence of other characteristics. By itself, a baby's
weight means nothing except the number you post on social media and in
your baby announcements. But being underweight or overweight at birth is
used to estimate what a child's risk is for something else, such as diabetes,
cardiovascular problems, or IQ decrease. A great number of studies have
linked birth weight to various outcomes: bigger babies are more successful,
really big babies have lower IQs, smaller babies have more asthma, really small
babies have slower development, and so on. But all these present a risk of
something; they aren't a guarantee.

Therefore, when you read that certain things will increase or decrease
the risk of high or low birth weight, you're passing that through two filters:
having gestational diabetes increases the risk of a large baby (macrosomia)
and being a large baby increases the risk, according to some studies, of a
lower IQ. Does that mean having gestational diabetes will affect your child's
IQ? Not at all. For one thing, the studies linking high birth weight to IQ are
flimsy, and for another, you have two layers of risk there—the risk that gestational diabetes leads to a big baby *and then* the risk that being a big baby
leads to some other outcome. Furthermore, it's not that birth weight *causes*

anything. Babies born small for gestational age, or underweight, can be up to 40 times more likely to die in infancy. This isn't because they're small. It's because being small is a result of other factors, such as being born very preterm, that accounts for the outcomes.

So what are the outcomes associated with being overweight or underweight at birth? As noted above, mortality is higher for the smallest babies. Some studies show mortality as being slightly increased for the largest babies, but most reviews find no increased risk. For large babies, both large for gestational age and those with macrosomia, the risks are generally related to birth: cesearean section risk doubles (though that does not mean those surgeries are all medically necessary), postpartum hemorrhage risk doubles, and the risk of shoulder dystocia (one shoulder becomes stuck) increases by at least 7 times (depending on size). Gestational diabetes increases the risk that a baby will be born LGA or with macrosomia, but any baby with a high birth weight (even if not related to gestational diabetes) has a higher risk of having above-normal blood sugar, becoming obese, or developing metabolic syndrome. Metabolic syndrome—a risk factor for type 2 diabetes, heart disease, and stroke—is diagnosed when someone has three of these five symptoms: high blood pressure, high blood sugar, excess abdominal fat, too little good cholesterol, or too much bad cholesterol.

It's the babies on the low end of the spectrum who face the greatest health and developmental risks, partly because most underweight or low-birth-weight babies are preemies or had experienced some other problem in the womb, such as growth restriction. Sometimes this problem is due to an exposure during pregnancy, such as smoking, and sometimes it's due to chromosomal abnormalities or an infection in the uterus. Sometimes there is no known cause. As birth weight decreases, even starting at 6.6 pounds (3,000 grams), the risk of infections, illnesses, motor delays, behavioral problems, cerebral palsy, learning disabilities, poorer cognitive function, stuttering, ADHD, and other developmental delays increases. The vast majority of low-birth-weight and SGA infants, however, will be fine—it's as a group that they show these greater risks, and the particular challenges each child may or may not face will depend on individual circumstances. What links all these outcomes to infants small for their gestational age isn't simply that they're small—it's whatever caused them to be small in the first place. Whatever that cause is, the more severely small it made them, the more severely it's likely to affect other outcomes. Unsurprisingly, birth weight tends to correlate with income—higher-income moms give birth to heavier babies—because they have access to more resources, better nutrition, and good-quality prenatal care.

Birth Practices: Vitamin K, Eye Drops, and Cord Clamping

Vitamin K: The Shot You Don't Want to Skip

If we had written this book even a decade ago, we might not have thought to include this subject, because vitamin K has been such an uncontroversial standard-of-care intervention since the AAP began recommending it in 1961. But the past several years have seen increasing numbers of parents skipping the shot. Still, a very small minority of parents turn it down: somewhere between 0.5% and 3%, depending on geography, though the rate is up to 7 times higher among birthing center births and home births. But if the numbers continue to grow, the result won't be small at all. In short, we'll see more babies dying or having serious long-term problems from severe brain bleeds and/or abdominal hemorrhaging.

Vitamin K is a fat-soluble vitamin that's actually named after what it does: *Koagulation*, the German word for "coagulation." It activates the molecules (clotting factors) that allow our blood to clot. If our vitamin K levels drop too low, though the threshold varies from person to person, we can spontaneously bleed internally. We get about 90% of our vitamin K from diet (mostly leafy green vegetables) and about 10% from bacteria in our intestines.

But it's metabolized and stored in the liver—not free-floating throughout the body—so almost none of a pregnant woman's vitamin K crosses the placenta. All babies are therefore born vitamin K deficient, putting them at risk for uncontrolled bleeding if their vitamin K levels drop too low and they have not received a dose to hold them over until they're eating solid foods (and their livers have developed sufficiently to extract and use the vitamin K in food). Yes, such hemorrhaging is really rare—but the results can be catastrophic. Any vitamin K deficiency bleeding can result in gross motor skill deficits; long-term neurological, cognitive, or developmental problems; organ failure; or death.

The three types of vitamin K deficiency bleeding—early, classic, and late—can occur in the brain or in the gut. Approximately 0.25% to 1.7% of newborns who don't receive vitamin K at birth will experience classic or early vitamin K deficiency bleeding. Classic is within the first week after birth; early is in the first 24 hours. However, nearly all early vitamin K deficiency bleeding is secondary, which means the newborn has an underlying disorder or was born to a mother who was taking medications that inhibit vitamin K, such as antiepileptic drugs, some antibiotics, tuberculosis drugs such as isoniazid, or blood thinners such as warfarin (Coumadin).

Late vitamin K deficiency bleeding, occurring when a baby is between 2 and 24 weeks old, affects an estimated 4 to 10 of every 100,000 babies who don't receive vitamin K at birth. About 1 in 5 babies who develop late vitamin K deficiency bleeding die, and 2 of every 5 who survive have long-term brain damage. Because it's rare and internal, it's always easy for the bleeding to go undiagnosed for too long, which probably contributes to the high mortality and long-term effects. The treatment for the bleeding is vitamin K.

Babies who are exclusively breastfed are at higher risk than formula-fed babies for vitamin K deficiency bleeding because most formula is fortified with vitamin K (about 55 mcg/L). A breastfeeding mother, however, does not transfer much vitamin K through her breast milk (about 1 mcg/L)—no matter how many supplements she might take—because, again, it's stored in the liver instead of being transported freely throughout the body. In fact, nearly all babies who experience vitamin K deficiency bleeding today are exclusively breastfed.

To almost entirely reduce this risk (nothing is 100%, but this comes darn close), babies receive an injection in their muscle of 0.5 to 1 milligrams (depending on birth weight) vitamin K after birth. Oral vitamin K is an option for those not wanting the intramuscular injection, but there are several reasons to choose the shot over oral administration: first, the oral option requires three carefully timed administrations, which are easy to forget, especially in the hectic first weeks after a newborn's arrival. Second, oral vitamin K is less effective than the shot—particularly for late vitamin K deficiency bleeding—because the shot's vitamin K is absorbed more easily and lasts longer. Anywhere from 1 to 6 of 100,000 babies who receive the oral vitamin K will still develop late bleeding.

What about side effects? Vitamin K is one of the very few interventions that has practically no risk of side effects except the temporary pain of an injection. Again, nothing is 100%, but the only documented possible effects are bruising at the injection site. After all, it's an essential vitamin. So what happened before vitamin K administration was standard? Is this some new deficiency of the modern era? No. Babies have always been deficient—vitamin K deficiency bleeding used to be called hemorrhagic disease of the newborn when it was first described in 1894. But the condition was so rare compared to the many other risks for newborns that it didn't garner much attention or resources until neonatal care improved enough for it to become an unacceptable risk and we learned (in 1944) how to prevent it.

Parents typically cite up to three reasons for declining the shot: they don't think it's necessary, they fear ingredients ("toxins") in the injection, or they fear the shot might cause leukemia. Regarding its necessity, the risk for vitamin K deficiency bleeding is highest in the first week of life. As far as ingredients, aside from the vitamin K, the preservative-free shots contain polysorbate 80, propylene glycol, sodium acetate anhydrous, and glacial acetic acid—all safe, standard ingredients that help the vitamin K dissolve, maintain the shot's moisture, or adjust the pH. Fears about leukemia stem from a relatively small case–control study (fewer than 800 children) with results that have never been replicated. A year after it was published in 1992, two *much* larger studies (1.4 million children and more than 50,000 children) found no link to cancer or any other conditions. Neither did eight more studies done later.

Eye Drops

Erythromycin eye ointment is administered to nearly all newborns for one reason: to prevent a type of pinkeye called ophthalmia neonatorum or neonatal conjunctivitis, which causes blindness in 3% of babies who have it. The primary causes of this type of eye infection are the sexually transmitted infections gonorrhea and chlamydia. Until the 1880s, about 1 in 10 babies developed ophthalmia neonatorum, which meant 3 of every 1,000 went blind from it. Today, erythromycin is used to prevent it instead of silver nitrate, which prevents only gonorrheal pinkeye and was used in the 19th century.

Erythromycin is just as effective as (and less irritating than) silver nitrate in preventing gonorrheal pinkeye infections and further reduces the risk of chlamydia-caused infections by 30%.

If a mother does not have gonorrhea or chlamydia, however, a baby isn't at risk for ophthalmia neonatorum, and there's no evidence to show that erythromycin prevents any other kind of eye infection besides this type of pinkeye. Babies who do develop it and didn't receive erythromycin can be cured with antibiotics before blindness develops. The babies that primarily benefit from the eye ointment are those born to mothers who aren't screened for gonorrhea and chlamydia, who get false-negative test results, or whose sexual partners infect (or reinfect) them after screening.

The risks of erythromycin are eye irritation and temporarily blurred vision, and it has a 20% failure rate in preventing gonorrheal pinkeye infections. One study also found that it contributes to antibiotic resistance, a bigger issue relating to overall antibiotic usage. However, about two-thirds of US states require the administration of the ointment, so it may not be something parents can opt out of. It's also worth checking to be sure your baby is actually receiving erythromycin and not an untested alternative; a 2009 shortage of erythromycin led some providers to use gentamicin, which hadn't been tested in newborns and caused some adverse effects, such as eyelid swelling and, in more severe cases, skin blistering.

One safe alternative is povidone-iodine, a non-antibiotic disinfectant that's just as effective at preventing gonorrheal or chlamydial pinkeye, but it's not yet available in the United States. Babies born by cesarean section would be unlikely to develop ophthalmia neonatorum if their mothers' water never broke.

Cord Clamping

Sometimes an intervention becomes common practice because it's thought to reduce a specific risk, but by the time it becomes clear that the intervention doesn't actually reduce that risk, it's already standard practice—and then it's harder to change. So it has been with delayed cord clamping until very recently. Throughout most of human history, there was no rush to cut the umbilical cord, which often remained attached for several minutes or longer, and certainly long enough for blood to stop pulsing through it. But for various reasons, including simple speed and efficiency in medical settings and the belief that early cord clamping reduced the risk of postpartum hemorrhage in mothers, cutting the cord immediately after birth became standard practice.

Research now shows that when the cord is clamped has no bearing on hemorrhage risk or on newborns' risk of death. But the past decade or so of research has also shown pretty clearly that waiting to clamp the cord for 2 to 3 minutes, rather than in the first 10 seconds after birth, carries a number of pretty significant benefits with very little risk.

In short, blood circulation continues through the cord in the minutes after birth, and about a third of a newborn's total blood volume is still in the placenta at birth. Guess what happens to all that (iron-rich) blood if you wait to cut the cord? It flows into the newborn, giving babies anywhere from 20 to 40 additional milliliters of blood volume than if the cord was cut right away (within 5 to 10 seconds). How fast this birth-blood transfusion takes place depends: about half is transfused in the first minute, and about 90% has been transferred 3 minutes after birth; but a complete transfusion may require up to 5 minutes if a baby is immediately placed skin-to-skin on a mother above the placenta, thereby forcing the blood to pump against gravity.

So what are the benefits of all that extra blood? Most important, it's rich in iron, the mineral essential for hemoglobin to carry oxygen throughout the body. Iron deficiency, which exists in about 10% of US toddlers (the proportion is higher among some demographics), is linked to poorer attention, memory, and overall cognitive development. Severe deficiencies can even interfere with children's social and emotional development. The iron stores a baby has at birth need to last until she begins getting iron through solid foods, usually at around 6 months old, unless she's otherwise getting iron supplements. And even though most infant formulas are fortified with iron, breastfed babies are at higher risk for iron deficiency without supplements. About 20% of exclusively breastfed babies have an iron deficiency by 9 to 12 months old.

Waiting 2 to 3 minutes to clamp the umbilical cord means approximately 30 to 35 milligrams more of iron, which can add an extra 2 to 4 months' worth of iron stores to a baby's blood. Delayed clamping also increases hemoglobin and the proportion of red blood cells in a baby's blood up to 6 months later and cuts an infant's risk of anemia in half. Although this boost is most beneficial for smaller babies or those born to iron-deficient mothers, even full-term babies following low-risk pregnancies have a lower risk of iron deficiency when the cord is clamped later than a minute or so. For babies who may be exposed to lead, that extra iron also reduces their risk of lead poisoning since iron inhibits the body's ability to absorb lead. Finally, delayed cord clamping makes for a smoother cardiopulmonary transition between the uterus, where a baby's oxygen comes from the cord, and the big wide world, where a newborn's lungs must start providing the oxygen: it's like getting a final "gasp" of oxygen-rich blood before the lungs fully take over.

For preterm babies, the benefits of delayed cord clamping are even greater since iron storage particularly builds up in the last 8 weeks of a full-term pregnancy. Most studies have focused on preemies and found that delaying clamping by even 30 to 45 seconds reduces the risk of brain bleeding and bacterial infection; reduces the likelihood of needing a blood transfusion; and increases brain oxygenation, circulating blood volume, and red blood cell concentration. One study found delayed cord clamping in preemies to be linked to a slightly reduced risk of motor skills delay or disability.

The main risk some studies have found with delayed cord clamping is a higher risk of jaundice or need for light therapy, though the data are contradictory on this, and the risk may not exist. Several studies also found a higher risk of polycythemia—an excessive concentration of red blood cells—but the condition resolved and did not lead to any actual problems.

What if a baby is struggling to breathe or needs immediate attention at birth? On one hand, struggling babies whisked off for help almost immediately receive fluids and oxygen—the very things that last bit of cord blood gives them. Ideally, the extra few minutes attached to the placenta should be just as good as whatever they're getting without the cord, which the studies on premature babies somewhat reinforce. That said, studies have not looked at these situations, so there isn't evidence one way or the other looking at delayed cord clamping in babies needing resuscitation or other emergency care. Furthermore, asking doctors to follow an unfamiliar procedure rather than their training may introduce mistakes.

What about those delivering by cesarean section or those who want to bank or donate cord blood? It is possible to delay cord clamping in cesarean deliveries (in fact, it's standard with some practitioners), and it's also possible to collect enough cord blood to bank or donate while also clamping the cord later. Check with the cord blood bank on the procedure your care provider should follow to do this.

Mother-Baby Separation

This subject might not be as broadly relevant as it was even 10 years ago, but because childbirth practices still remain less than optimal in some areas, we felt that the evidence around keeping mother and newborn together after birth, in the absence of medical reasons indicating otherwise, is worth presenting. First of all, we bring you the AAP, which states in its breastfeeding guidelines for hospitals that just after the birth, hospital staff should:

> Dry the baby, assign Apgar scores, provide identification bracelets to mother and baby, and perform initial physical assessment while the newborn is with the mother. The mother is an optimal heat source for the neonate. Normal newborn care such as weighing, measuring, bathing, needlesticks, vitamin K, and eye prophylaxis should not delay early initiation of breastfeeding. Newborns affected by maternal medication and primiparous mothers may require assistance for effective latch-on and initiation of breastfeeding. Except under special circumstances, the newborn should remain with the mother throughout the recovery period.

The evidence base for keeping mother and infant together is compelling. The authors of a Cochrane Review from 2012 concluded that they could find no evidence supporting mother–baby separation. In their review, which targeted the effects of separation versus rooming-in on breastfeeding duration, the authors found only one study that met their inclusion criteria. That report on 176 women found that mothers who were separated from their infants after the birth were 42% less likely to be exclusively breastfeeding at day 4 postpartum. That's a pretty rapid effect of mother–baby separation.

Regarding the longer term, such as 1 year, a 2009 study of 176 Russian mothers found that having mother-to-infant skin-to-skin contact or early suckling for 25 minutes up to 2 hours was associated with positive mother–baby interactions a year later. They confirmed their findings using videotape. The contact and suckling was important within the first 2 hours in this study; even a 2-hour separation seemed to influence the 1-year outcome even if infants otherwise roomed-in with their mothers.

Another Cochrane Review confirmed the importance of early skin-to-skin contact for outcomes like breastfeeding. In a 2012 review, researchers evaluated 34 randomized controlled trials of mothers and their infants and found positive benefits of early skin-to-skin contact (placing the newborn naked and prone on the mother's chest and covering the infant's head with a little hat and back with a blanket). This early contact was associated with benefits for breastfeeding and decreased crying, better heart rate stability in late pre-term infants, and improved early blood sugar levels. Interestingly, a small 2013 study of infants who were briefly separated from their mothers, followed by skin-to-skin contact, found that the cesarean-delivered babies cried less during the maternal separation than those born by vaginal delivery. Babies who cried longer had higher cortisol levels, but the study involved only 31 infants, and oxytocin was used in the vaginal deliveries, which suggests a couple of major limitations.

Thus, the evidence supports the AAP recommendations for immediate skin-to-skin contact between mother and infant as long as no medical situation demands otherwise.

Getting Over Baby Bonding Guilt

Here are a few things that did *not* happen when Tara had her son in June 2010: angels did not fly into her room singing, and fireworks did not go popping out her window. She and her husband also did not weep tears of joy and love, and she did not fall madly in love with the creature in her arms, suddenly realizing in a flash that her entire world had changed. In fact, he wasn't even in her arms. He was clumsily placed beside her head in a tightly wrapped bundle, while she waited for the placenta to make its exit (it never did—she needed an emergency surgical extraction). The point is that she didn't experience that wave of love washing over her that she had read about. (And actually, the retained placenta might have partly accounted for that since its release triggers some of the hormones that contribute to that sensation.) One moment there had been a cantaloupe-size head lodged in her vagina while she impatiently waited for the doctor, and the next, there was the tinny cry of a newborn in the room, but nothing else was really different.

Over the next few weeks, she felt similarly detached. In fact, the strongest emotion she experienced was guilt at *not* feeling enough for this strange, needy little critter. She didn't have postpartum depression, she didn't dislike him, she thought he was cute, his cries brought her running and seeking ways to calm him, and she quickly responded to his needs. But when she looked at him, she felt as she might about a new little puppy: bemused affection for a cute, clumsy, odd sort of creature who relied on her for everything.

But here's the thing: *none of this is abnormal.* And none of it means bonding wasn't occurring or wouldn't occur. And none of it meant her son wouldn't develop the attachment that becomes so critical in his first 2 years for later development. In fact, several studies on attachment have found a child needs to bond with only one of his parents—the second is just gravy—for healthy development. It's lacking attachment from both parents that's linked to more behavioral problems. Regardless, feeling that awkward weirdness and not hearing muses whispering love sonnets in your ear in the first hours or days (or weeks) after birth is not a red flag guaranteeing that you won't develop that attachment. Certainly, if you experience warning signs of postpartum depression, beyond the crying that might accompany the roller coastering "baby blues," you need to seek help. But not feeling an intense bond right away doesn't jeopardize the gradual bonding you will develop. Tara and her son have a wonderful attachment bond now, and her lower expectations about that wave-of-love thing with her second probably helped her relax and actually enjoy his arrival a bit more.

That inner conflict over whether she would ever bond with him enough is something two motherhood researchers, Mira Crouch and Lenore Manderson, explored in a 1995 paper called "The Social Life of Bonding Theory," one of the few pieces of research that actually delves into this issue. They trace the idea of maternal–infant bonding from its early popularity in the late '60s through the early '90s, discussing how the loaded meanings of the term "bonding," whether used scientifically, culturally, or popularly, have shifted—and even been used to make women feel guilty (perhaps to "keep them in their place"?) as the feminist movement raged and then settled a bit.

For example, they quote a 1980 undergraduate textbook whose unequivocal description of a "sensitive period" immediately after birth would lead any new mom to feel inadequate:

An intimate psychological unit between mother and infant can be achieved in the hours and days after delivery. Such a relationship has profound beneficial effect on the child . . . and for the mother. The opportunity for creating this bonding exists only in the immediate puerperium [period after childbirth] and should anything interfere with its establishment then the bonding will be at best inadequate, at worst non-existent.

Except, fortunately, that's not what the evidence shows. It's even possible that the love-at-first-sight phenomenon popularized in women's magazines and on parenting websites is cultural, but whether it is or isn't is irrelevant. Many mothers feel that instantaneous love, and many mothers don't. Many fathers feel it, and many fathers don't. What matters is basically that parents fake it till they make it: attachment begins by responding to your infant's needs, and certainly in the beginning, that doesn't require you to ooze love from your every pore. It means feeding, holding, changing, and feeding some more.

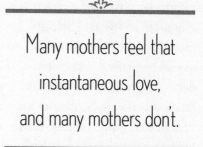

Many mothers feel that instantaneous love, and many mothers don't.

Infants do, however, need more than just food, warmth, and protection—they need interaction with other human beings, such as looking at faces and hearing live human voices, and they do better when sleeping close to their primary caregivers, in the same room. We know that skin-to-skin promotes bonding, though the mechanics aren't fully understood, and we know that depression in fathers or mothers (but particularly mothers) can interfere with bonding. Poor sleep in infants can also interfere with bonding because it negatively affects babies' primary brain functioning. But there is no evidence that sparks must fly within some magical 24- to 48-hour window of opportunity to assure a healthy relationship with your child.

What We Did: Emily thought her sons were very cute when they were born, but with her first, especially, it took her at least a few weeks to get comfortable with the idea of having this level of responsibility for another human

being, which definitely precluded unmitigated doting on him. She found them precious but new, and in each case, she and her son simply needed some time to get to know and understand each other. She is now very close with each of her sons. Tara did not feel immediately "bonded" to her first son, but she developed a strong bond with him over time. She felt more attached to her second child from the first days, and that attachment also strengthened over time.

Breastfeeding Blues

Although about 8 in 10 newborns started to breastfeed in 2011, only half of infants born that year were still breastfeeding at 6 months old, and just over a quarter at 1 year. Exclusive breastfeeding rates that year were 41% at 3 months and 19% at 6 months. For mothers who planned to formula-feed or to stop breastfeeding before a year, that's fine, but a large proportion of those decreases reflects mothers who aren't meeting their own breastfeeding goals. A 2014 study of more than 2,300 women who planned and started to breastfeed found 12% of those women experienced problems related to breast pain, low milk supply, or infant latch. That group weaned at a median 1 month, compared to 7 months among those without breastfeeding interruptions. That means 1 in 8 women didn't reach the breastfeeding goal they set for themselves due to some of the most common problems nursing moms experience. Another study found that almost a third of moms didn't meet their goal of breastfeeding at least 3 months, largely but not exclusively because they had to return to work. Yet another found that the top reasons for stopping breastfeeding were sore nipples, inadequate milk supply, the baby's difficulties, or believing a baby wasn't satisfied. These challenges aren't limited to first-time moms either. Another study in New Jersey found that only 7 in 10 moms who exclusively breastfed their first child also exclusively breastfed their second.

Study after study finds that breastfeeding moms need support to reach their goals—support from their partners, families, care providers, pediatricians, and communities—and evidence summarized by the Cochrane Collaboration finds that both lay and professional support increases breastfeeding rates, but many women lack access to professional support. The same CDC report card that provided those 2011 numbers also reported an average 3.8 Certified Lactation Counselors and 3.5 International Board Certified Lactation Consultants per 1,000 live births. Given how poorly trained pediatricians and ob-gyns are to address breastfeeding difficulties and these low numbers of lactation consultants (LCs), that's not nearly enough professional support to go around. It's no coincidence that breastfeeding is more common among women with higher incomes and more education: they have more access to support and resources.

What we'll address here are some of the most common problems nursing mothers face and an overview of the research relating to those challenges and to primary and secondary "lactation failure." (While we recognize the problematic nature of the term "lactation failure," we use it for lack of a better commonly understood term.) This section cannot serve as a complete troubleshooting guide for the many concerns you might encounter while breastfeeding, but it will hopefully give you a starting place for the questions to ask in seeking out help, ideally from a lactation consultant, and help you realize what is and isn't normal.

First, three important points: (1) No, not all women can breastfeed. (2) Whether you do or don't breastfeed, formula is not "evil" and will not harm your child. (3) Despite how "natural" breastfeeding may be, that doesn't mean it comes "naturally" to the majority of women or their newborns, and difficulties can often lead to (or arise from) nipple pain. And yes, all three of those are abundantly clear from the evidence base.

Not All Women Can Breastfeed

Trying to pin down the proportion of women who are unable to breastfeed is no easy task. The best data available are based on small studies and extrapolated estimates, and it depends on how "unable to breastfeed" is defined. The two types of lactation failure are primary and secondary. Primary lactation failure refers to women who physically cannot produce milk or whose milk does not come in. The best US estimate for its prevalence—up to 5% of women—comes from a single study in the 1980s of 319 married, college-educated, mostly white first-time mothers who had at least $35,000 in annual income and were highly motivated to breastfeed. Given those demographics—women with access to quality healthcare and nutrition—the 5% estimate is probably on the low end. The conditions most likely to cause primary lactation failure are insufficient glandular tissue (IGT, not having enough of the tissue needed to make milk) and previous breast lumpectomy or surgery (reduction, enhancement, or cancer-related), though an infection or retained placenta can also cause it. Women with IGT share several recognizable characteristics: at least 1.5 inches of space between their breasts, breasts that are more "tubular" than "full" and have an unusually small base circumference, and breasts that didn't grow during pregnancy. In a different study, only 1.7% of women did not experience their milk coming in a week after delivery, but this study did not follow the women to see if they ever produced enough milk. (Someone with primary lactation failure might produce *some* milk and be misclassified as not having primary failure.)

Secondary lactation failure, also called secondary lactation insufficiency, is much more common: something interferes with milk production or breastfeeding early on and irreparably damages a woman's milk supply. Unlike primary lactation failure, in which the breasts are incapable of producing milk (or any substantial amount of it), those with secondary insufficiency usually (though not always) start out making enough milk, or they would if the baby took in enough. But lactation is a supply-and-demand endeavor. Without sufficient demand, supply drops. Medical conditions, illnesses in mom or child, breastfeeding problems, or other issues can get in the way, and with secondary lactation failure, by the time the issues are managed, the breasts have already adapted to making less milk.

Among the long list of medical conditions that can contribute to secondary insufficiency are Hashimoto's disease, polycystic ovary syndrome, hyperthyroidism and other endocrine disorders, pieces of retained placenta (prolactin production is stimulated by the ejection of the placenta), postpartum hemorrhage, obesity, diabetes, high blood pressure, a breast infection, and certain autoimmune conditions. But other factors can contribute as well, such as a stressful delivery (including unscheduled cesarean sections), emotional stress, severe calorie restriction, certain medications, and infrequent breastfeeding or a delay in starting, especially if mother and baby are separated for 12 to 24 hours after birth. Secondary failure can also result from an undiagnosed tongue- or lip-tie, an underweight or preterm baby, multiples, or newborns with Down syndrome or another developmental or medical condition. Babies born in the 36th or 37th week of pregnancy (late preterm) may not be able to nurse well or pull out enough milk because of a "disorganized" suckle caused by neurological immaturity or weak mouth or tongue muscles. Even full-term babies might have disorganized suckles due to tongue- or lip-ties, poor coordination, or above- or below-average muscle tone.

There is debate over the extent to which stress or depression can contribute to an insufficient milk supply. Animal studies have found reduced milk supply in response to stress, but it's not clear if that happens in humans or, if it does, how often. Severe physical or mental stress can reduce oxytocin, which can delay or impair the let-down reflex, and it's possible repetitive let-down delays could prevent babies from emptying the breast, which will gradually decrease supply. A smattering of other studies have suggested that extreme stress might affect prolactin and that depression may cause a drop in milk volume (though skin-to-skin and regularly expressing milk may help), and then other studies find no evidence for stress affecting lactation. Certainly women in war zones and after natural disasters continue breastfeeding, though an old case study described two women whose milk and colostrum abruptly dried up after a 1985 earthquake in Mexico City. Really, though, we just don't know much about the link between stress and lactation.

Regardless, secondary lactation insufficiency from any cause is more common than many women—and even healthcare providers and LCs—might realize. That same small study above found an additional 10% of women never produced enough milk for their babies (aside from the 5% with primary lactation failure), and that was, again, a fairly healthy, upper-income, well-educated group. The problem is that women, or their care providers, might not recognize this problem, especially if breastfeeding "seems" to be going well. Among women who feel strong pressure to exclusively breastfeed—from medical staff, themselves, or their family or social group—accepting the possibility of secondary lactation insufficiency can be difficult and accompany feelings of shame, inadequacy, and depression, despite the fact that it's not uncommon, not the mother's fault, and caused by so many possible factors. Mothers who hear that "only 5%" of women can't exclusively breastfeed don't realize that figure leaves out this second form of lactation failure. As breastfeeding researcher Alison Stuebe has said, trying to separate biology and environmental factors (including but not limited to insufficient support) as factors is like trying to separate how much type 2 diabetes is caused by "biology" versus "the environment."

Tara experienced secondary lactation insufficiency, and the feelings of inadequacy and "failure" she felt because of it contributed heavily to her postpartum depression. Her second child, born early in the 37th week, seemed to nurse fine, but he was falling asleep too early at the breast and wasn't waking easily or long for feedings. His nursing was disorganized, and he never pulled out enough milk to reach the fattier hind milk, which caused her to make less milk and deprived him of the calories he needed . . . to nurse well enough long enough to reach the hind milk. It required her firm but compassionate pediatrician and an experienced lactation consultant to realize supplementing with formula was the right thing for her son, who only regained a few ounces in his first 2 weeks.

Not recognizing secondary lactation insufficiency can seriously endanger infants, putting them at risk for insufficient weight gain, dehydration, and failure to thrive. One study found that among 3,700 hospitalized newborns in Pittsburgh, 1.7% had hypernatremic dehydration—an imbalance of electrolytes with high sodium levels—that had resulted from insufficient milk intake that was missed. In severe cases, not realizing a baby isn't getting enough milk can result in seizures, kidney failure, or death. Risk factors among mothers for an infant's insufficient milk intake include flat or inverted nipples that affect a child's latch, excessive or unrelieved breast engorgement, cracked or bleeding nipples or severe nipple pain, birth complications, chronic illness, a delay in milk coming in, no previous breastfeeding experience, and being older than 37. Warning signs that babies may not be getting enough milk include difficulty latching, excessive sleepiness or non-demanding behavior (often needing to be woken up for feedings), a weak or unsustained suck, irritability or dissatisfaction after feedings, constant crying and rooting, excessive pacifier use, weight loss greater than 10% of birth weight, no stools or fewer than six wet diapers by 4 days old, fewer than four stools a day before age 1 month, and not surpassing birth weight by 2 weeks old.

SIGNS YOUR BABY IS GETTING ENOUGH MILK

1. Your milk comes in within 4 days postpartum, and your breasts feel full at the start of feedings and softer afterward.
2. Your baby breastfeeds 8 to 12 times per 24-hour period.
3. Your baby latches well, sucks for at least 10 minutes on each breast, and seems satisfied or "milk drunk" after feedings, often falling asleep at the second breast.
4. Your baby has at least four mustard-yellow, seedy, cottage cheese–like stools a day by 5 days old.
5. Your baby has at least six wet diapers a day.

Formula Isn't Evil

It's true that mothers who plan to exclusively breastfeed should generally avoid formula, because it's a child's suckling from the breast that stimulates the breast to make more milk. Anything the child doesn't get from the breast is usually a lost opportunity to stimulate more milk production. However, the idea that mom's colostrum will always, without fail, be sufficient until mom's milk comes in is flat-out false, especially if it takes a few more days than average. One study of more than 400 first-time mothers found that 44% experienced a delay in their milk coming in, defined as more than 72 hours after birth.

And the idea that giving newborns a small amount of formula in the early days will always derail a breastfeeding relationship is not gospel. In fact, one randomized controlled study—albeit very small and not yet replicated—found the opposite: 40 exclusively breastfeeding moms, all with newborns who had lost at least 5% of their body weight, were assigned to continue exclusively breastfeeding or to give their baby 2 teaspoons of formula after each feeding until their milk came in. A week later, 10% of the early-formula group were receiving formula compared to 47% of the moms who didn't give their babies any formula in those first few days. Three months later, 15 of the 19 babies (79%) in the early-formula group but only 8 of the 19 control group babies (42%) were exclusively breastfeeding with no formula supplementation.

This study caused big waves when it came out, but it definitely calls for caution because it's so small. It's important that babies get all they can from the breast first to stimulate sufficient milk production (and reduce the risk of secondary lactation insufficiency). But it provides food for thought. Along the same lines, a single drop of formula will not "contaminate" your child. The new area of research into gut microflora—the configuration of bacteria in the digestive system—is exciting and interesting, but there is no definitive evidence that formula somehow irreparably "corrupts" this microbiota with drastic lifelong consequences. In fact, breast milk has its share of contaminants anyway: plenty of environmental pollutants gather in the fatty tissue of the breast and pass into your breast milk, and reading a list of them would probably give most women a heart attack.

Nipple Pain Is Common but Also Commonly an Indication of Problems

The idea that "breastfeeding should never be painful, ever" is false, which research plainly shows. One small study of 100 women, for example, found 96 women experienced nipple soreness in the first week of breastfeeding, and various expert commentaries note that typical nipple soreness peaks toward the end of the first week of nursing. Perpetuating the idea that "proper breastfeeding should never hurt" may lead some women to quit early because they think they can't ever do it correctly when, in reality, it may just take longer for the soreness to fade. For example, a study of more than 300 Australian women found that nearly 80% of them had nipple pain at hospital discharge. Over the next 8 weeks, more than half had experienced nipple damage, and almost a quarter had had vasospasms, where blood vessels in the breast contract suddenly and cause extreme pain. By the end of those 2 months, 1 in 5 women still had nipple pain and 8% still had nipple damage.

On the other hand, it's also true that severe pain or pain beyond the first week usually, albeit not always, indicates a problem. Therefore, women with pain should seek help sooner rather than later, because nipple pain can interfere significantly with daily activities, mood, and sleep. Vasospasms, as women in the study above experienced, can be treated, and so can most other problems that cause pain. In fact, several reviews of nipple pain treatments found that not much helps with nipple pain except fixing the underlying problem causing the pain.

The most common causes for nipple pain are an improper latch from the baby or poor positioning of your baby, both of which a skilled LC can help with. Another common cause of nipple pain is a sucking or tongue problem in the infant, again usually requiring the help of an LC or an occupational or physical therapist. Tongue- or lip-ties, discussed later, can cause pain, and other causes include thrush (yeast infection), clogged ducts, mastitis, vasospasms, or Raynaud's phenomenon.

If the pain is not from any apparent cause, however, a wide range of treatment options has been assessed in several systematic reviews: warm water compresses, tea bag compresses, heat, expressed breast milk, lanolin, vitamin A, hydrogel therapy, glycerin gel therapy, moist dressings, prescription drugs, vitamin moisturizers, prescription creams, breast protection shells, phototherapy, and antibacterial sprays. Of these, rarely did one topical agent blow the others away, but lanolin and breast milk seemed a little more effective than other treatments, sometimes with breast protection shells. A Cochrane Review didn't find much evidence for anything other than expressed breast milk in helping nipple pain.

Raynaud's Phenomenon and Vasospasm. Raynaud's was previously thought to be rare, but more recent reports estimate up to 20% of women experience it. It's basically recurrent vasospasms—which can be excruciating—that are triggered by cold or stress. Raynaud's phenomenon is often misdiagnosed as thrush, since the two conditions share the symptom of nipple discoloration, but with Raynaud's, the nipple turns white and then blue (and sometimes then red) as blood returns. Treatment includes avoiding cold and avoiding drugs that constrict blood vessels (including smoking) and using the prescription drug nifedipine, which is considered safe during breastfeeding.

Thrush. In infants, this yeast infection usually looks like white patches in the baby's mouth, interspersed with reddened tissue. In mothers, thrush may involve red, sore nipples or an itching, burning, or shooting pain in the breast—or it may not involve any pain at all. A red, shiny, peeling areola or one with white patches might also indicate thrush. Risk factors include diabetes, steroid or antibiotic use, immune deficiency, cracked nipples, and using plastic-lined breast pads, which trap moisture. Treatment has to include mother and child and involves prescription antifungal drugs (oral or creams) or gentian violet. Thrush shouldn't be confused with eczema, which can share some of these symptoms but usually features crusting or oozing and calls for a dermatologist.

Clogged Ducts. When a milk duct becomes clogged, often from positions that don't empty the breast or from underwire bras, it causes a tender lump. Treatment with massage, warm packs, and position changes to fully empty the breast can prevent a plugged duct from becoming mastitis.

Mastitis. This excruciating infection, occurring in 5% to 10% of mothers, occurs most commonly in the first month. The breast is usually warm or hot to the touch, and the skin is usually red and/or shiny with a hard area, about the size of a pea, under the skin. If it's a bacterial infection, it usually involves a fever and flu-like symptoms, and treatment requires antibiotics. But not all mastitis is bacterial. Without the fever and flu-like symptoms, rest, massage, fully emptying the breast each feed, and fluids are sufficient. About 3% of mastitis cases can develop into an abscess that might require draining with a needle.

Tongue-Tie or Lip-Tie

Though previously dismissed by many practitioners, more and more pediatricians are finally recognizing what lactation consultants have been aware of for much longer: a tongue-tie can seriously derail breastfeeding. A tongue-tie refers to a thickened, tightened, or shortened frenulum, the narrow membrane of skin that runs down the middle under the tongue, connecting the tongue to the skin on the bottom of the jaw. When the frenulum is too tight, thick, or short, it prevents a baby from getting enough of the breast tissue in his mouth, which prevents a good latch and seal. Tongue-tie, or ankyloglossia, occurs in 3% to 11% of babies, most often males, and is possibly inherited.

Tongue-ties can cause nipple pain or tenderness, bleeding nipples, and poor weight gain because the baby isn't getting enough milk, and several studies have found moms of tongue-tied infants quit breastfeeding earlier than they wanted. Yet the treatment is fast and simple with very little risk: a healthcare provider snips the frenulum with a pair of sterile scissors, a surgical procedure called a frenotomy or frenulotomy. (The procedure can also safely be done with a laser.) No anesthetic is necessary, and the only complication is bleeding. In several randomized controlled studies (including a couple of blinded ones in which a "sham frenotomy" was performed), the improvement in latching, feeding, milk uptake, and pain relief was immediate and almost

100%, especially for a posterior tongue-tie but also for an anterior one (in which the membrane is less prominent). In one of those randomized trials, the group not receiving frenotomy received 48 hours of intensive lactation support, but breastfeeding improved for only one of the babies. After those 48 hours, the mothers were offered a frenotomy, all accepted, and all but one saw improvement.

Of course, a frenotomy isn't helpful if a tongue-tie isn't causing the problem. And if tongue-tie is a problem and a frenotomy doesn't fix it, three other possibilities remain: the cut wasn't made far enough up under the tongue, the membrane healed too quickly and reattached, or there's a different problem going on. An ENT who specializes in tongue-ties and related breastfeeding problems, Dr. Bobby Ghaheri, has proposed that lip-ties can also interfere with a baby's latch if the baby cannot fully project her upper lip outward to get a good seal. Unfortunately, there is extremely little research on lip-ties (a couple of articles only) and no randomized trials.

Other Breastfeeding Concerns

For information on pacifiers, see page 162. No peer-review evidence offers guidance on biting during nursing, and there's no evidence that a pierced nipple interferes with breastfeeding, as long as the piercing itself is removed.

Dysphoric Milk Ejection Reflex (D-MER)

This uncommon issue refers to negative feelings that occur during let-down and last from 30 seconds to 2 minutes. Although the feelings can include wistfulness, anxiety, agitation, anger, or even self-loathing, they are physiological, not psychological. D-MER appears to result from a brief drop in dopamine that occurs at let-down, temporarily leaving mom with a dopamine deficit. Because breastfeeding is a supply-and-demand system, if D-MER leads mom to nurse less often or she doesn't receive early support, it can prevent her from establishing a sufficient supply early on. D-MER hasn't been studied much, and there is no known treatment, but it passes quickly, so simply knowing what it is and that it's physiological may make it easier to tolerate. (If these feelings persist throughout nursing and afterward, they are more likely symptoms of postpartum depression.)

Milk Production

Though less common than other problems, oversupply can lead to regular (painful!) engorgement, mastitis, and regurgitation in infants that can be misdiagnosed as reflux. Offering one breast per feeding can gradually decrease stimulation and thereby production.

Low milk production goes along with secondary lactation insufficiency discussed on page 136, but many women still worry about low production and want to know ways to boost it. A Cochrane Review didn't find evidence that drinking extra fluids boosts milk production (though dehydration can hurt it). As for the old wives' tale about beer drinking, one review found that barley, an ingredient in most beers, can stimulate prolactin, the hormone that stimulates the production of breast milk, but alcohol can inhibit the letdown reflex, so the effects might cancel each other out. (We don't know.) For more on the effects of caffeine and alcohol on production, see page 146.

Listening to music while pumping or breastfeeding, relaxation techniques like deep breathing or massages, and having pleasurable food or drink have all been shown to help a little bit with milk supply, most likely because they all reduce stress. Some hormones have been tested for increasing milk supply, such as oxytocin and human growth hormone, but data on effectiveness and safety are thin.

For women who have a diagnosed insufficiency, the prescription drug metoclopramide can increase prolactin levels, resulting in up to 1.5 ounces more milk per feeding, but it should be used only short term, no more than 3 weeks. It can cause gastrointestinal side effects, anxiety, or sedation in moms, but there's no evidence of effects in babies. (Another similar drug, domperidone, isn't approved in the United States.)

And then there are the herbal remedies, and lordy, there are a lot! Unfortunately, there isn't much reliable research, but plenty of problems exist with what little research there is. Studies are usually small, with 10 to 75 people, and aren't often well controlled. The women aren't necessarily representative of all women, and dosages are all over the map. Because herbs are not regulated in the United States, supplements aren't standardized, and it's hard to know how much of an herb is in a capsule and what other ingredients are in there. We'll run through the most popular herbs here, but keep in mind that none of them has a strong evidence base, and all the studies discussed are very small. The ones with the "best" evidence (which isn't saying much) are fenugreek, milk thistle, and torbangun.

Fenugreek. A trial using tea with fenugreek against a placebo group and a control group led to double the pumped milk from the fenugreek tea group compared to the other two. The best dosage, based on a poorly described anecdotal account of 1,200 women, is 3 capsules (580–610 milligrams) 3 times a day, and if it's going to work, the effects should appear within 2 to 3 days.

Possible side effects include nausea, diarrhea, flatulence, and smelling like maple syrup (seriously!). Fenugreek can also interfere with some medications and increase the risk of bleeding in women taking blood-thinning medications, and it may cause congenital anomalies if taken while pregnant. Those allergic to chickpeas, soybeans, or peanuts may have an allergic reaction to fenugreek since it's in the same family.

Milk Thistle (*Silybum marianum*/St. Mary's Milk). A placebo-controlled trial of 50 Peruvian women found a 64% increase in milk production among women taking silymarin (the commercially available form), compared to a 22% in the placebo group after a month. At 2 months, the silymarin group experienced an 86% increase, compared to 32% in the placebo group.

Shatavari (*Asparagus racemosus*). One trial found a 33% increase in prolactin levels and a 16% increase in babies' weight in women taking this herb, compared to a 10% prolactin increase and a 6% baby weight increase in the comparison group. Possible side effects are a runny nose or red eyes during preparation, and it may cause congenital anomalies if taken while pregnant.

Torbangun/Spanish Thyme. After a month of use, mothers' milk volume increased 33% compared to a 15% drop in two comparison groups, one of which was taking fenugreek. Torbangun may increase the risk of bleeding in mothers using blood-thinning medications.

All the Rest. Fennel, blessed thistle, chaste tree seed, goat's rue, raspberry leaf, basil, black seed, anise, caraway seed, alfalfa, and stinging nettle have all been tried or suggested, but no data exist on them. Chaste berry or chaste tree seeds may cause congenital anomalies when taken while pregnant. Blessed thistle may increase bleeding risk if taken with blood-thinning medication, and fennel may interact with some drugs' effectiveness.

Bottom line: experiment, but caveat emptor.

Caffeine, Alcohol, and Marijuana

Pathetically little research has looked at how consuming caffeine might affect a breastfeeding baby or at how caffeine might affect milk supply. A study from the 1980s compared 11 mothers' infants during 5 days when the mothers drank 5 cups of decaf coffee and then 5 days when they drank 5 cups of coffee containing 100 milligrams of caffeine each. Although their breast milk contained a small amount of caffeine (1.6–6.2 mcg/mL) at the end of the 5-day, 500 milligrams per day caffeine period, no caffeine was detectable in the infants' blood, and the children's heart rate and sleep time didn't change across the different periods. A handful of equally old studies similarly found no effects from caffeine on nursing infants. Another more recent study of Brazilian women found that consuming more than 300 milligrams of caffeine a day had no influence on how frequently their babies, almost half of whom bed shared, woke up in the night. A review from the mid-1990s also found no measurable effects from caffeine on infants and, surprisingly, concluded that caffeine can stimulate milk production, though the evidence was pretty weak. And there is no evidence, by the way, that caffeine reduces milk production.

Alcohol, on the other hand, can reduce milk supply, at least temporarily, because it inhibits oxytocin, which is needed for the let-down reflex, according to 2013 review of 41 studies on breastfeeding and alcohol. In one of the studies reviewed, women expressed about 9% less milk 2 hours after drinking the equivalent of about 2 standard drinks. Another found that babies drank 20% less milk in the first 4 hours after their moms drank alcohol—but then they nursed more often and made up for it 8 to 12 hours later.

The good news is that the same review and other studies have consistently found that having a few drinks does not mean you have to "pump and dump." Your blood alcohol level is basically your milk alcohol level, and newborns metabolize alcohol at roughly half the rate adults do—*but* the actual amount of alcohol your baby gets through breast milk is only 5% to 6% of the weight-adjusted amount you get. Although there have been a smattering of reports in which infant behavior or sleep changes slightly after moms drink and nurse, there's no consistent evidence to suggest that a couple of drinks will have much effect on a breastfeeding baby. There was one study in 1989 that found slightly slower motor development among 1-year-old children who breastfed from mothers who had 1 daily drink, but the same researchers couldn't reproduce their findings in another study of 18-month-old children.

If you do drink, even to tipsiness, you could wait until you sober up, or you could just nurse anyway: the review found "even in a theoretical case of binge drinking, children would not be subjected to clinically relevant amounts of alcohol." Or, to throw some math at you, even if you breastfed right after doing 4 shots, when your blood alcohol level was highest, your baby's blood alcohol level would never exceed 0.005%. Even better, acetaldehyde, the toxic product resulting from your liver's metabolism of alcohol (and which contributes to hangovers), never passes into breast milk. So your baby neither gets drunk nor has a hangover.

Marijuana is a different story, but we have so little evidence on the correlation between cannabis and breastfeeding that it's hard to know what any true effects are. Within the few studies that have been done, marijuana use almost always accompanies tobacco smoking and alcohol use (and other drugs), and often all these or just marijuana were used during pregnancy, so it's hard to separate the effects. Furthermore, the studies always involved smoking marijuana and no other methods. We do know that THC (tetrahydrocannabinol, one of the predominant physiologically active chemicals in marijuana) makes its way into breast milk at approximately 0.8% of what the mother takes in from a single joint, adjusted for weight differences, and that it accumulates: infants exposed to pot-laced breast milk excrete THC metabolites for 2 to 3 weeks, according to one review. There is some evidence from animal studies only that marijuana can possibly limit milk production, primarily by interfering with prolactin levels, but no human studies exist. As far as effects, some scant evidence suggests a baby will become sleepy, may experience growth delay, and may have poor sucking, but there's very, very little evidence overall. In the only two substantial studies that looked at children's development, one found no differences for children exposed to marijuana in breast milk, and the other found a decrease in motor development at 1 year old—but there are no longer-term studies, and that one study's finding doesn't mean the marijuana caused any delays (that delay could go away or be related to something else). In fact, any baby exposed to pot in breast milk might also be exposed to pot smoke in the air or tobacco smoke, and the baby's relationship to mom could play a role too. So the short version? We don't know much.

What We Did: Emily had every breastfeeding complication possible (or so it seemed), including thrush, mastitis, poor latch because of tongue-tie, inability of one son to suck, and with each son, horrible, teeth-gritting pain as a result of these complications. For thrush, she successfully used gentian violet but had to suffer through an alarming amount of purple staining all over everything. With each son, she used a Medela breastpump to create a supply for her absence. She drank neither coffee nor alcohol. Tara experienced excruciating nipple pain with her first son that was never explained but faded after a couple of weeks. She experienced partial secondary lactation failure with her second son. She took fenugreek, milk thistle, and Mother love supplements, and her husband baked her oatmeal-and-brewer's-yeast-filled "lactation cookies" (despite the scant evidence for either). She has no idea if those cookies or supplements made any difference, but the cookies were yummy. She used a hospital-grade pump for 2 weeks to keep her supply up while working in Mozambique when her second son was 7 months old. She drank coffee and wine and nursed, but her husband hasn't forgiven her for that one time she had a Red Bull and nursed even though no one can prove her son's next 3 hellish hours of fussiness were caused by it.

CHAPTER 5

The First Weeks

More Than Baby Blues

Postpartum Depression

If the 1 to 2 weeks after giving birth are a roller coaster ride, then postpartum depression is a twisted amusement park, where you hop from a stomach-churning zero-gravity spaceship to a submarine that plunges you to the bottom of the ocean. Postpartum depression doesn't always develop immediately after giving birth. It can take several months to show up for some women, so women shouldn't dismiss creeping feelings of worthlessness or resentment toward their baby just because it's been several months since they gave birth. As noted earlier, Tara struggled just after her second child's birth, then felt better, then experienced postpartum depression and anxiety symptoms for which she sought treatment.

Like so many mental conditions, scientists don't fully understand what causes postpartum depression, and it's most likely a combination of factors anyway. Hormones almost certainly play some part, as well as too little sleep, anxiety about motherhood, a demanding baby, other stressful events in your life, and other physical changes in your body from pregnancy or delivery.

There's some weak evidence that postpartum depression could be related to nutrient deficiencies during pregnancy, such as too little vitamin D, but the data on that are fuzzier, and there's not much evidence that popping extra vitamins or other supplements will help considerably (though a balanced diet may help some).

How do you know if what you're experiencing might be postpartum depression? Healthcare professionals mostly use the Edinburgh Postnatal Depression Scale to screen women for depression, and diagnosis is based on experiencing at least five key symptoms—see the box on page 151—that last 2 weeks or longer and prevent you from being able to function well. The tricky part is that several of those symptoms are par for the course with a new baby. Decreased energy? Insufficient or fragmented sleep? Changes in your weight? Mommy guilt? Decreased concentration? All those may continue throughout the first year after giving birth, but postpartum depression also tends to involve persistent feelings of worthlessness or extreme guilt and an inability to enjoy pleasurable activities.

More than half of women with postpartum depression have obsessive thoughts related toward harming their baby even though they are extremely unlikely to do so. In fact, the shame and guilt women might feel about those thoughts may prevent them from divulging them to a professional even though that's precisely what they should do. Women might also experience "passive suicidal ideation," which means they don't think about plans to kill themselves, but they might feel a desire to die without any clear method.

Consider the list of symptoms in the box, and if even a handful of them sound like a description of your day in between feedings and diaper changes, it's important to talk to your care provider about how you're feeling, especially if you're finding it increasingly difficult to function. Most likely, your doctor will want to do lab tests to eliminate the possibility of a thyroid disorder, since the symptoms are similar. If you do have postpartum depression, it's more likely to get worse without treatment, and it affects more than just you. It can interfere with breastfeeding and, more problematically, affect your attachment to your baby. Women with postpartum depression are also less likely to use healthy feeding and sleeping practices with their baby, to be attentive or sensitive to their baby, to continue breastfeeding, to talk to or play with their infant, to show their child books, and to follow routines. The children of depressed mothers may be at risk for being less attached to their mothers or for greater behavioral problems, and they may be at higher risk for depression in the teen years.

However, it's important to keep in mind that some of these concerns may be outside a mother's control whether she is treated or not. Depression itself has a genetic component, and some children's behavioral or mood difficulties, while young or as teens, may be related to inheriting a bit of mom's mental health, to oversimplify it a bit. The good news is that long-term cognitive development does not seem to be affected by depression, but it *is* affected by poor mother–child interactions in the first year and a half of life, which depression might contribute to.

POSTPARTUM DEPRESSION SYMPTOMS

Most postpartum depression symptoms are the same as depression symptoms, but several are unique because they relate specifically to your baby. Also, keep in mind that several of these—fatigue, poor sleep, feelings of inadequacies as a parent—are normal and common, but when they're accompanied by the other symptoms, they should be considered a symptom.

- Change in appetite
- Unusual weight loss or gain
- Insomnia, excessive sleepiness, sapped energy or extreme fatigue (more than the normal walking-zombie mom state!)
- Inability to smile, laugh at jokes, or enjoy pleasurable activities
- Feelings of shame, guilt, worthlessness, or inadequacy (more extreme than the standard-issue mom guilt and inadequacy)
- Trouble bonding with your baby
- Thoughts of harming your baby or yourself, even if you don't act on them or consider them seriously
- Feelings of incapablities in caring for your child
- Excessive anxiety, fear, or worry about your child or in general
- Any other ongoing negative feelings toward your baby
- Feelings of exceptional irritability, anger, or quick temper
- Severe mood swings

- Withdrawal from family and friends
- Difficulty concentrating or making decisions
- Frequent feelings of sadness and/or frequent crying
- Loss of motivation
- Feelings of being out of control of your life and/or "like you're going crazy"

Postpartum Psychosis

Postpartum psychosis is rarer than postpartum depression, occurring among 1 to 2 women out of every 1,000 who give birth; but that statistic still means several thousand women experience it every year. It's also very serious and requires immediate treatment, often hospitalization. Onset is usually within the first few weeks after birth, and women with bipolar disorder are at much higher risk for postpartum psychosis—by some estimates a hundredfold more likely than women without bipolar disorder. Symptoms include thoughts, desires, or attempts to harm your baby or yourself; hallucinations, such as hearing voices; intense anger toward your baby or yourself; bizarre and/or unpredictable behavior; paranoia; disorganized thinking; impulsivity; severe agitation; and mania. Treatment can involve psychotropic drugs (including antidepressants, antiepileptics, and others), hospitalization, psychotherapy, and, in some cases, electroconvulsive therapy.

Postpartum Anxiety (Panic) Disorder

Like prenatal depression, postpartum anxiety disorder is less known to most people, but it can be just as debilitating as depression, and the causes and risk factors are thought to be similar. Up to 10% of women experience the symptoms, which include, as you'd expect, extreme anxiety and panic attacks, including a racing heartbeat, agitation, shortness of breath, or chest pain. Dizziness, nausea, and ongoing insomnia are red flags too. Women with postpartum anxiety disorder may excessively worry or feel consumed by fears, especially fear of losing control, fear that they are "going crazy," and/or fear that they or their child will die. In addition to the risk factors for postpartum depression, a history of an anxiety disorder puts a woman at higher risk for this condition.

Another type of more specific but less common (but also underreported) postpartum anxiety disorder is postpartum obsessive compulsive disorder (OCD), which affects 3% to 5% of mothers. Although a history of OCD is a risk factor for this condition, it's not required, and other risk factors include unrealistic expectations of one's self as a mother and negativity toward motherhood. Similar to non–pregnancy-associated OCD, symptoms include repetitive actions—such as repeatedly giving a baby a bath or excessively changing her clothes or diapers—and obsessive thoughts, especially related to harming or even killing their baby. But women with postpartum OCD feel a sense of horror or embarrassment about these obsessions; unlike psychosis, they *recognize* that they are having bizarre thoughts and are not likely to actually harm their child.

The treatments for postpartum anxiety disorders are generally similar—therapy and psychotropic medications—to those for prenatal and postpartum depression.

Paternal (or Partner) Depression

Just because dad—or another partner—isn't incubating the baby (or even if neither of you did) doesn't mean the experience cannot affect your partner's mental health as well. Paternal (or partner) depression affects approximately 1 in every 10 fathers, though some estimates put it at 1 in 4 fathers during the period of 3 to 6 months postpartum. A father may be at higher risk for depression if the mother is experiencing depression already. One study found that younger men, under age 29, were up to 2.5 times more likely to experience postpartum depression, and other risk factors included a low educational level, low income, financial worries, or a poor relationship with their partner. As with mental health concerns among moms, a father's mental health may affect his children. A depressed father is less likely to engage in enriching activities with his child, such as reading, singing songs, and telling stories.

It's tough to juggle everything after a baby arrives, and it's even tougher to care for yourself at the same time that you're caring for a brand-new tiny human. But ignoring the signs of any of these mood disorders is likely to interfere with caring for that tiny human. Taking care of yourself is one of the ways you also ensure that you are taking care of your child.

Antidepressants While Breastfeeding

Regardless of what you did or didn't take while pregnant, you may want to reassess your decision if you will be breastfeeding. Any medications you take will generally end up in breast milk in some concentration, but it's often low enough not to have an effect on your child. No large studies have consistently shown any problems in babies to be linked to antidepressant use while breastfeeding. Most adverse effects that have been seen that might be related to taking SSRIs while breastfeeding have come from case reports, which means they are rare and it can't be confirmed that the medication actually caused the symptoms.

The symptoms described in those case reports have included uncontrollable crying for long periods, irritability, poor feeding, insomnia, or weight loss; so if you are taking an antidepressant and your child experiences these symptoms, the best thing to do is contact your pediatrician and discuss whether the symptoms might be related to the medication. Because the research literature is constantly being updated with new information, the National Institutes of Health has created an incredibly helpful website called LactMed, a drugs and lactation database where you can look up any medication to find out the most recent research related to its safety while breastfeeding (online at Toxnet.nlm.nih.gov/cgi-bin/sis/htmlgen?LACTMED).

In light of all these contradictions and the low rates of what increased risks have been seen, the most important thing to consider in discussing your medication use with your doctor is the benefit you might receive from it. If the benefit is negligible, it may be best to skip the meds. If the benefit is significant and the risks are low and unproven, it could be riskier not to take the medication.

What We Did: Emily had a prolonged period of postpartum depression and some very concerning moments, but her ob-gyn was not responsive to her concerns, so Emily did what she could to self-treat with outdoor time, work, and support from her husband. Tara experienced postpartum depression with her second child. She contacted her ob-gyn office to help her find an appropriate therapist, and her antidepressant dosage was slightly increased.

Why Babies Cry

When we are helpless, the ability to communicate needs to those around us becomes critical. Infants are helpless: they cannot feed or care for themselves, they aren't even mobile, and they cannot gesture or sign or otherwise control their communications to their caregivers. So they cry. This communication from an infant requires recognition for the infant's need—hunger, pain, fatigue—to be addressed. That means that a caregiver must have the tools to recognize and respond to this communication.

The opening salvos in this communication exchange can be awkward. Parents have to learn to recognize what these nonverbal but very expressive ways of informing mean and how best to respond to them. All the infant knows is the feeling that triggers his sounds. A good feeling sets off a tiny giggle, even in sleep. A bad feeling, like gas pain or hunger, sets off wails.

Given how critical this early understanding is and its role in parent–child bonding, you might expect a fairly large literature addressing how to interpret a baby's cry. It's not large, relatively speaking. Maybe it's because even the call of research can't drown out the pain of listening to a baby cry, a sound that any airplane passenger can tell you is among the most disturbing a human can make. It urges action, flipping the switch in some primal core and lighting up our nerve endings, abuzz with the need to Make. It. Stop.

Eventually, parents come to understand a child's cry, just as they come to understand when a toddler's wail is "I really just want some more cookies" versus "Yes, I am bleeding and it hurts." But how do parents, especially first-time parents, navigate the world of early infant communication without a translation guide?

First of all, it's best to pay no attention to old wives' tales of how a baby is "trying to manipulate" you with crying. No. Babies don't have the long-term memory or cortical wherewithal to do that. So what does all the crying *mean*? A few studies have looked at how to interpret infant crying. One group of Spanish researchers identified some critical features of anger crying versus pain or fear crying. Pain crying, they concluded in a 2012 paper, involves rapidly escalating weeping to "maximum intensity" and eyes squeezed shut. Anger and fear crying usually come with eyes open (baby has "angry eyes"), but with anger, the crying builds gradually to a peak, just like anyone working themselves into an angry fit, while fear crying hits a rapid peak just as pain crying does. Angry eyes are half closed (the infant side-eye?) while fear eyes are open, with what the researchers describe as a "penetrating look" and the head moved backward—just as any human experiencing fear might do. In other words, infants are people and communicate the way people do.

This group's measure of pain crying finds confirmation in another study from 2004 that examined the quality of the crying sound relative to an infant's level of pain. In a study that seems near the border of ethical practices, infants were subjected to heel pricks under different numbing techniques, and each level of numbing was associated with a presumed pain level. The authors recorded the sound frequencies and analyzed them. Not surprisingly, the highest level of pain elicited an immediate high-pitched crying that was maintained and repeated, like a "siren." So if your baby sounds like a siren, that likely indicates some pretty intense pain.

But no such interpretations are infallible. Part of the natural process of forming a relationship with a new human being is understanding the nuances of each other's communications. Infant communication isn't only about crying. Adults and babies learn to talk with each other without words by imitating one another's sounds, almost musically. They each attune to the other through sensitive registries of change in voice pitch and volume and through learning each other's facial expressions.

All of which is to say that no science or summary in a book will help you understand your infant as much as just being and communicating face-to-face with your baby. At least until the teen years, anyway.

The Art and Science of Baby Soothing

In researching this book, Tara already was a bit biased in terms of seeking out research on soothing babies, because she had relied heavily on Harvey Karp's Happiest Baby on the Block methods for calming her first newborn, and she found his methods to work brilliantly for both of her children. Karp's method involves the five S's: swaddling, side/stomach, swaying, shushing, and sucking. Side/stomach refers to placing babies on their sides or their stomachs, swaying is quite literally swaying or rocking with a baby, shushing means creating white noise with a loud *shhhh* sound, and sucking could be on a finger, a pacifier, or a nipple. Swaddling, of course, is the art of wrapping up your baby like a burrito.

But Tara's kids are anecdotes at best, a single case study at worst; so what does the evidence say? Unfortunately, not much published research has assessed these five strategies as a single intervention. Several papers presented at conferences have shown the combination to effectively reduce crying and colic symptoms, and more than a half dozen studies are underway to assess them as a single method, but only one (poorly conducted) randomized controlled trial has tried to assess Karp's method to reduce crying. That study showed no difference between a control group of mothers and mothers told to watch Karp's instructive video on his method, but there was no validation that the mothers actually watched the video, only 35 women participated, and half were lost to follow-up.

Fortunately, however, each of the strategies Karp espouses has been studied individually, primarily in studies on pain relief for newborns. After all, one of the best ways to learn what soothes babies is to see what lessens their experience of pain using pain scale assessments based on behavioral clues and measuring physiological responses such as heart rate, breathing rhythms, and cortisol levels. One such study did evaluate Karp's five-part method for relieving pain from vaccinations. The randomized controlled trial involved 230 infants and found that babies receiving the five S's cried less and experienced less pain compared to babies who didn't. Interestingly, even though sugar water is perhaps the best studied, most effective known pain-relief option, the babies who received sugar water and the five S's were no different from those who got the five S's without sugar water. The rest of the research overall finds varying levels of support for each of the strategies Karp recommends and a handful of others.

Shushing and White Noise

Fetal hearing is developed by about 26 weeks, and overall sound environment of the womb has been estimated to range from 72 to 88 decibels, or up to 111 decibels with a voice at a mother's abdomen, though that's based on a single study in 1990 that measured the sound levels with a microphone inside women's uteruses. While we don't have any other womb-volume estimates to go from, those of us who have had an ear against a growling stomach can attest that internal bodily sounds are likely louder than we might expect. It stands to reason, then, that a completely quiet room might feel eerily unsettling to a newborn, and a handful of researchers have tried to test what millions of parents will anecdotally swear to: white noise helps calm down their babies and helps them sleep.

One trial of 40 newborns did find that 80% of babies exposed to white noise (about 70 decibels a foot away) fell asleep within 5 minutes, compared to only a quarter without the noise. Another trial compared 120 newborns while they received heel pricks: one group sat on their mother's lap, one sat on their mother's lap while listening to white noise, and a third listened to white noise while in a crib. The infants who cried the least and showed the least behavioral response to the pain (changes in breathing and heart rates) were actually the babies listening to white noise in their cribs, followed by those listening to white noise on their mother's lap. But these comprise just about all the research on the possible benefits of white noise on babies; it just hasn't been studied much (though the mountains of anecdotes are admittedly convincing in this case).

Regarding harms, you may have heard of a study that supposedly claimed white noise could damage an infant's hearing. The researchers assessed 14 infant sleep machines from about 1 foot, 3 feet, and 6 feet away and found that 3 of the 65 sounds made from them exceeded 85 A-level decibels (about the volume of a hair dryer) when turned up to full volume and measured a foot away. But the study didn't actually involve any babies, so it couldn't show noise harmed them. The only real takeaway was not to blast a sound machine at full volume a foot from your kid's head. A significant body of research has looked at background noise in NICUs, but much of that focused on quiet time for premature babies so they could sleep. The responses of premature babies to sound can't necessarily be extrapolated to full-term babies, but a review of those studies found no direct evidence of physiological harm from noise to newborns anyway. In fact, we know almost nothing about the possible effects of white noise on infants or even on animals in rat studies.

Meanwhile, emerging research has begun pointing to moms' singing as an effective way to soothe babies. Some older, limited evidence has found short periods of music reduce babies' pain response (under 15 minutes to avoid sensory overload), but a more recent small study found preemies' heart rates stabilized and their mothers had lower anxiety when the mother sang during kangaroo (skin-to-skin) care. But then, most parents don't need a study to tell them the value of singing lullabies to their children.

Skin-to-Skin Contact, Breastfeeding, and Breast Milk

Though not one of the "official" five S's in Karp's method, skin-to-skin contact has emerged in the past couple of decades as a highly effective therapy for helping very preterm infants thrive, and it appears effective at soothing any term newborn. A 2014 Cochrane Review of 19 mostly high-quality studies, involving more than 1,500 infants, found skin-to-skin care to be effective for pain relief, whether alone or combined with other methods, such as breastfeeding or sugar water. The only two studies that compared skin-to-skin with an infant's mom versus someone else found no difference between the two. A similar Cochrane Review of 20 studies looked only at breastfeeding and breast milk and found both effective, compared to placebo or no intervention, for pain relief, but also found sugar water to be just as effective.

Sucking and Swaying

It shouldn't surprise anyone that non-nutritive sucking might soothe babies when you recall that the most common item for such sucking is called a pacifier. But regardless, a large review of non-medication pain-relief methods found strong support that sucking without sustenance calms babies, slows their pulse, increases their attentiveness, and decreases their crying.

Swaying, rocking, and other calming movements have not been specifically studied, but "Rock-a-Bye-Baby" dates back to at least the 18th century, and the multibillion-dollar industry of baby swings, rockers, bouncers, and gliders implies that movement is a winner for most kids.

Positioning on the Side or Stomach and Facilitated Tucking

Only a small amount of research has specifically looked at positioning babies on their sides or stomachs to calm them. Much of those findings show this positioning to help reduce pain, but a couple found no effect. It's well established that babies sleep much better on their stomachs, but that's actually what makes stomach sleeping a risk factor for SIDS, discussed on page 180.

Another method found to be mildly effective in the review on pain relief, called facilitated tucking, is really just pulling in and holding your infant's legs and arms close to his torso to keep him from flailing. More recently, a study of 42 infants found that this method reduced pain in preterm infants during a blood draw, but another study of 71 babies found it considerably less effective than sugar water.

Swaddling

Swaddling a baby, perhaps the most ancient and enduring of infant care practices, has likely been studied the most of these strategies, and most of the findings are positive with a couple of caveats. Overall, swaddled babies wake up less often during sleep, startle less, and sleep longer (we discuss more about swaddling in the sleep section on page 183), and one trial of nearly 400 babies found swaddling decreased crying in babies under 2 months old. Another small study of babies with head injuries found swaddling more effective than massage in reducing their crying. Swaddled preemies appear to self-regulate better and show better motor organization and neuromuscular development as well as lower physiological stress. No evidence shows positive or negative effects from swaddling on children's motor development, but developmental dysplasia of the hip—basically a slightly dislocated hip joint—can occur if babies' hips are kept flexed for long periods. But this generally occurs only when a baby is strapped or swaddled to a cradleboard; if the knees and hips can freely bend and flex, hip dysplasia is not a concern. Most research shows the benefits of swaddling wear off by an infant's third or fourth month.

PURPLE Crying and Shaken Baby Syndrome

Before Tara was discharged from the hospital with her second son, she and her husband were required to watch a video on shaken baby syndrome. The main message was clear: never, ever, ever shake a baby. Decades' worth of strong evidence has shown that violently shaking infants, particularly those under 1 year old, can cause blindness, brain damage, or even death. The most common symptoms from shaken baby syndrome include retinal bleeding as well as swelling and bleeding in the brain, but these do not always occur, and each of these symptoms can sometimes individually occur due to other conditions. Most of the time, however, the combination of them, especially alongside other injuries such as bruises or broken ribs, indicates a baby has been severely shaken.

In recent years, a small group of neurologists, pathologists, and medical examiners have questioned whether shaking a baby can produce those characteristic symptoms or even kill a child. Conveniently, nearly all these doubters also earn money traveling the country to testify for the defense in shaken baby court cases. As anti-vaccine advocates have done, these defense experts point to cherry-picked, discredited, or poorly conducted studies to question the validity of shaken baby syndrome, yet their objections cannot overcome the consensus of the evidence: dozens of studies, some involving validated confessions, clearly establish the danger of violently shaking a baby. The AAP stopped using the term "shaken baby syndrome" in 2009 and instead began using "abusive head trauma" to encompass any form of abusive head injury, whether caused by shaking or not.

So why mention this information here? The majority of individuals who shake babies do not intend to harm the child. Rather, studies have shown they become overwhelmed, no doubt exacerbated by sleep deprivation in many cases, with an infant's nonstop crying. Desperate to stop the wailing, they suddenly find themselves shaking the baby. While that level of frustration and desperation is understandable, the key is recognizing it in time to remove one's self from the situation before tragedy occurs. Nearly all infants go through a developmental stage that includes bouts of seemingly endless crying. Developmental pediatrician Ronald Barr coined the term "PURPLE crying" to describe the features of this period: it "peaks" between 2 weeks and 4 months old; the crying is "unexpected"; the baby "resists" soothing and makes a "pain-like" face; the crying is "long-lasting," stretching for hours; and it occurs more often in the "evening." Parents can learn more at the website PurpleCrying.info. Knowing that this stage, often labeled colic, is common and not abnormal may help parents cope. Most important, however, knowing it exists may encourage parents to seek help when they feel themselves reaching a breaking point—before they find themselves desperately shaking a child to quiet him.

Plain Talk About Pacifiers

Even 3 years after Tara's oldest son had last used a pacifier, she continued to find Soothies stashed in random places—office drawers, car glove box, an old camera bag. Conservatively, she estimates she bought more than a dozen in her son's first 6 months, trying to account for the ones that got lost, dropped, and left behind while also ensuring one was always in easy reach, regardless of where she was. Because Soothies worked—for her first son. The second? Not so much. In fact, he wasn't very interested in any type of pacifier except his hands, which served the same self-soothing purpose. Emily's experiences were similar: her first and third sons couldn't live without a paci for years while her middle son never cared about them at all. And if the research is any guide, these boys will not necessarily have any particular advantage or disadvantage for having used or not used a pacifier. The studies show pacifiers to confer both benefits and risks, in differing amounts depending on the child's personality, age, and frequency of use.

The Goods on Sucking

The most established benefit is relief from anxiety or pain. Sucking, with or without eating, helps infants comfort themselves and gain control when feeling stressed. The calming effect of pacifiers is solidly established, as is their effectiveness as pain relievers for all sorts of medical interventions: heel sticks, circumcision, immunizations, catheterization, punctures for IVs, and other such procedures. Using a pacifier dipped in sugar appears even better at pain relief, but no better than breastfeeding, which also works. For preemies in particular, non-nutritive sucking has been linked to shorter hospital stays and better bottle-feeding, and no studies that looked at preemie use of pacifiers found any harm. Babies not given a pacifier will often become thumb-suckers for the same soothing effects, which can be good—thumbs are always readily accessible—or problematic—taking away a pacifier is easier than taking away a thumb when it's time to break the habit.

Another clearly established benefit of pacifiers is a reduced risk of SIDS up through a year old, though it's not clear why. Routine pacifier use reduces SIDS risk by 15% to 30%, and using a pacifier "at last sleep" cuts SIDS risk in half. However, SIDS itself is still rare, and it's estimated that about 2,700 babies would need to go to sleep with a pacifier to prevent one SIDS death. Some of the theories for why pacifiers help are that they prevent obstruction to the breathing passages by encouraging a forward position of the tongue, they improve mouth breathing when nasal passages are blocked, they encourage back sleeping, and they increase arousal—but none of these has evidence to support them, and pacifiers could be a "marker" for another factor that reduces SIDS risk. We don't really know why they work.

What Are the Trade-offs?

Pain relief, comfort, and a very slightly lower likelihood of dying in sleep are certainly benefits, but what are you trading them for if your child uses a pacifier? The two clearly established possible risks for pacifiers are ear infections and dental problems. Evidence does consistently show that using a pacifier slightly increases the risk of ear infections, primarily after 6 months old. The increased risk was relatively small, such as one study in which recurrent ear infections occurred in 16% of pacifier users but only 11% of nonusers. And it's possible to strike a balance between SIDS risk reduction and ear infection risk: one study showed 21% to 29% fewer ear infections among babies whose parents were counseled to give their children pacifiers only at bedtime, compared to parents receiving no recommendations. As with SIDS risk reduction, however, it's not clear why pacifiers increase the risk of ear infections. The sucking might influence pressure in the middle ear, making it more susceptible to infections from reflux, or the middle ear may be affected by dental changes.

Which brings us to how pacifiers affect teeth. Bacteria, particularly *Candida* and *Staphylococcus*, can live on pacifier surfaces and tend to prefer latex over silicone, but there isn't strong evidence that pacifiers increase the risk of infection or tooth decay—unless you're dipping it in sugar or using your spit to clean it, which can transfer bacteria from your mouth to your child's. Pacifiers can, however, contribute to misalignment of the teeth, including open bite, crossbite, and overjet, though only after 18 months to 2 years old and with a good 4 to 6 hours of daily sucking. Many jaw changes will likely reverse naturally if the child stops using the pacifier while teeth are still coming in, and it's primarily 3-, 4-, and 5-years-olds who are at highest risk for jaw misalignment.

What About Breastfeeding?

The biggest worry many have about pacifiers is their influence on breast-feeding, and the evidence here is tricky. Generally, there isn't much to support breastfeeding worries, but we could do with more research in this area. Early studies found that women stop breastfeeding sooner when their infants use pacifiers, but these were all observational studies. Later, better randomized controlled studies found no effect from pacifiers—including one where babies started using them as early as 2 weeks old—so there's no current evidence pacifiers *cause* women or babies to stop breastfeeding sooner.

Instead, women may be actually using pacifiers to help wean, or women already having breastfeeding problems may be more likely to use a pacifier. Pacifiers may also be related to other factors that just happen to be linked to shorter breastfeeding. So why do professional organizations suggest avoiding pacifiers for the first 4 to 6 weeks? Most studies have investigated breastfeeding duration several months down the line, not the earliest days. Establishing successful breastfeeding is already challenging enough that professional organizations are cautious about a potential interference: there isn't strong evidence to show pacifiers are a problem (one study's results are barely significant, and others contradict them), but there isn't great evidence to show it *isn't* a problem in the first several weeks either.

Furthermore, pacifiers used specifically to postpone feedings can reduce milk production by reducing breast stimulation (since the child is sucking the paci rather than the breast)—but that's only if a mom is giving her child a pacifier instead of feeding a hungry child. There's not much to show that using a paci *between* feedings will cause any issues for mothers who are confident about breastfeeding, as long as moms recognize that the child truly is not hungry and her breasts are getting regular stimulation to induce milk production.

In fact, interestingly, one recent study offers the possibility that pacifiers might actually *support* breastfeeding. A hospital put pacifiers, but not formula, under lock and key (though parents could bring them from home) and compared breastfeeding rates before and after the restriction. To the researchers' surprise, exclusive breastfeeding dropped from 79% (out of 812 babies) to 68% (out of 1,278 babies) while the supplemental formula feeding increased from 18% to 28%, and exclusive formula feeding increased from 1.8% to 3.4%. It's just one study, but it's possible that exhausted moms who could keep crying babies at the breast for only so long were opting for formula when a pacifier wasn't available.

What about so-called nipple confusion? The way a baby physiologically sucks a pacifier or a bottle—the way she uses her tongue—is different from the way she sucks a breast. Nipple confusion, or nipple preference, refers to the concern that she will become too used to one way of sucking and then be unable or unwilling to suck on the breast effectively to get the milk. Yet the only evidence that exists for nipple confusion with pacifiers comes from anecdotes. (Bottles are a different story, since the concerns relate to how hard the baby has to work to get the milk out of a bottle versus a breast.)

Sucking is one of a handful of reflexes newborns have at birth, along with the grasping and startle reflexes. Long before birth, a fetus sucks on her hands, feet, arms, and whatever she can get into her mouth, and none of this interferes with her later ability to suck on a breast. While a baby can be uncoordinated, or "disorganized," in learning to properly latch and feed from the breast, there is no research evidence that using a pacifier or a bottle interferes with this ability. It's possible that a baby's struggles to latch or suck properly might accompany use of a paci, or that underlying problems with breastfeeding may be interpreted as nipple confusion, but no evidence shows that a paci or bottle *causes* the baby to be unable or unwilling to latch onto a breast properly.

Other Considerations

There's not much evidence that pacifiers affect speech development, but one possible area of concern is allergies for children with a family history of latex allergy. The risk of allergy plus the lower risk of bacterial and fungal growth on silicone make silicone a better choice. (Boiling new pacifiers for 5 minutes and washing them regularly helps too.) There's no evidence that any one pacifier shape or type is better than another, so it's pretty much baby preference.

There are also safety concerns regarding choking and strangulation. Although pacifier-related deaths have occurred, most happened before 1999, usually from pacifier cords or ribbons. Since 2008, the Consumer Product

Safety Commission requires testing for durability, safe design, and lead and phthalate limits. The few injuries that continue to occur result from nipple breakage or small parts breaking off pacifiers. To dodge those problems, avoid clip-on ribbons or strings and pacifiers with small parts or decorations that could become choking hazards. Pull on the nipples to make sure they're strongly attached (unless they are one complete piece as Soothies are) and check them regularly for cracks, tears, or swelling so you can toss pacifiers past their prime.

Bottom line: the benefits—pain relief, soothing, SIDS risk reduction—appear to be greatest leading up to 6 months old and then start gradually declining as risks slowly increase, first with ear infections and then, after 2 years old, with dental problems.

What We Did: Tara's first son loved Soothies pacifiers (and only those), but her second son had no interest in pacifiers at all. Emily's first and third sons both loved their pacis and were loath to give them up, but ultimately both voluntarily did so at about the age of 3. One has apparently had no consequences, but the other one had a near miss with a crossbite. Her middle son, who never used one at all, had the most severe and frequent ear infections of any of her children.

WHEN GRANDMA SAYS HE'S SPOILED

The short answer is no, babies can't be spoiled. Children don't come with a "use by" date. They don't rot morally or behaviorally from the inside out under the unwitting encouragement from parents who think they're simply fulfilling fundamental needs. Infants and toddlers, those who cannot feed or clean or support themselves, won't be spoiled by being fed and cleaned and supported physically and emotionally. Infants and toddlers are people, like you, but they don't have friends or other forged relationships to turn to for their emotional and physical needs. They just have you. Their requests for support and help are no more bratty than when you call a friend or reach out to a spouse for emotional support after a particularly trying day.

Some research suggests that a perception that an infant or very young child can be "spoiled" can lead parents to misread a child's needs and disregard them, to everyone's detriment. The AAP assures parents that babies cannot be spoiled by having their needs addressed. This recognition is important to ensure that parents don't ignore what a child needs out of fear of "spoiling" the child. That concern is very real, given that in a 1997 survey by Zero to Three, more than 50% of adults, including parents of young children, thought that a child who is only 6 months old can be spoiled. Even worse, 60% of grandparents and 44% of parents of young children in that survey of 3,000 adults thought that *picking up a 3-month-old* every time the child cries would spoil the child. Perhaps as a corollary to that, a 2009 Zero to Three survey of 1,615 parents of children from birth to 3 years found that most think that 6-month-olds don't feel sadness or fear. Obviously, these data show a generational gap, with grandparents being more likely to call "spoiling" on situations that aren't. The survey authors also found that household income was associated positively with the level of understanding about child development.

More specifically regarding infants, they don't have the neural networks in place to be "spoiled" or to manipulate you in any intentional (or even unintentional) way. They are as unmanipulative as anyone you're ever going to know, so enjoy it while you can, and, yes, "give in" to their basic requests for food, shelter, love, and comfort. Substitute "nurturing" for "spoiling," and you'll realize how critical it is that you do so.

Feeding by the Clock

How often should you feed a newborn—by watching the clock and sticking to a schedule, or when the infant requests it? Current best practices are to feed an infant when an infant requests it with the usual signs of rooting for a breast or becoming restless or distressed. According to the AAP, "crying is a late sign of hunger," and that bump in restlessness needs to be recognized as a communication about hunger. The AAP also offers that newborns should be wakened and fed if a certain time interval has passed between feedings, so the "schedule" concept can go both ways: making the infant wait or waking the infant who seems to be waiting too long. So what does the research say?

Not much. First, we can't find the concrete rationale for waking a newborn within certain time frames for feeding, but it seems to relate to blood sugar needs, and it's a practice that has been disseminated to hospitals, so be ready for it. Second, regarding the "make the infant wait" evidence . . . there's not much there, either. Most studies from this century focus more on breastfeeding versus bottle-feeding or length of breastfeeding, rather than on-demand versus scheduled feeding. Some studies that are probably older than many readers of this book have looked here and there at scheduling (no one seems to have considered demand feeding much), but our goal is to present recent findings. Only a couple of studies meet this criterion. One that looked at 19,419 children in the UK identified how babies were fed at 4 weeks old and looked at how mothers and children fared over the coming weeks, months, and years. When mothers followed a feeding schedule, they reported better well-being than mothers who fed on demand, except for the measure of depression. While the mothers who schedule-fed seemed to do relatively well, however, their children did less so on IQ tests over time compared to their demand-fed counterparts. But that "less well" doesn't seem huge—a 4-point difference in IQ scores at age 8.

The second study, of 2,834 children, looked at how feeding on demand or on schedule affected a child's weight up to 4 years old. Although longer breastfeeding in general was associated with less risk for being overweight or wanting unhealthy snacks, the authors found no effect of demand versus scheduled feeding on these outcomes.

With this dearth of recent findings from large studies and the mixed outcomes, what remains is to refer you back again to what the Cochrane Review describes as the current best practices: feeding when the infant is hungry if that is something you can do, especially in the earliest weeks.

Sling or Stroller or Both?

One of the biggest movements in recent years, "attachment parenting" posits that baby wearing is an essential part of building an attachment bond with your child. Other schools of thought that criticize attachment parenting argue that wearing your baby, or at least doing so for "too long," will make her dependent on you, that she won't effectively develop the independence to explore her world. In reality, there isn't much evidence for either of these positions. Attachment between a parent and child, as already discussed, is vital for healthy parenting. But it does not require baby wearing. It's about being responsive to your baby's needs and building a positive relationship, which can be done with your child in a sling or wrap or soft structured carrier, or can be done in myriad other ways without wearing her at all.

About the only research that comes close to assessing the impact of wearing babies are two old trials for crying, one in 1986 and one in 1991. Both tested whether more time spent carrying a baby reduced crying, and one found carrying or wearing an infant at least 3 hours a day reduced crying in 6-week-olds by about 43%. The other found no difference. Another 2002 study found wearing preemies and full-term babies in slings had no influence on heart rate, nose airflow, abdominal breathing, or movements.

The only evidence of harm that can come from baby wearing relates to improper hip growth. Hip dysplasia, when the hip socket doesn't fully cover the ball portion of the upper thighbone, is usually a condition individuals are born with, but it can be worsened when babies are kept with their legs and knees straight (extended) instead of in the relaxed, partially bent position. So a carrier that allows them to sit naturally, with their legs slightly bent, better supports hip development—but this is generally only a risk if the child is already prone to hip dysplasia in the first place. The best estimate for the frequency of hip dysplasia, after considering false-positives and misdiagnoses, is about 0.5%, perhaps up to 5%, of children.

There is evidence, as we also discussed in the soothing section on page 159, that kangaroo care, placing a child skin-to-skin with you, can soothe infants, ease their pain, and enhance bonding. Among preemies in particular, kangaroo care in the NICU supports regular heart rate and breathing, deeper sleep, more alertness, less crying, fewer infections, and better weight gain. This benefit exists primarily in the first month or so and is independent from whether you wear your child.

So, no, you don't have to wear your child to ensure a healthy attachment bond, but if you do, no, there's no evidence your child will be any less independent than any other child.

What We Did: Tara wore her first son in a Sleepy Wrap (now called a Boba Wrap) everywhere. She also used an umbrella stroller as he got older. She didn't go as many places with her second son, and he hated the Sleepy Wrap. He did better with the Beco Gemini soft-structured carrier when traveling, but at home he loved being walked around the neighborhood in a stroller. None of Emily's sons were particularly interested in being worn in a wrap, although she did give it a try. A Baby Bjorn was a huge success in the early months.

CHAPTER 6

Now I Lay Me Down to Sleep

The Science of Sleep Deprivation

If you haven't experienced it, no simple description will capture the feeling of deep, dizzying fatigue that can accompany the first few weeks with a newborn. By the third child, Emily was wishing for an infant boarding school that could keep her son for those first few weeks of constant night waking and return him in a semi-regulated state at about 8 weeks. Well, not really, but the thought might have crossed her admittedly addled brain at 3 a.m. on several successive nights.

We know why we're awake—blame the baby, right? But what does all that sleep deprivation do to us, if anything, in the short and long term? Are we taking years off our lives with this stuff when we haven't even gotten to the teens yet?

You might think that mothers, being the ones with the breast milk, have it the worst. But science seems to indicate otherwise. For example, one 2013 study of 21 mother–father pairs enjoying their first infant experience found that fathers actually got less sleep than the mothers and experienced more confirmed sleepiness, as measured using wrist trackers. The study authors also found that even though the mothers got more sleep, their sleep was disturbed more often, which makes sense given their role in feeding. Both parents reported feeling about the same level of tiredness, but mothers scored worse on neurobehavioral testing (all those awakenings). Amusingly, the authors compared these 21 pairs of new parents to 7 pairs of childless couples and found, not even remotely surprising, that the new parents were sleepier and had more sleep impairments, which, even if you are sleep impaired, would be pretty obvious.

Lest you think that maybe that study, with its small sample, was a one-off, a 2004 study of 72 couples during the first postpartum month also used wrist trackers and also found that fathers had objectively less sleep than mothers. Sleep was measured throughout the day, though, and the mothers appeared to play catch-up during daytime hours, when fathers were unable to do so. The authors noted that work factors played a role in the level of sleep disturbance, which seems like yet another bit of evidence in favor of family or parental leave for both parents. Not unexpectedly, both mothers and fathers were tired, and both parents were a lot more sleep disturbed and fatigued during that first month with an infant than they were in the last month of pregnancy.

The allure of the studies that include fathers is that much of the earlier research focused only on mothers and their level of fatigue. But of course, a family with a newborn typically involves a parental partnership of some sort, and the role of the non-birthing partner can be critical. As the above studies indicate, the non-birthing partner experiences considerable sleep deprivation and fatigue—but does it go unrecognized by his birthing partner? A 2011 study of 21 new parent pairs suggests as much and that this lack of recognition of sleep-deprivation problems goes both ways. Mothers overestimated how well fathers slept (the study looked only at mother–father parenting pairs), and fathers overestimated mothers' disturbed mood. In other words, the women didn't think the men were as sleep deprived as the men felt, and the men thought the women were moodier than the women felt. Just one more reason that a good partnership is foundational for surviving the stresses of parenting an infant.

In fact, a 2009 review takes on the reasons for what the authors call a "robust decline in marital satisfaction across the transition to parenthood." The term "robust decline" sounds rather dire, and these authors point to sleep deprivation and disruption as having a role in this fraying of the partnership following the arrival of the bundle of joy.

In addition to these short-term effects on function and mood and potentially long-term effects on partnership, sleep deprivation can have more acute consequences. Again, fathers bear the brunt. A 2012 study of 241 new fathers found that even though they got fewer than 6 hours of sleep a night—interrupted sleep, at that—they still worked "long hours." The fathers, completing a questionnaire when their infants were 6 and 12 weeks of age, were tired, and that fatigue seemed to feed into reduced vigilance about safe behaviors in the workplace. Without the ability to compensate for lost sleep during the day, these fathers simply rode out their fatigue while working. Again, more evidence supporting a need for family/parental leave, not only for social reasons but also for safety reasons.

Mothers who stay at home also need relief, and science supports them in that. A 2014 cross-sectional study of women in Taiwan, for example, found that women whose daily housework duties were reduced experienced better sleep quality in the postpartum period. That suggests that even unofficial jobs, such as maintaining the home front, require relief in the form of parental leave as well.

Of course, in special cases such as a mother recovering from a cesarean section, sleep deprivation can be even worse. One study comparing women who'd had cesarean sections with those who'd had vaginal deliveries found that the women who'd delivered by cesarean section got less sleep (4.5 hours a night) than those who'd had vaginal deliveries (6 hours a night). The study was tiny, with only 6 women who'd had a cesarean section and 15 who had had a vaginal delivery, and all the infants spent time in ICU just after birth, but the results do suggest some extra support is needed for women who have had the major surgery that is a cesarean section.

Twins are another special case, and not only because they change the parent-to-baby ratio from 2:1 to 1:1. Here again fathers take the bigger hit: in a 2008 study of 8 parent pairs of full-term twins, the dads got less sleep, whether measured for only the night or for the entire day. The good news is that things got better over time.

That's the message we leave behind here: in general, things do get better over time when it comes to parental sleep deprivation. But don't underestimate the dangers of sleep deprivation, especially in those early days. Studies have shown that sleepy driving can be as dangerous as or worse than drunk driving. Plus, plenty of research links insufficient sleep to various health problems and to irritability, higher stress levels, and reduced patience, all of which can be dangerous for an infant if the parent is severely sleep deprived. For those with a history of mental illness, sleep deprivation can cause relapses. Meanwhile, tend to your partnership, and if you have the opportunity, don't refuse to take family or parental leave if it's offered. And that includes you stay-at-home moms who want to do it all yourself. Let grandma, uncle, aunt, sister, nephew, neighbor help you if it's offered.

WHAT DO YOU DO WHEN YOUR INFANT WAKES YOU?

You'd hope that being armed with information might help you problem-solve postpartum sleep deprivation. Sadly, not so. Some researchers have looked at parent education in the hospital involving nurse advice and brochures along with follow-up phone calls in the weeks following the birth. Unfortunately, according to a 2013 study, being well armed with information didn't seem to improve sleep for the mothers compared to women who received only follow-up phone calls in the postpartum period.

That might make you wonder what possible good this chapter can do you, then, but we do have a little bit of, er, enlightenment for you. Actually, it relates to endarkening, as in when women whose infants wake them spend their wake time using a computer or watching TV, they're more likely to be awake longer compared to women who do not. The 2014 study that yielded these findings involved 201 women who responded to an online survey, so a bias toward computer use in that population is possible. Having a night-light or other light source on did not seem to influence how long the mother was awake, but women who formula-fed rather than breastfed were less likely to fall asleep while feeding their infant, which supports findings from other studies that women who breastfeed exclusively wake more often but still get more sleep. Younger infants were more likely to be awake longer but not more likely to wake more frequently. We hope these findings at least give you some actionable way to try to address nighttime sleep deprivation.

Infant Sleep

Our experience as parents was that the first question many, many people asked us when they learned we had an infant was, "How does he sleep?" (We can say "he" because all our children are boys.) A question that at least one of us asked herself pretty much every night of the first 6 weeks or so with each of her sons was, "Will he ever sleep?" One of our sons slept through the night—9 hours! The brass ring of early parenting rewards—when he was 11 weeks old. Another of our sons didn't really sleep a full night until he was 4 years old.

In other words, "normal" when it comes to infant and child sleep doesn't really exist. Cultures also vary in how much sleep infants get, with infants in some Asian countries going to sleep later and sleeping less than their Western counterparts. Circadian rhythms can be very idiosyncratic. And human infants emerge earliest in their development and most helpless of any primate: in addition to not being able to cling to you or anything in the early weeks and months, they also have yet to develop a rhythm internally or externally that syncs with the outside world. Getting into that sync—with people, feeding, light and dark, smells, touches, sounds—takes time and habituation. They also have sleep patterns that are the same as an adult's patterns. They're programmed to sleep lightly more than they sleep deeply, and they tend not to do either in very long spurts in the beginning.

Add in some substantial early growth and metabolic requirements, and then try to imagine how well you'd sleep under similar circumstances. Of course, many parents don't sleep much during this period, either, as we discussed on page 171 addressing parental sleep deprivation, with fathers experiencing more sleeplessness than you might expect. But sleeping patterns aside, how much infant sleep is not enough or—is this even possible?—too much?

A 2012 systematic review of observational studies around the globe found that, on average, infants slept about 13 hours a day and that infants ages birth to 2 months woke up between 3 and 3.5 times a night. As with all things parenting, your mileage may vary.

There is, however, an average arc that infants follow when it comes to sleep habits. A newborn will sleep in little bursts of a few hours at a time but accumulate a total of 13 or more hours in a 24-hour period. As time passes, the bursts become more predictable blocks of time. Of course, that doesn't mean little Camilla won't grab a half hour here or there when you really wish she'd take 3 hours, or sleep for 6 hours right when she's due for her first visit to the pediatrician. These are all averages, not expectations.

Eating is the great sleep inducer in babies, but it doesn't always do the trick, and you might find yourself awake at 3 a.m., awash in postpartum hormone waves and fatigue, wrangling an unhappy, unsoothable infant. For the first-time parent especially, this nightly trial can seem like it has no end, but infants do eventually begin to develop what are called self-soothing skills and demand less input from you to feel comfortable. The 3-month mark is cited as a time of pretty distinct transition to a more regular sleep habit, but the variation around that is large.

The reality is that those early weeks can be a serious adjustment period. You're adjusting to an infant. Your infant's adjusting to being an infant and to everyone and everything. Your body's just been through the process of pregnancy and birth. Hormones are not necessarily your friend. And, as we might have mentioned, you're sleep deprived. We write all this because it helps us make a point about infant sleep and how research says it relates to expectations of parenthood: parents who have unrealistic expectations might feel like failures if little Jaden doesn't sleep through the night by 2 weeks old or if you feel a little resentful about the fact that you are dizzy with fatigue thanks to little Jaden's night waking. These feelings can pile on an already overloaded emotional state and create a giant, crushing snowball of parenting shame. If you have an understanding that expectations about infant sleep are, in general, unrealistic and that infant sleep is unpredictable and largely under the infant's control, perhaps you can shake some of the stress of even trying to control it yourself.

That recognition matters for a number of reasons. Studies suggest that one problem is the pervasiveness of the perception that a night-wakeful infant is problematic instead of pretty common. Some research indicates that a mother's ability to adapt to her infant's sleep habits is a critical factor in overall perception of how problematic an infant's sleep habits are. The nature of that adaptation can be important. Mothers who choose to cosleep with their infants (more on cosleeping on page 184), for example, find their infants' sleep behaviors to be less problematic than mothers who cosleep with their infants in response to perceived problems with sleep.

In other words, it's not the sleep behavior that's a problem—it's the perception of the behavior and parental expectations built around it. These perceptions can be profoundly important. If a mother thinks her infant has a difficult temperament, for example, she is more likely to perceive her child as having sleep problems even if the infant's sleep habits are within the average.

The Science of SIDS and the Safety of Bed Sharing

If it's not every parent's greatest fear, it's darn high on the list—that your baby will die in his sleep. Part of that fear arises from powerlessness because we don't know if we can ever completely prevent it or even get a warning that it's coming. Part of it arises from the fact that infant sleep deaths are, in fact, a leading cause of infant deaths in general, even if they aren't frequent. About 4,000 babies die in their sleep each year in the United States, and a little over half of these deaths (about 2,300) involve SIDS. That number is just small enough for us to recognize the rarity of the occurrence—about 6 of every 10,000 babies—but just large enough to cause anxiety.

Equally nerve-racking, however, is the fear that we might actually cause our babies to die in their sleep through accidental suffocation or strangulation, which comprise the majority of the other infant sleep deaths and generally fall under the umbrella term "sudden unexplained infant death," or SUID. That brings us to the cosleeping, or bed sharing, debate: Does it decrease the risk of SIDS but increase the risk of suffocation? Or increase the risk of SIDS too? And what's a breastfeeding mom in particular to do when cosleeping makes breastfeeding so much easier? Multiple studies have found mothers who cosleep also generally continue breastfeeding their infants for longer, but it's not clear that cosleeping causes longer breastfeeding; the causation might run both ways. (By the way, throughout this section, we use "cosleeping" and "bed sharing" interchangeably to refer *only* to a baby and a parent sleeping together on the same bed, mattress, or floor—not a couch or any other surface. Cosleeping can also refer to having a baby sleep in her own bed in a parent's bedroom, but we will refer to that as in-room sleeping.)

Let's first review what we know about SIDS and the challenges of distinguishing it from other infant sleeping deaths. Then we'll discuss the risk factors and protective factors for SIDS before finally diving into that thorny cosleeping question.

An Overview of SIDS

Although we still don't know exactly what causes SIDS, we've learned a lot more in the past two decades, and it appears the condition results from a combination of biological, genetic, environmental, and behavioral or cultural factors. The most likely biological mechanism is a baby's inability to arouse when she stops breathing while asleep or when some other challenge to her system occurs. The dysfunctional cardiorespiratory or arousal response might have a genetic cause or relate to the environment in the womb or both. Several genes have been identified that may predispose infants to SIDS when they're in an environment that makes it more difficult for them to basically fight off death—such as secondhand smoke or lying on their stomachs.

One theoretical model for understanding how SIDS occurs is the "triple-risk model," the idea that death occurs at the intersection of a "vulnerable infant," a "critical developmental period," and "outside stressors." A vulnerable infant could be one with an unidentified genetic anomaly, with exposure to nicotine or alcohol during pregnancy, with any kind of current infection or chronic health condition, or born preterm or with a low birth weight or growth restriction. One study found that preemies with a history of apnea or reduced heart rate, infants exposed to prenatal smoke, and infants with a recent infection had decreased arousability. Although evidence is building that babies who die of SIDS have a genetic predisposition, there's no evidence it's inherited. Emerging, tentative evidence suggests that babies' gut microbiomes may influence their risk of SIDS. *Staphylococcus aureus* bacteria are more often seen in the guts of SIDS infants, particularly those sleeping prone. Interestingly, however, no major differences in gut bacteria have been seen between breastfed and formula-fed infants who died of SIDS.

The critical development period refers to those first several months of life, when the cardiorespiratory and/or arousal systems are still immature, which explains the erratic breathing patterns of your newborn. Then, when newborns sleep, their heart rate slows and their blood pressure drops. If something environmental decreases the oxygen immediately available to the baby, her blood oxygen levels may drop and her lungs may not fully remove carbon dioxide from the body. A buildup of carbon dioxide increases the acidity of her blood, and this respiratory acidosis might be one contributing factor to SIDS. Environmental stressors could be her sleeping position, an airway obstruction, a poorly ventilated room, or being overbundled, as examples. Whatever the malfunctioning arousal mechanism is, babies appear to grow out of it. About 90% of SIDS cases occur before a baby is 6 months old, with cases peaking between 1 and 4 months old.

Distinguishing Between SIDS and Suffocation

The conclusions of a study are only as reliable as the data analyzed in them, and when it comes to infant sleeping deaths, the data we have and how they've been interpreted are all over the place. For a long time, any infant sleeping death without a clear explanation was considered SIDS, even though it may not have been true SIDS. Many studies have therefore linked bed sharing, for example, to SIDS when many of those deaths may have been (and likely were) suffocation deaths. SUID deaths are often coded as SIDS, but SUID can refer to a number of different situations, from SIDS to suffocation to strangulation to "we just don't know what happened"—which could even include underlying conditions (such as an undiagnosed heart condition) unrelated to SIDS, suffocation, or strangulation.

Experts have spent at least the past decade trying to define SIDS and SUID in meaningful ways, but distinguishing between the two is harder than you might expect. SUID cases usually aren't witnessed and often occur in "unsafe sleeping environments," regardless of what actually caused the death. Not all infant sleeping deaths are investigated the same way, and no standardized definitions or specific biological signs exist for clearly distinguishing between SIDS and suffocation, making it harder to know actual trends and risk factors for different SUID types.

The CDC created a new SUID registry, which began collecting data in 5 states in 2010 (now up to 9 states) and does standardize different definition categories, but it will take a while before the data set is large enough to provide the data needed to really tease out factors related to safe and risky sleeping practices beyond what research has already explored.

SIDS Risk Factors

Parents can't control every SIDS risk factor—a premature birth or low birth weight is out of your hands—but fortunately we do have control over the majority of them. The two single biggest risk factors for SIDS are the baby's sleeping on his stomach or side and the presence of smoking, which includes a mother's smoking cigarettes during pregnancy and secondhand smoke in the home during pregnancy or after birth. Other factors include overheating, soft bedding, and inadequate prenatal care.

Sleep Position. Stomach sleeping increases the risk of SIDS anywhere from 2 to 13 times that of back sleeping. Why? While the link is not fully understood, some evidence points to a baby's nervous system having more trouble managing the cardiovascular system while sleeping on her stomach, which results in less oxygen reaching the brain—a risk that peaks between 2 and 3 months old. Stomach sleeping also increases the risk of overheating and, separately, makes it more likely she'll rebreathe her exhaled air, which can increase the proportion of carbon dioxide and decrease the proportion of oxygen she inhales. Lying on their sides is just as risky because it's easy for babies to roll onto their stomachs. In fact, more babies may be dying from SIDS after being placed on their sides than on their bellies. Once a baby can roll on his own, however, there's no need to move him to his back if he rolls onto his stomach.

For those worried that babies will choke or aspirate—especially if they have reflux—the gag reflex prevents this, and studies show no increase in aspiration when babies are moved from stomach sleeping to back sleeping. Elevating a baby's head in the crib doesn't help reduce reflux and might increase the risk the baby will slide down. Parents may also lament that their children don't sleep as well on their backs—but that's exactly why the position may prevent SIDS. As much as the idea of long periods of heavy sleep from our babies sounds divine, babies need to be able to wake themselves up when their bodies face any physiological or

> Children don't sleep as well on their backs—but that's exactly why the position may prevent SIDS.

environmental difficulties, and that's easier to do while back sleeping. Two potential drawbacks of back sleeping are an increased risk of a flat spot on their heads and slowed motor development, but research shows that tummy time helps with both of these.

Sleeping in car seats, strollers, swings, infant carriers, and slings also puts children at risk because their oxygen saturation levels drop several percentage points when sleeping in the upright position. (Parents of preemies may recall the car seat challenge their child had to pass before leaving the hospital. This challenge tests a preemie's ability to maintain high enough blood oxygen levels in the upright position of a car seat.) The drop in blood oxygen levels appears related to the way the head sits on the neck with an underdeveloped jaw. When a child's head is slumped forward with her chin on her chest, the chin bone puts pressure on the airway, possibly partly obstructing it.

Smoking and Other Prenatal Factors. Prenatal smoke is a risk factor in nearly every study ever done on SIDS. It's hard to separate this from smoking exposure after a child is born—a separate risk factor because it makes it harder for a baby to arouse—but prenatal smoke plays a bigger role. Approximately one-third of all SIDS deaths might be prevented if all smoking during pregnancy were eliminated. Exposure to nicotine may affect development in areas of the brain stem related to autonomic function—the nervous system's automatic regulation of bodily processes such as breathing, heart rate, and digestion. Basically, poor autonomic function makes it harder for a baby to wake up when the body is crying "Danger! Danger! Wake up!" One small study showed that babies born to smoking mothers had impaired arousal, and prenatal tobacco smoke exposure has been linked to a greater increase in blood pressure and heart rate when breathing in more carbon dioxide. While randomized controlled trials would be unethical, the evidence strongly points to prenatal smoking as being a contributing cause of SIDS, especially since it's dose-dependent: more smoking translates to greater risk.

There isn't much evidence one way or another regarding thirdhand smoke (smoke in furniture, clothing, etc.). Though less data exist, prenatal drinking, binge drinking, and first-trimester drinking during pregnancy also appear to increase SIDS risk. Most studies looking at opiates, cocaine, and other drug use during pregnancy did not control for smoking and alcohol use, but one study did and found a two- to threefold risk of SIDS for babies exposed to methadone, heroin, and cocaine during pregnancy.

Sleeping Surface. Babies are more than 20 times more likely to die from SIDS if sleeping on their stomachs on soft bedding, such as pillows, comforters, and quilts. Even with back sleeping, a too-soft bed may force the baby's head forward a little, again putting chin pressure on the chest or partly obstructing the airway and increasing SIDS risk. The sleeping area should also have no loose bedding or soft objects, even blankets or thin sheets that might cover a baby's head.

Sleep Location. Sleeping in a room away from caregivers slightly increases the risk of SIDS. One study found higher levels of cortisol, a hormone linked to stress, in babies who slept in a separate room from their parents compared to those sharing a room with parents.

Crib Bumpers. One of the largest studies to look at crib-related injuries found that the risk of suffocation or strangulation with crib bumpers was much greater than any benefit from bumpers in preventing minor injuries. Major injuries weren't prevented, but suffocation against them, entrapment between the pads and the crib or mattress, and strangulation from the bumper ties have all occurred.

Positioners. There is no evidence that wedges or sleeping positioners decrease reflux or the risk of SIDS, but they have been implicated in both suffocation and in SIDS deaths.

Overheating. Although overheating is a risk factor, this seems mostly linked to the amount of clothing or blankets on a baby. Evidence related to bedroom heating or using a fan is sparse and weak.

Sibling Bed Sharing. No solid evidence shows benefits from putting twins or other multiples together, and doing so may increase risk of SIDS (though evidence is weak).

Non-Risk Factors for SIDS

Immunizations Are Safe. It's been definitively shown that vaccines do not cause SIDS. Whether they help prevent SIDS is less clear. Babies up-to-date on their vaccines have a lower risk of SIDS, but that may be because babies who were already sick skipped their vaccines, something called the healthy vaccinee effect, and having an infection might increase the risk of SIDS. Only one study has used babies as their own "controls" to try to figure out if vaccinations are actually protective or if there are simply differences between vaccinated and unvaccinated babies that affect risk. The answer appears to be the latter: immunizations do not really affect the risk of SIDS either way, but those babies who are typically vaccinated are also the babies who share some other characteristics (not fully understood) that reduce their risk of SIDS.

Swaddling Is Fine. Swaddling increases SIDS risk only if the baby sleeps on her stomach, not if she sleeps on her back. One study claimed a whopping thirtyfold increase in SIDS risk with swaddling—but didn't take sleep position into account and is therefore worthless. The trick with swaddling is to achieve the Goldilocks wrap: not so tight that it makes breathing more difficult but not loose enough that it starts to cover the head or a bit of wiggling releases enough for possible suffocation or strangulation. Interestingly, swaddling appears to reduce startling and increases sleep time, yet it doesn't appear to affect arousability, the best of both worlds. However, once a baby starts rolling, swaddling becomes risky: recent studies have shown swaddled babies who roll onto their stomachs are at high risk for death.

Environmental Contaminants Pose No Concern. No studies have found a link between silver, cadmium, cobalt, lead, mercury, or nitrate exposure and SIDS. There's also no evidence that gases released from mattresses, such as antimony, phosphorus, or arsenic, are related to SIDS or that wrapping mattresses in plastic protects against SIDS.

Finally, a child's hearing screening results are not related to SIDS risk.

Protective Factors Against SIDS

You can do a number of things to decrease a child's risk of SIDS:

- Providing regular, quality prenatal care
- Avoiding tobacco smoke
- Sharing a room cuts the risk of SIDS in half compared to solitary sleeping
- Breastfeeding, especially exclusively, cuts an infant's SIDS risk in half. This benefit actually appears to be causal based on the number of studies, the other factors those studies account for, and physiological studies finding that breastfed babies arouse more easily from sleep. The immune benefits of breastfeeding might also play a role in this—that's less clear—but the primary reason is that babies tend to sleep more deeply when they've been fed

formula, while breastfed babies arouse like little birds chirping for more food. Breastfed babies also have lower rates of diarrhea, upper and lower respiratory infections, and other infections that might increase a baby's vulnerability. Levels of immunoglobulin A—important for fighting bacterial and viral infections—are low in infants ages 2 to 4 months, but breast milk contains a little IgA and some cytokines that reduce inflammation. (Cytokines are proteins that can promote or reduce inflammation.) No studies distinguished between nursing and expressed milk.

- Using pacifiers cut the risk of SIDS by a third to almost a half, but no one knows why or even whether it's the pacifier itself or other factors associated with a baby who goes to bed with a pacifier. Maybe the sucking helps the autonomic nervous system with arousal. Or helps keep the airway stronger. But then we don't have the same evidence for finger-sucking, and the protective effects remain even when the pacifier falls out. The mechanism for this effect remains unclear.

What Doesn't Help?

- Although overheating is considered a SIDS risk factor, it's a difficult one to quantify, and only one small, poorly conducted study found that a fan reduced risk, so fans may not help much.
- There is no evidence that cardiorespiratory or other kinds of baby monitors reduce SIDS risk or help you "get there fast enough."
- Evidence that bed sharing is protective against SIDS is pretty weak and likely outweighed by the risks in some situations.

Cosleeping and Bed Sharing

This is where things get sticky. Every single sleep environment carries risks, some greater than others. It is impossible to create a sleeping environment in which SIDS will never occur, so knowing that there is no "safe" environment means making risk–benefit decisions about the options.

As noted above, no good evidence suggests that bed sharing reduces SIDS risk. Although Japan—where many parents sleep with their babies—has one of the lowest SIDS rates in the world, their rates of all unexpected infant deaths, including those classified as "other sudden death, cause unknown," are similar to those of other developed countries. Therefore, their low SIDS risk is most likely a quirk of how deaths are classified. A fascinating body of research, mostly led by James McKenna at Notre Dame, suggests a baby can better regulate her heart rate, breathing, and other autonomic processes when sleeping with her mother, implying a lower risk of SIDS with bed sharing. However, other sleep labs have not attempted to replicate McKenna's findings, and it's unclear whether sleeping right next to mom on the same bed is necessarily any better than sleeping a foot or two away in a bassinet in the same room, something we already know reduces SIDS risk.

The real question, however, is whether bed sharing increases risks. There are definitely very unsafe ways to share a bed with your baby that increase her risk of SIDS or suffocation. But that's far from the whole story, and claims that sharing a bed *always* increases the risk are simply not supported by the evidence. The majority of published research investigating bed sharing and SIDS (and SUID) risk shows an increased risk of death with bed sharing, but none of the studies finding that association controlled for every other possible risk factor, including parental smoking, mother's use of alcohol or drugs (legal or prescription), prenatal smoke exposure, premature or low birth weight, breastfeeding, and others. Even the handful of studies that did control for all the major factors just mentioned did not consider whether the parents planned to bed share or knew (or attempted) ways to reduce bed sharing risks. In fact, some of the earlier studies counted sleeping together on the couch in the same category as sharing a bed, and there is no question that sharing a sofa with an infant is extremely risky. One 2014 study investigated nearly 8,000 infant sleep deaths in 24 states over 8 years and found 13% of them were sofa-related—of these approximately 1,000 deaths, about three-quarters were newborns and 90% involved sharing the sofa with another person. Overall, 2 in 5 died due to suffocation or strangulation, a third had an undetermined cause of death, and a quarter died from SIDS. In that same study, only 1 in 5 deaths occurred in a crib, but half occurred in an adult bed.

Yet in some of the only studies that come close to controlling for enough other factors, the increased risk of SUID from bed sharing is negligible when those factors are considered. In fact, two case–control studies reveal the possible danger of telling parents "never" to bed share, no matter what. In one, 7 infants died when their parents fell asleep on the couch while feeding their children in the middle of the night, and 2 parents said they went to the couch because they had been warned against bed sharing. In another, half of 16 parents whose babies died on the couch said they fell asleep there by accident. They're not alone: a survey of almost 5,000 mothers in 2010 found just over half of them fed their babies at night on chairs, recliners, or sofas specifically to avoid bed sharing, and almost half these women (44%) admitted falling asleep with their babies in these places. These sad examples of unintended consequences reveal how challenging it is to give parents advice on safe sleep while taking into account, well, real life.

The reality is that bed sharing can allow many families to get sleep that they otherwise cannot get. There are also undeniable benefits to bed sharing. One small study of 56 moms found most planned to room share (but not bed share) when they left the hospital but instead ended up bringing the baby to sleep with them in bed. Their main stated reason? Bed sharing helped them soothe nighttime fussiness. Breastfeeding rates also tend to be higher, and the breastfeeding relationship tends to last longer among moms who bed share. It's not clear whether bed sharing necessarily promotes or better enables breastfeeding or whether moms who breastfeed are simply more likely to bed share for other reasons, such as parenting philosophy, but at least some research suggests that bed sharing facilitates breastfeeding. And then there is the intimacy of the practice: many parents want to snuggle up with their babies and keep them well within an arm's reach. The question is whether that can be done relatively safely.

Before we address that question, though, consider the possible risks for some parents of *not* bed sharing. If sharing a bed is the only way a parent gets sleep, and not bed sharing means insufficient sleep, that parent won't be terribly functional during the daytime. In fact (Anecdote alert! Confirmation bias alert!), that's what Tara experienced with her first son. From day one, he absolutely would not sleep alone. Her exhaustion became so great that she eventually ditched her no–bed sharing rule and bed shared. She finally got sleep, her son got sleep, she was a better functioning mother in the daytime, and she was probably a whole lot less likely to rear-end another car because she wasn't driving through bleary-eyed exhaustion. We never found a study that directly compared the risk of drowsy driving with the risk of bed sharing deaths, of course, but plenty of research shows poor sleep and drowsiness increase the likelihood of a car accident, and sleep deprivation overall contributes to poor decision-making and functioning.

Still, a stack of studies calls the safety of bed sharing seriously into question, and there are all sorts of ways bed sharing can be hazardous: overheating, a possibly higher risk of rebreathing exhaled air, airway obstructions, head coverings, and exposure to tobacco smoke, for starters. One study videotaped parents and babies as they slept, for example, and found bed-sharing babies' heads were covered much more often than those of the solo sleepers. Parents' beds are also usually much softer surfaces than cribs, and sinking a bit into the mattress or comforter may push a baby's head forward a little, putting that chin pressure on the chest that slightly obstructs the airway. And that aforementioned fatigue works both ways: overtired parents might be sleeping so deeply that they smother their babies or don't wake up in time to stop their babies from suffocating. But therein lies the rub: nearly all parents of newborns are going to be excessively tired, and as we noted earlier, not bed sharing may increase that fatigue even more for some families. (We know—you can't win.) Yet a couple of studies have found breastfeeding mothers get more sleep when bed sharing, and others have shown bed-sharing moms tend to be lighter sleepers who awake more frequently.

So where does this leave us? Well, in the few studies where researchers did account for other risk factors, the link between bed sharing and SIDS often vanishes, or at least drops below measurable significance. For example, a 2012 meta-analysis of 11 studies found an overall increased SIDS risk with bed sharing, but when they looked only at babies whose mothers didn't smoke, the slightly increased risk didn't reach statistical significance. Furthermore, babies at least 12 weeks old had no increased risk. Most SIDS and bed-sharing studies have found the higher risks of bed sharing with babies under 3 months old, even when controlling for most other factors, though, again, no study has controlled for all factors. A recent study of more than 1,700 infants, including 400 who died from SIDS, found that even with these younger babies, the overall sleeping environment makes a bigger difference than whether the child is bed sharing. Cosleeping on a sofa or bed sharing with an adult who had at least two units of alcohol increased an infant's risk of death 18 times, and babies under 3 months old were 9 times more likely to die from SIDS if bed sharing with a smoker. But older infants didn't show a higher risk sleeping beside a smoker, and none of the infants were at higher risk for SIDS while bed sharing after other risk factors had been accounted for. In fact, as long as the sleeping environment itself was not hazardous—no smoking, no alcohol use, and especially no sofa—bed sharing was found to be mildly protective against SIDS among infants older than 3 months.

Another study in Alaska, where almost 4 in 10 moms slept with their babies during the time period of the study, shows how important it is to consider all the other factors that can make bed sharing more dangerous. Researchers investigated 126 babies who died while bed sharing. Of these, 99% had at least one risk factor for SIDS, and a third had at least three risk factors: most often a smoking mom or one who used alcohol, tobacco, or drugs the night the baby died. A quarter of the babies slept on their stomachs. Yet 60% of the bed-sharing moms whose infants did not die had no risk factors. The authors concluded that these babies' likelihood of death was not related to bed sharing but to all the other risk factors present.

Still, some studies have controlled for most risk factors and found higher rates of SIDS among bed-sharing babies. What those studies did not take into account—very, very few studies ever have—is whether bed sharing is routine for a family. The handful that considered whether bed sharing was routine (and therefore intentional) found no increased risk for SIDS—except among families who bed shared when it wasn't routine. No studies have surveyed parents on whether they intended to bed share and what precautions, if any, they took in doing so, and it's therefore impossible to know whether carefully and conscientiously planning to bed share carries significantly greater risks than crib sleeping.

Despite this shaky evidence base, the AAP and many other public health agencies state that it's never, ever safe to sleep with a baby. One controversial ad campaign in Milwaukee actually featured sensationalistic photos of babies sleeping with butcher knives to convey the dangers of bed sharing. Putting aside, again, that no sleeping arrangement is ever 100% safe, this "abstinence-only" policy might, tragically, contribute to some deaths. Consider this analogy: abstinence-only policies for teen pregnancy aren't simply ineffective; they actually increase teen pregnancy rates. Teens continue having sex regardless (as they have for millennia), and data have shown that telling them not to without also providing education on contraception and STI prevention only increases how many become pregnant or infected with an STI. Yet sex

education, combined with promoting abstinence, does decrease teen pregnancy and STI rates. Similarly, parents who bed share are going to continue
bed sharing—one study found approximately one-third of mothers shared a
bed with their infants despite current recommendations. They may simply
do it secretly and lie to their pediatrician to avoid a lecture (as Tara did, with
both sons). And meanwhile, their babies might end up at higher risk for death
because they might not know how to make the sleeping environment safer or
how important those precautions are. Or they may try to avoid bed sharing
but fall asleep accidentally, either on a couch or on a bed, in a much more dangerous position because they did not plan ahead. (It's pretty tough to plan
ahead when you're exhausted.) Or again, if the only way a parent gets sleep is
to share a bed with her fussy child, will public health officials then recommend parents shouldn't drive? In short, forcing abstinence when some parents clearly opt anyway to bed share for the sake of a halfway decent night's
sleep and other reasons doesn't help anyone and leaves many parents who do
bed share uneducated and unprepared regarding best practices.

So far, no solid evidence exists to show that bed sharing, breastfeeding,
nonsmoking mothers who have not used a substance that would make them
drowsy (alcohol or illegal or prescription drugs) and are not overtired put
their babies at any greater risk for SIDS or suffocation than if those babies
slept alone in the same room. There may be an increased risk, but it's so
small it hasn't been detected. Adding some of the factors below can increase
bed-sharing risks, at which point parents will need to assess the risk–benefit
calculation for their family.

Factors That Increase Risk When Bed Sharing

A number of factors increase the risk of infant death to varying degrees
while sleeping with a parent:

- Waterbeds, couches, armchairs, and sofas carry the highest likelihood of suffocation, smothering, or SIDS deaths, sometimes up
  to 50 times greater risk.
- Any smoking in the household increases SIDS risk, but this is
  particularly true while bed sharing, with two- to seventeenfold
  increased risk. Babies exposed to prenatal smoking are also at
  greater risk for SIDS while bed sharing.

- Multiple bed sharers (such as having a sibling in the bed) increases the risk 5 times, though no studies took into account the positioning in a multi-child family bed (such as if the infant is on the edge beside only the mother as opposed to being in the middle of the bed).
- Excessively tired parents doubles the risk.
- Use of a pillow or blanket doubles to quadruples risk of death, and placing an infant on a pillow or thick bedding also increases risk.
- Premature and low-birth-weight infants have a much higher risk of death while bed sharing.
- Use of alcohol may increase risk of death (up to twice as much), as does use of illegal drugs, sedatives, or other prescription drugs that can cause drowsiness.
- Infants have a higher risk of death sleeping next to anyone other than a parent.
- Evidence regarding a parent's obesity is inconclusive: we don't know if it increases risk or has no effect on it.
- Exclusively formula-fed infants already have a higher risk for SIDS and sleep more deeply and often for longer than exclusively breastfed infants. Mixed-fed babies fall somewhere in between but generally closer to the odds for exclusively breastfed babies, possibly due to positioning. Some of McKenna's research has suggested breastfeeding mothers usually place babies below their shoulders, away from pillows, and sleep facing their infants, making rolling less likely.

Reducing the Risk

If you want to make bed sharing as low risk as possible—recognizing that you cannot remove risk entirely—the following conditions should be met:

- Use a firm mattress away from the wall and other furniture.
- The baby sleeps on her back without pillows, blankets, or comforters near her or any covering on her head, including the mother's clothing.
- No strangulation hazards (cords, draperies, etc.) nearby, including the mother's clothing.

- The infant can't fall out of bed but can't get trapped, either.
- No one in the room is a smoker, and mom isn't impaired by alcohol, drugs, or exhaustion.
- Mom is neither a heavy nor a restless sleeper.
- Only the mother shares the sleeping surface with the child.
- The baby isn't at risk for overheating.

What We Did: Emily's first son slept in a cosleeper next to her bed. She coslept with her other two sons on a flat, queen-size futon bed with only a half sheet covering her legs and nothing else. Tara anxiously and begrudgingly bed shared with her first son out of desperation. (She swears that kid is allergic to sleep.) Her second slept in a cosleeper beside her bed for half the night but often ended up in her bed halfway through during breastfeeding, but intentionally so. By 4 or 5 months old, he mostly bed shared. With both children, Tara used only a sheet or comforter wrapped tightly around her and far from her children.

Sleep Training: The Help or Harm of "Cry It Out"

In planning this book, we knew that some topics would be especially controversial: home birth, circumcision, organic versus conventional foods, and vaccines certainly sit at the top of the controversy list. But the one that can lead to shouting matches on the playground is sleep training, the tactic of using behavioral interventions to "train" an older infant or toddler to develop a regular sleep schedule. To some parents, behaviorally training a child to adjust to a presumably parentally imposed sleep schedule is tantamount to child abuse, while to other parents, this approach to early childhood sleep is rational, in keeping with the child's developmental needs, and good for the child and the parent.

The concept of sleep training does not apply to young infants in their earliest months, when they experience unpredictable spurts of needing sleep or food, and a schedule is simply not feasible. For the discussion that follows, we're talking about older infants, 4 to 6 months old and beyond, and toddlers. Newborns start out with getting many, many hours of sleep each day, but those hours are spread out in chunks, some as small as a half hour, and some as long as 4 or 6 hours (eventually). But as time passes, most infants start to stitch those sleep periods together into increasingly larger stretches, at increasingly predictable times (morning nap, afternoon nap, nighttime). They're forming this wake–sleep predictability by building their own circadian rhythms, or daily sleeping and waking clocks.

Some aspects of nighttime rhythm are inherited. Emily and some of her family members slide naturally into a rhythm of 1 a.m. to 9 a.m. when left to their own devices. Emily suspects that one of her sons would do exactly that if left to his own schedule. But her husband and some of his family members pop awake with the dawn, and two of her sons are naturally early risers as well. These anecdotal examples find support in studies showing the role of the aptly named "clock" and "period" genes in determining our daily rhythms. The influence of these rhythms extends far beyond our sleep–wake cycles, with research suggesting a role in immunity, heart disease, and other conditions. Indeed, our circadian clock operates under the influence of our body's various adjustments to maintain homeostasis, and vice versa. Twin studies also provide evidence for a strong genetic component to the development of nighttime sleep habits.

Thus, in addition to a genetic component, internal and external environmental cues play a role in our daily patterns of sleeping and waking, cues that these genes mediate for us. At a basic level, light keeps us awake and alert and boosts our cognitive function whereas dark—for most people—does the opposite. Emily is not one of these people, and Tara isn't either. Darkness brings on a second wind for both of us, and always has, something our mothers would readily confirm.

In the first few weeks of parenting an infant, you might feel that a regular cycle is never, ever going to develop. In some cases, people do remain idiosyncratic for their entire lives (ahem, Tara and Emily), and certain developmental and neurological conditions may underlie those idiosyncrasies. But for most people, some kind of pattern does develop . . . eventually. One study of 7 babies tracing their patterns of rest and activity from the newborn period to 1 year found that some of the babies already had some inkling of the 24-hour day in terms of rest and activity, while others showed steady increases in patterning to this time period over their first months of development. However, the authors of that 2006 study also note that the infants showed a large variability from baby to baby. Indeed, a 2012 study of 1,200 infants showed that most of them woke only 1 night per week by the time they were 6 months old, but . . . always a but, 34% of them didn't come to that point until age 24 months.

All of which is to say, some people might be more trainable than others or trainable at different ages or developmental periods, and some people might be more amenable than others to being behaviorally adapted to a "normal" rhythm. So with any research citing an average, keep in mind, for this topic and many others, that an average isn't a dictate for individual performance or expectations.

The main goal of sleep training is to leave a child to his own devices during wakings so that, ultimately, the child learns to wake and then self-soothe back to sleep. The question is whether the older infant or toddler whose parents engage in this kind of intentional behavioral modification experiences negative short-term or long-term outcomes. That question arises because sleep training is often used synonymously with the term "cry it out," which brings on images of a lonely, abandoned infant wailing away in the crib to a background noise of the clink of highball glasses and party music as the responsible adults in her life willfully ignore her cries. In reality, it is intended to be an intentional and careful approach to "extinguish" nighttime behaviors that seem frustrating for the infant or the parents.

But what about those outcomes? Several randomized controlled trials have found that sleep training is effective in the short term. Now that these approaches have been studied for a longer period, recent reports have described longer-term results. In one trial of 326 infants randomized at 7 months old to either a behavioral intervention (a sleep-training method) or no behavioral intervention, the researchers found no differences between the two groups on any measures at 5 years of follow-up—not emotion or conduct of the child, sleep problems or habits, parent- or child-reported psychosocial functioning, parent–child relationship, stress, attachment, parent mental health, or how authoritative the parent was. It may well be the longest string of "no significant findings" we've ever seen in a publication. The take-home from that 2012 study seemed to be that it doesn't matter which course you choose, on average; intervention or no intervention, there were no adverse effects or benefits one way or the other over the long term.

An earlier review in 2006 presented results from 52 studies of behavioral interventions for night waking in infants and toddlers. According to that review, these therapies produce "reliable and durable" changes (durable in the short term, anyway) and are effective in about 80% of children. Whether the "extinction" intervention was rigid or graduated or involved a presumably gentler "fading" approach, they were still effective overall in adjusting sleep patterns. Notably, a 2015 review led by the same author found that toddlers fall asleep more quickly, stay asleep longer, and wake less often when the family follows a regular bedtime routine each night. In a sense, this is a different kind of sleep training that families can customize to their needs.

If your child is a terrible sleeper, that doesn't seem to be associated with IQ, according to a 2013 study following pregnant mothers and then their children from infancy to age 5 years. However, in that study, more highly stressed mothers were more likely to try helping infants settle during wakings and to have infants with poorer sleep in the long term. Children who had poorer sleep at age 5 also were more likely to be anxious or show aggression, but their early infant sleeping habits didn't predict their sleep problems at age 5.

So intervention during a nighttime waking might signal a mother who is being as fussy as the infant or toddler, but research also shows that what the mother (always the mother in these studies) does at bedtime can influence whether nighttime wakings happen at all. As you'll find all over the web and as confirmed in controlled studies, a regular series of "getting-ready-for-bed" behaviors is recommended from early on so that the child receives the building environmental cues that sleep time is coming and physiologically reacts accordingly. But possibly just as critical in behavioral outcomes might be the mother's emotional availability at bedtime—how well she reflects and is sensitive to the child's emotional needs at that critical period. A 2010 cross-sectional study of 45 families with babies under age 24 months showed a strong negative relationship between how emotionally available moms were at bedtime and the level of sleep disruption their babies showed. In other words, the more responsive the mother to the child's emotions, the less sleep disruption her baby experienced, especially younger babies. No specific bedtime practice seemed to matter as much as this responsiveness to a child's emotional needs. The feeling of safety and security that this responsiveness gives a child leads to a better overall quality of sleep, the authors suggested.

The nature of the child–parent interaction and relationship emerges as an overriding factor in other studies of infant and child sleep quality. One study of 55 mother–child pairs found that mothers who saw their children as having an insecure resistant mode of attachment (meaning that the child clearly depends on his caregiver but also may show a sort of angry resistance to her) also thought their children had more sleep troubles even if they didn't.

The idea is that security at falling asleep, as seen in children who have a secure attachment relationship with their parents, will help with settling when the child awakes alone in the dark because that sense of security will persist. A 2009 study that looked at the parent–child dynamic also found a link between resistant attachment and poor sleep quality. The success of a sleep-training intervention thus might depend in part on the nature of the parent–child relationship.

What We Did: Emily didn't try sleep training on her children. She was too tired. Tara tried it only with her older son—the one who was allergic to sleep and led her to cosleep in desperation—and indeed he was in that 20% for whom sleep training of any sort just didn't work. Her nanny even stayed over several nights to help—no dice. Some nights Tara drove her older son around for an hour to get him to fall asleep. By age 3 or so, he was a great sleeper. By 5, he even stayed in his own bed all night long. Tara's younger child was magical: he slept through the night from day one and had to be awakened for feedings.

CHAPTER 7

⸎

The Joys and Pains of Feeding

Why We Care So Much About Feeding

Parental—and, let's face it, mostly maternal—obsession about "feeding," as the sociologists call it, begins early, at least at birth if not before. If you didn't give up caffeine or alcohol or Twinkies during pregnancy on behalf of your child, then for whom did you give them up? Once a child is born, the worry and incessant consideration about feeding kick into high gear. Breastfeeding starts it off. As Gill Thomson and other researchers put it in the title of their 2015 paper on breastfeeding, it's "Shame If You Do—Shame If You Don't." As we discussed in the breastfeeding section on page 91, the title references the guilt and blame heaped on women who don't breastfeed and the shaming targeted at them when they try to breastfeed in public. These authors collected narratives from 63 women about their earliest experiences feeding their children, and it's clear that social pressures drive much of the emotional responses women in particular have around feeding their children—including persistent feelings of guilt and inadequacy about giving their children proper nutrition.

Judgmental messages about feeding our children come at us from everywhere: mother, child, father, grandparents, friends, playground mothers, online sources, news stories, books, TV commercials, grocery stores, magazines, radio, movies, religious communities, and probably even the family dog, who gets to eat what little Stella sneaks to him.

In addition, mothers today face uncountable messages about how their children's early nutrition will catch their little ones up in the "obesity epidemic" plaguing the Western world, adding to the already existing angst about balanced meals and concerns about sugar intake, portion size, and snacks. Playing into these choices are factors like culture and socioeconomic status, especially with data showing that obesity affects children from disadvantaged households more than other children. The availability of time for food shopping and preparation and how children react emotionally to foods offered to them also are important. Suddenly, with all these variables feeding into the issue of feeding, it's no wonder that from birth onward, parents spend a lot of time thinking about their children and their food. So we spent some time gathering information about feeding and nutrition, and we hope that evidence serves as a shame shield and possibly as earplugs against some of these nattering and judging voices of our society.

Terrible Teething and the First Trip to the Dentist

Teething seems to have a whole mythology attached to it, from symptoms to treatment, perhaps because parents perceive it lasting for so long once it begins, which is typically between 4 and 7 months of age (though earlier or later isn't uncommon). But much of the wisdom passed down through generations has little to back it up. In fact, one of the most persistent beliefs—that teething causes fevers—has absolutely no evidence, despite the fact that a majority of parents and even many healthcare professionals believe it. The danger here is that a parent might dismiss a fever as being related to teething when it's actually an indication of some other condition. Most other symptoms attributed to teething, such as rashes and diarrhea, are also not usually related to teething.

One of the first studies to rigorously test for all the popular teething symptoms collected data on 236 "tooth days" for 21 children, ages 6 to 24 months. They measured a variety of symptoms for the day a tooth came in as well as the 5 days after that day and the 5 days leading up to it, all referred to as "tooth days." When they compared "tooth days" to "non-tooth days," they found no evidence that fever, irritability, drooling, sleep, diarrhea, strong-smelling diapers, red cheeks, or rashes occurred more often on the tooth days—even though all the parents reported many of these as teething symptoms their children experienced.

However, those researchers might have defined "tooth days" too broadly. A more recent study had a similar design but checked children's temperature and symptoms every single day for 8 months, during which 47 Brazilian children, ages 5 to 15 months, had 231 teeth come in. They found a very small increase in temperature (taken in the ear) on the day before, the day of, and the day after tooth eruption—but it was equivalent to about 0.2 degrees Fahrenheit, far below what most would consider a noticeable increase in temperature. But they did find increased salivation, sleep difficulties, rash, runny nose, diarrhea, loss of appetite, and irritability to be more likely the day the tooth erupted or the day before or after, just not other days leading up to those 3. Still, the increases were all very small. Another large study found similar symptoms associated with teething: irritability, wakefulness, ear rubbing, facial rash, decreased appetite for solid foods, and mild temperature elevation (again, almost undetectable), as well as more biting, drooling, gumming, and sucking than normal. However, they didn't find any difference in diarrhea symptoms, sleeping problems, congestion, cough, non-facial rashes, fevers more than 102 degrees, or vomiting. In fact, more than a third of the children experienced no symptoms at all on the day a tooth arrived or the day before or after. The other symptoms varied greatly, so teething clearly affects individual children differently.

So despite what your mother, aunt, and grandmother have told you, or what you remember from your niece, nephew, or previous child, most of the symptoms you think are caused by teething probably aren't, or if they are, they're mild and only on the day the tooth comes in, immediately before or immediately after.

So what do you do about it? Well, even though there are about a dozen studies on attitudes and beliefs about teething, there's very little on how to ease teething pain beyond good ol' cold teething rings. None of the research reviewed using acetaminophen or ibuprofen (though both of these are safe in appropriate dosages) or any other pain-relief methods except lidocaine, the active ingredient in many numbing tooth gels. Several deaths have been attributed to lidocaine, and there is no strong evidence to support it as effective.

Teething Necklaces

In one of only two studies about amber teething necklaces in all the literature, interviews with 29 parents revealed that 73% of the parents believed the necklace would soothe their infants. The rest thought of it as a birth accessory, a pretty necklace, a protective amulet, or serving some other therapeutic purpose. Yet 92% had not received information about the risks of an infant necklace when they bought one. Teething necklaces carry a significant risk of strangulation, and there is zero evidence to show they soothe babies or reduce teething symptoms.

When to First Visit the Dentist

Not much high-quality evidence about the best time to first visit the dentist exists, and asking five dentists might get you five different answers. That might be because the benefit of early dentist visits varies based on a child's risk profile for tooth decay. A study of almost 20,000 children on Medicaid—and therefore low income and at higher risk for cavities—found that only children at the highest risk for tooth decay benefited from a dentist visit before 18 months old. For most children, visiting before age 3 made no difference on later dental outcomes.

Some parents may head to the dentist during toddlerhood simply to normalize the experience for the child, ask questions about children's dental hygiene, and ensure no major concerns are showing up. That's not a bad idea. There just isn't evidence to show it makes any significant long-term difference on the child's dental health until late preschool. A more recent study found that preventive dental visits did result in fewer non-preventive dental visits (in other words, visits where kids need fillings or other dental work), but it grouped together all kids under 8, so there's no way to know at what early age preventive visits start paying off.

But at least parents can make a determination based on a little knowledge of what makes a child a high risk for cavities. Whether cavities develop depends primarily on the various aspects of five factors: bacteria in the mouth, saliva, pH levels, diet, and genetics. We're not going to get into the weeds on all these, but let's just say the common wisdom on candy rotting out your teeth has some strong evidence behind it. Lots of sugar—especially from foods that remain in the mouth awhile, such as a lollipop—can greatly contribute to tooth decay. Here are the other risk factors for newborns up to 3-year-olds:

- The mother or primary caregiver has cavities (some bacteria that can cause cavities can be transmitted to others, and poor dental hygiene during pregnancy increases an infant's likelihood of cavities)
- A lower socioeconomic status
- The child has more than 3 snacks or drinks containing sugar in between regular meals
- The child has special healthcare needs
- The child goes to bed with a bottle containing natural or added sugars

Ways to reduce the risk of cavities are drinking fluoridated water or taking fluoride supplements if local water isn't fluoridated, daily brushing with fluoride-containing toothpaste, and getting a fluoride varnish from a health professional. The evidence for benefits from a fluoride varnish, applied by a pediatrician or dentist once every 3 to 6 months after teeth appear, is pretty strong. If you're fretting over a child's risk of cavities from going to sleep with a bottle, fluoride is your hero. (But don't go overboard, or your hero leaves you with light browning on your child's teeth, called fluorosis, discussed on pages 204 and 266.)

When Breastfeeding Should End

When it comes to the question of when breastfeeding should end, the answer can generally be summed up in five words: when you want it to. Women stop breastfeeding for a variety of reasons, sometimes by choice and sometimes by circumstances. One study found that the number one reason cited by more than 1,300 mothers for stopping breastfeeding was a perception that their infant was not satisfied by breast milk alone. Other reasons women stop include concerns about nutrition or milk supply, needing to return to work or school, fatigue, inconvenience, biting, and believing their baby has "lost interest" in nursing.

We address many of these concerns in "Breastfeeding Blues" (page 134), but the one we don't address there is nutrition and what the evidence shows regarding how the benefits of exclusive breastfeeding relate to how long you nurse. A Cochrane Review analyzed 23 studies (out of a couple thousand) and found that exclusive breastfeeding for 6 months has three main benefits over exclusivity for 3 to 4 months: lower risk of gastrointestinal infections in babies, weight loss in mothers, and delay in a mother's next pregnancy. A couple of studies have found limited evidence for fewer ear infections and lower risk of pneumonia in babies breastfed to 6 months, but collectively, the highest quality studies don't find reduced risks for allergies, obesity, dental cavities, cognitive or behavioral problems, or any infections other than gastrointestinal ones. Since that review, one study of 600 babies found that infants already at high risk for becoming overweight had a slightly more stable rise in their weight gain (that is, not a fast rise) when they were breastfed for longer than 4 months, compared to those breastfed fewer than 2 months. The effect was small but not insignificant and applied to babies who were at higher risk of obesity because of their mother's weight, education, smoking status, level of social support, and postpartum stress.

Beyond exclusivity, however, the AAP recommends continuing to breastfeed to at least 1 year, and the World Health Organization (WHO) recommends continuing for at least 2 years. Many moms may continue breastfeeding their children past toddlerhood into the preschool years. For extended breastfeeding, most people want to know two things: the benefits and the potential harms of extended breastfeeding.

Despite the many websites promoting big benefits for continuing to breastfeed into toddlerhood, the references provided to bolster those claims don't actually show the benefits the sites claim they show—with one exception. The research makes it clear there is no evidence of harm—nutritional, emotional, developmental, or otherwise—from breastfeeding beyond 2 years, even into later preschool years. There is no evidence of psychological harm, no evidence that children will be any less independent than other children, and no evidence that the breast milk doesn't remain healthful in providing calories, fat, and nutrients. There also is no evidence that prolonged breastfeeding is "unnatural" in any way. Trying to pin down the "natural weaning age" of human primates is a rabbit hole all its own, especially since evolution (including our own) is an ongoing process. The best anthropology can tell us is that an average length of breastfeeding in humans has traditionally hovered around 30 months, depending on environment, culture, and other factors, and has ranged from 12 months to 66 months.

Somewhere after a year or so, however, at least in the resource-rich countries of the developed world, the actual measurable benefits of breastfeeding become a matter of diminishing returns, though we never know when (or if) they ever reach zero. That certainly doesn't mean there is no upside. The most frequently cited reason that mothers chose to breastfeed past 12 months in one study was that "breastfeeding was a special time for mother and baby that the mother was not ready to give up." But if breastfeeding your 3-year-old appears to comfort them and strengthens your bond with them, you don't need a population-level study on bonding to tell you that's worthwhile, and there is nothing out there to say you're causing problems for your child down the line. We also know that the act of sucking itself (at any age, actually) is comforting and can reduce blood pressure, heart rate, and breathing rate, so breastfeeding can be pain-relieving and comforting.

But the claims that breastfeeding into the second year provides huge nutritional, immune, and other health benefits to children are overblown, relying on studies in populations from low-income countries in Africa and Asia that are not generalizable to children in the West. In low-income countries, the nutritional value of breast milk into the second year and beyond can be substantial, especially since the fat content and calories in breast milk increase 15% to 20% in the second year of lactation, but that's because mothers don't have access to the clean water and foods available in richer countries.

What about immune benefits? As a child's immune system matures, it begins taking over the role of fighting off infections on its own, and the helpfulness of mothers' antibodies becomes less clear. There are a number of studies showing all kinds of antibodies in breast milk past the second year of nursing. But whether children can actually use those antibodies—we just don't know. There's no evidence so far to say they can.

Finally, there is evidence that longer breastfeeding benefits the health of mothers, typically in the form of reduced risk of type 2 diabetes, rheumatoid arthritis, osteoporosis, cardiovascular diseases, and ovarian, uterine, endometrial, and breast cancers. However, these reductions in risk tend to be very modest, such as 15% lower per year of breastfeeding for up to 2 years for type 2 diabetes. Furthermore, most of these studies did not control for other factors, such as weight, diet, or exercise, and none analyzed outcomes past 2 years of lactation. Therefore, we don't know if these benefits accrue for longer than that. Even if they do, a healthy diet and exercise will garner more gains, and we would be hard-pressed to find a mom who will say she's breastfeeding her 4-year-old to reduce her own risk of osteoporosis and breast cancer.

POST-WEANING DEPRESSION

Regardless of when you wean your child, your body will undergo many changes as it stops making milk. Some women experience post-weaning depression during this time. Very little research has looked into depression following weaning except two old studies and a recent review that hypothesizes that the mechanism is similar to postpartum depression. As oxytocin and prolactin levels drop and other changes occur in the endocrine and reproductive systems, mood changes might accompany all these chemical changes. If you experience a drop in mood that becomes depression or that you can't overcome, seek help as you would for postpartum depression.

What We Did: Emily breastfed her first until he was 8 months old, when he self-weaned in favor of the interesting visual world around him. She breastfed her middle son until he was about 6 months old, when her milk supply fell to almost nothing even though she was pumping at work. Her third son could not breastfeed, so Emily pumped around the clock for him until he was 4 months old and then during days as much as she could until he was 6 months old. Tara breastfed her first son until he was about 3.5 years old. She stopped when her second pregnancy made breastfeeding uncomfortable. She was still breastfeeding her second son at 1.5 years old as she finished writing this book.

The Best Form Formula Can Take

About Formula

As remarkable as we find it that a human can live for at least 6 months and longer only on something we can squirt from our boobs, sometimes, we know from personal experience, nature's little food plan just doesn't work out. Luckily, we have a backup in the form of formula that provides the nutrients a baby needs and has undoubtedly been a lifesaver, a time-saver, and a support system for women who couldn't or didn't want to breastfeed and for their babies. Indeed, with Emily's first child, whose growth was always off the charts, at one 3 a.m. newborn wake-up in which breastfeeding just wasn't doing the trick, Emily's husband disappeared, returned with 4 ounces of formula the hospital had sent home, and administered it to their 2-week-old. The formula was gone in minutes, and their boy sank blissfully into a satisfied sleep. "I think I stunned him," was her husband's observation. Emily was just grateful for those 4 ounces. It was one of many rescue executive decisions her husband has made over the years.

As you may already have discovered, formula comes in three forms: a powder to mix with water, a concentrate to dilute with water, or already diluted and ready to feed. For the former two, one consideration for parents is whether the water should be boiled or filtered or can come straight from the tap. According to the CDC, a potential risk of water straight from the tap in the United States is fluoride, which can lead in some cases to fluorosis, or very small white spots on the tooth enamel. The CDC describes this condition in children who strictly formula-feed as being "mild" if it occurs at all and suggests that periodic dilution of tap water with low-fluoride types of bottled water can reduce the effects. The formula itself is already low in fluoride. The FDA says parents can use regular tap water if it's been boiled for a minute, with the caution that any boiled water must be cooled before use for an infant.

The FDA in 2014 consolidated some standards for manufacturing infant formula that included testing products for nutrient content at different stages, including at the end of the product's shelf life. The FDA doesn't approve (or disapprove of) formulas, but all formulas marketed in the United States have to meet federal nutrition requirements. The AAP recommends that formula-fed infants be fed iron-fortified formula, which contains 12 milligrams of iron per liter.

In some cases, formulas are made to meet specific nutritional needs of infants in special populations, such as the so-called elemental formulas, which can serve infants who have nonspecific gastrointestinal issues and are a high allergy risk, among other things. An elemental formula consists of amino acids in units rather than strung together into proteins. These broken apart—or hydrolyzed—proteins are supposed to make it possible for an infant to obtain these necessary building blocks for growth even if the machinery to break down proteins is lacking. But how effective are these more expensive formulations of formula?

A 2013 randomized controlled trial of infants fed an elemental formula versus a regular formula found no difference in a number of measures, including growth and weight, number and quality of poops (important!), and a blood biomarker of protein intake. A 2006 Cochrane Review found "limited evidence" that using a hydrolyzed formula for infants who can't exclusively breastfeed might help prevent allergies in childhood and infant milk allergy in some cases. A 2014 systematic review of 74 studies, however, found that using these hydrolyzed protein formulas for infants up to age 4 months who are at high risk for food allergy could be beneficial. "High risk" translates as having a parent or sibling with a documented allergic condition of some kind (food allergy, eczema, asthma). Also of note, the most recent AAP publication addressing these formulas, from 2008, points out that they are not all the same and don't all offer similar protection against "atopic" disease—asthma, allergies in the common understanding of "things that make you sneeze," and dermatitis. Some of these formulas are extensively hydrolyzed whereas others are partially hydrolyzed. The appropriate choice for your child if such a formula is indicated is a discussion topic for your pediatrician.

What We Did: All of Emily's sons received a mix of (mostly) breast milk and (some) formula from infancy. The hospital refused to release her first son until he took formula and had a blood sugar reading that satisfied them. Her middle son breastfed exclusively until Emily returned to work, when he was

4 months old, and her milk supply decreased, in spite of pumping. Her third child was unable to nurse; Emily pumped milk for him and supplemented with elemental formula because of digestive complications he had. Tara's first son received formula only on his first night home from the hospital, but her second needed formula supplementation from his second week because he wasn't gaining any weight, and (as she later discovered) his inadequate suckling meant her production was too low. She used a popular cow's milk powdered formula fortified with iron and brought along ready-to-feed servings when the family traveled.

When to Start the Spoon

It's the question that can start a food fight over baby's breakfast: When can your baby start solid or "complementary" (as in, complement to breast milk or formula) foods? A check of the changing guidelines over the years and across institutions and nations is sufficient to get across the take-home message that no one's quite sure. For example, the WHO guidelines in existence when Emily's oldest child was born would have suggested introducing complementary foods as early as 4 months old. The latest set of guidelines, though, shifted that recommendation to 6 months at the earliest. If he had been exclusively formula-fed, there were no guidelines that would have addressed his needs at all.

Two considerations underlie the deep interest in the question of when to introduce solids. One relates to nutritional need and developmental readiness while the other is about later health, such as allergies or obesity. Regarding readiness, as might be obvious, a baby needs to be able to swallow the food successfully. Being able to sit up, open the mouth, and have the motor control required to take the food and swallow it are all critical to successful complementary food ingestion. There are averages for achieving these milestones, but children can wander away from the average as a result of certain conditions or an idiosyncratic developmental pace. As far as nutritional needs, entire books are available that discuss infant nutritional needs, and some have asserted that a baby can breastfeed through 1 year, at least, with no need for other foods.

For this section, as with most of this book, the discussion centers on children in the United States. This caveat is especially important in light of the extremely differential access children globally have to food, clean water, and adequate healthcare, which affects the relevance of exclusive breastfeeding and its duration. In the United States, the AAP, like most Western institutions with an interest in this subject, also now supports exclusive breastfeeding to 6 months old, but evidently, the switch from "no complementary foods" to "needs complementary foods" is a sudden one. After age 6 months, solid foods are recommended because of concerns about nutritional deficiencies. We were not clear about how a child can go from not needing solid foods at 5 months and 29 days to needing them at 6 months and 1 day. So we tried to find the evidence base, laying down the evidence about whether complementary feeding is helpful or harmful or neither and what timing has to do with it.

First, the latest Cochrane Review (2014) took a look at eight (mostly) randomized trials of breastfeeding alone versus breastfeeding plus other tasty eats and treats (solids or liquids). They analyzed data covering 613 infants and mothers from six of these trials. As is almost always the case, comparisons across trials were difficult because no two author groups conduct studies of the same research question the same way, ever, anywhere in the universe. Thus, the Cochrane Review could look only at weight change for their combined analysis, and the evidence quality even for this comparison was low. For this reason, their conclusions are not all that conclusive, but overall, they found no evidence supporting divergence from the current widespread recommendation that, where possible, exclusive breastfeeding to age 6 months is best. They did look at three trials that had evaluated adding foods at 4 months versus 6 months, a relevant comparison given a 2013 study of 1,334 mothers showing that 40% start adding in foods even before age 4 months, despite recommendations. Even with this comparison, the Cochrane Review found no evidence of benefit from adding foods at 4 months versus 6 months, but they didn't find any risks (for example, weight gain or health), either. Their finding agrees with that of an earlier Cochrane Review of 23 studies, half of them from developing nations.

The aforementioned 2013 study showed not only that 40% of mothers introduce complementary foods before age 4 months but also that the source of earliest nutrition is a factor. A quarter of mothers who exclusively breastfed introduced solids early on whereas half the mothers whose infants had formula plus breast milk or formula only did so. Type of food source is not the only influence on this choice. A 2011 study found that 62% of parents had introduced a solid food to their infant between ages 4 and 6 months, still before the end of the recommended period of exclusive breastfeeding. But mothers who were African American, English-speaking Latina, or white with only a high school degree were less likely to do so, in addition to all mothers who were breastfeeding at 4 months or later.

The conclusions of the 2014 Cochrane Review notwithstanding, one randomized controlled trial comparing infants breastfed exclusively to 6 months old and infants who were breastfed but also received complementary food starting at 4 months old found one tiny benefit: of the total group of 100 infants who completed the trial, the babies who had earlier complementary food had a slightly better iron status at 6 months old. That said, this slightly higher iron level did not translate into differences between the groups in conditions related to iron deficiency, such as anemia. The study authors themselves say that the clinical relevance of this finding is elusive; add in that the study population consisted of infants in Iceland, and any broad relevance of this outcome is also rather elusive. Obviously, iron levels are typically no concern at all for infants consuming iron-fortified infant formula.

Studies like the above that randomize babies into two different nutritional groups, one that doesn't reflect current recommendations, are probably pretty tricky to pull off in terms of ethics approval and recruitment. But how about a study of infants and nutrition that uses meat—just meat—as the complementary food? A 2014 study in the *American Journal of Clinical Nutrition* did just that. The authors cited research suggesting that the cow's milk protein in formula is associated with weight gain and increased "adiposity," or fatness. They wondered if the type of nutrition mattered and what effect meat-derived protein would have on otherwise breastfed infants. The infants were all 5 to 6 months old and were randomly assigned to having cereal as their complementary food or to having "commercially available pureed meats," aka baby food. The infants in each group then dined on breast milk and their assigned complementary foods for about 5 months while researchers tracked their growth and dietary intake. The carnivores got more protein than the cereal-vores, and at 9 months, the carnivores showed a steeper growth rate for length and weight whereas the cereal babies showed a very slight average flattening of their trajectory. In spite of their greater growth, the meat-fed babies maintained their weight-for-length scores, indicating that they weren't simply getting wider rather than taller. The open question is whether the breastfeeding and meat protein in combination somehow prevented the "adiposity" previously observed in infants fed cow's milk formula even though animal proteins were present in both diets. The most optimal protein in terms of amount, timing, and content simply remains "debatable," according to a detailed review in *Current Pediatric Reports* in 2013.

Obesity as it relates to early feeding experiences is a big research question, at least for children in developed nations. But coupled with this concern is the fact that young children need fat in their diets for appropriate brain and overall health. In fact, while only 3% of toddlers in the United States have too much fat in their diets, about a quarter of US toddlers don't get enough fat. As an infant moves from exclusive formula or breastfeeding to other foods, fat intake can decline steeply. According to current understanding, the recommendation is for 30% to 40% of infants' or toddlers' calories to be from fats, including fish and vegetable oils.

In addition to maintaining fat intake as an infant shifts to complementary foods, the issue of iron and zinc sufficiency comes to the fore. According to some studies, iron deficiency at about 6 months old becomes a serious concern for breastfed infants, which is why that age is the current recommendations' dividing line for introducing complementary foods. This recommendation is based on calculations of average iron in human breast milk and of iron turnover and needs through the first year of life. A newborn has relatively limited iron needs of about 0.27 milligrams per day whereas the older infant, ages 7 to 12 months, has considerably greater need, about 11 milligrams per day, in part because the rapid growth means a greater need for iron.

How severe is iron deficiency in the United States? One national survey identified a rate of about 9% in the general population, with a rate of the more severe iron deficiency anemia of 2.1%. Two small studies, one with 88 infants and the other with 45 babies, showed a rate of iron deficiency of 30% to 40% in 9-month-old infants who were exclusively breastfed. This risk increases from age 6 months. Iron is a big deal; deficiency alone is associated with long-term negative effects on neurodevelopment, and iron deficiency anemia has a number of adverse outcomes, including potentially boosting intestinal absorption of lead.

So that explains the 6-month recommendation.

What about the obesity question? Ah, obesity. If only there were one simple factor we could identify as causative. But there's not. Different early life experiences have been associated with increased risk of obesity, but no single factor will cause or prevent it. Timing of complementary foods is no exception—the findings are all over the place. One 2013 prospective cohort study of 847 children followed up through age 3, for example, found that children who were breastfed at 4 months old did not have increased odds for obesity at 3 years old that was associated with when solid food was introduced. Formula-fed infants, however, had sixfold greater odds of obesity at age 3 *if* they were fed solid foods before 4 months. But not all studies find similar results. What else goes into these outcomes?

Another 2013 study examined several factors that might be relevant to obesity in preschool children. In that work, involving 3,610 white children in the Netherlands, the authors found showed associations between obesity risk and having a parent with a high BMI, a low-income household, and a high birth weight. Maternal factors related to a child's obesity in preschool included smoking, greater weight gain during pregnancy, and lower education level. Obesity in the children also was linked to early rapid growth, including *in utero*, leaving open the question of whether food intake affected growth or growth dictated food intake. Introduction of solid foods after the age of 6 months was associated with a reduced risk of obesity when compared to introduction before age 6 months, but breastfeeding was not.

A 2012 systematic review confirmed the association of greater infant birth weight and rapid early growth with a child's later becoming overweight. These authors also found a 15% decrease in the likelihood of childhood overweight among ever-breastfed versus never-breastfed infants but describe the evidence as "mixed." In addition, they identified a link between maternal smoking during pregnancy and a child's risk of being overweight. Four of the five studies they evaluated for breastfeeding duration found no association with overweight status in childhood; the fifth found that breastfeeding for more than 6 months was protective against overweight status in childhood compared to breastfeeding for 3 months or fewer.

As far as early introduction of solid food, results were, again, mixed. One study reported a modest 12% increased odds of later overweight status for children who started solids before age 4 months compared to those starting after age 4 months. Another found a sixfold increased risk for childhood over-weight status in formula-fed infants receiving solid food before age 4 months compared to those receiving it between ages 4 and 5 months, which seems like a very narrow window. Another author group found a link between later intro-duction of solid food and less overweight and obesity in childhood, but yet another study found no link between early solid food introduction and later childhood overweight status. It's important to note that "overweight" and "obese" are not the same thing, clinically or otherwise, and these studies did not all look at the same end point. In addition, BMI, especially as it applies to children, has plenty of drawbacks. As you can see, it's difficult to draw a clear consensus from the variety of findings on these questions.

A factor related to complementary feeding that some parents might not consider—because aren't there enough factors to consider already?—is par-ent attitude about feeding. For example, zinc is a critical nutrient that might become deficient in exclusively breastfed infants when their need kicks into high gear halfway through their first year. The symptoms of a zinc deficiency are a slowdown in normal weight gain and a poor appetite. This latter symp-tom can trigger strong parent concerns about feeding, which can disturb the entire process of infant feeding, worsening the problem. We know from research that it's more important that parents feed a child when the child is hungry, deferring to what the child wants to eat, than to impose a parent's will on what the child eats—within obvious limits (since we can't all just eat cotton candy every day). Negative parent attitudes about feeding—including with introduction of complementary foods—can result in disrupted feeding behaviors and patterns in the child, and these have been linked to later prob-lems, including obesity. A couple of studies have found that educating par-ents to help them understand these issues has helped improve children's outcomes, at least through the preschool years, although both are in the same group of children by the same author group.

A wonderful review of the allergy question as it relates to timing of com-plementary food introduction was published in the *Canadian Family Physician* journal, authored by Elissa Abrams and Allan Becker. Our favorite part is where Abrams and Becker summarize the history of why official recommen-dations once cautioned against early solids because of allergy fears but then did an about-face and suggested early introduction might be protective. The two physicians write: "Confused? So are we. And so are our patients." And then they do what we find isn't done enough: they tackle the complexity. They state what is a central theme of this book: depending on dose, frequency, type, age, and genetics, your mileage is going to vary considerably in terms of outcomes. There is no early feeding "formula" that guarantees a slender, allergy-free, healthy child.

But what *do* we know when it comes to food and allergies? Peanuts. As in, peanuts were thought to be a food for which an early introduction may be risky, although recent research suggests a link between early introduction of peanut protein in high-risk children and reduced allergy prevalence. Indeed, in August 2015, the AAP endorsed a recommendation that infants with a high allergy risk actually be given foods containing peanuts in their first year of life. Once developed, a peanut allergy is risky in a big way, given that the reaction to peanuts can be fatal and that, unlike allergies to eggs or cow's milk, a peanut allergy persists into adulthood in the majority of people who have one. Abrams and Becker write that when a child has a sibling with a peanut allergy, the baby's risk is increased sevenfold. Everything else, they note, will have to be individualized. We address this question more in the allergies section on page 230.

What We Did: Emily's sons started on solids at around age 4 to 6 months. Tara's first son started at about 5 months, and her second started around 7 months because, well, they sorta forgot to get around to starting them.

The Scientific Skinny on Childhood Obesity and Diabetes

When it comes to helping your child maintain a healthy weight and develop healthy nutritional and physical activity habits, you're often fighting an uphill battle against your environment, depending on where you live and the social norms around you. Obesity is a complex animal, influenced by everything from genetics to metabolism to medical conditions to psychological and emotional wiring, but more than anything else, it's environmental influences, from the womb onward, that affect the extent to which we gain (or lose) pounds. Smoking during pregnancy, for example, increases a child's risk of later obesity, but so might air pollution (the evidence is emerging but not definitive). We have control over the former but not the latter. Fortunately, as we'll discuss below, there is a tremendous amount about your children's immediate environment that you can engineer to reduce their risk of gaining too many pounds.

It's not news that childhood obesity has been steadily increasing and recently reached "epidemic" levels. But this increase has not resulted from radical drops in children's activity levels or from a massive increase in fast-food consumption. Research shows children's activity levels have dropped slightly, but not by much (just minutes per day), and certainly not by enough to account for the widening of waistlines we've been seeing. The strongest evidence in this area reveals that it's not so much inactivity that leads to obesity—it's more complicated than that—but that individuals with obesity become less active. Fast-food consumption is also up, but again, blaming McDonald's and Pizza Hut ignores the many other significant changes in our environment that have occurred in the past 50 years.

Two influential voices in this area are obesity physician Yoni Freedhoff and researcher Brian Wansink, both of whom have raised awareness of the "obesogenic environment" in which children are now growing up. An obesogenic environment refers to the way our living spaces, on both large and small scales, contribute to excessive caloric intake and insufficient energy expenditure. In short, our environment makes it easy to eat more but harder to burn it off. Freedhoff's blog highlights those influences—from pizza parties in preschool to lollipops given away in the bank drive-through—and Wansink's work has explored nearly every dimension imaginable that influences how many calories children take in each day. As Freedhoff told us, "The problem is that it's stupidly difficult to prove which of the dozens, if not hundreds, of changes we've made to our environment and the way that we live are causal or most important. No single raindrop is responsible for the flood, and yet many studies are designed to try to evaluate single raindrops." Consider some of those raindrops: reduced sleep, more restaurants, fewer family dinners, sugar-sweetened beverages, the decline in cooking from scratch, the rise of fast-food and convenience stores in walkable distances from schools, nutritional and caloric illiteracy, advertising that targets kids, other changes in marketing (the amount, sophistication, targeting, and use of cross-promotions and celebrities), screen time, the rise in the prescription of psychiatric medication in kids, supersizing of portions both in and out of the home, sugar-sweetened milks, and the advent of sports drinks.

And that's a short list.

Again, though, some of those things parents have complete control over: if you don't keep soft drinks in your house, your kids will drink fewer of them. Others you can't control: Tara couldn't stop a McDonald's from being built smack between her house and her son's preschool. (It's not that ever eating at a McDonald's is "bad," but it's also true that her older son has had more McDonald's dinners than he would have had it not been built because the convenience of its proximity and her son seeing it every day increase how often they end up stopping.) So we've approached this with a twist on the Serenity Prayer and provided the things you can't change and the things you can change. We also provide a list of things you have moderate but not complete control over; you'll have to exercise the wisdom to pick your battles there. Finally, we present a framework promoted by Wansink for how to set up your own household to discourage behaviors that increase weight gain.

Things You (Arguably) Can't Change

- Genetics and medical conditions are first on this list, but there is no point in listing all the possibilities. Suffice it to say that genetics definitely plays a role, but environmental effects can play a larger part in nearly all situations.
- Children are more likely to become overweight if they had a high birth weight or if their mothers were overweight before becoming pregnant.
- ADHD increases the risk of being overweight, though it's not clear why. It could be related to boomerang effects of stimulant medications after children stop taking them, but even those without medication are at higher risk, so it could also result from the decreased inhibition associated with the condition.
- Air pollution may play a role in increasing obesity risk, but again, it's not clear why. You could arguably move into the nice, clean country air, but this isn't practical or possible for many families.
- The number of fast-food restaurants and food and drink outdoor advertising, such as billboards, is linked to a higher risk of obesity among the area's residents. Sure, you could move, but that's rarely a real option.

Things You Can Potentially Help Change

You can't control society at large, but you might be able to exert some effect over your smaller community, such as your child's school, sports teams, friends' parties, if you choose. For example, a 2015 study found children take in an excess of calories on the days they eat pizza. Homemade pizza can be healthy, but most pizza that kids eat comes from school cafeterias and parties. Completely avoiding all pizza parties probably isn't a great (or practical) solution, but offering to bring something else to those parties, joining the planning committees at school, or talking to teachers and school administration about the "reward" food offered at functions may make a difference. If you can't avoid driving past or living near fast-food restaurants and billboard advertising, you can distract your child from seeing them with conversation in the car, and you can avoid normalizing them by making fast-food meals a rare "treat" instead of a norm.

Things You Can Change

Now you can take control—but not too much, because being overly controlling about how children eat is actually a risk factor for obesity itself. Children need to exercise self-regulation—remember the bottle studies we discussed on page 90—and actions like requiring children to "clean their plate" can actually override their self-regulation and lead to weight-gain behaviors. (One study found preschoolers told often to clean their plates asked for more food when away from home.) Here are some other big-picture ideas gleaned from research:

Smoking. Children have almost 50% greater odds of becoming overweight if their mothers smoked during pregnancy.

Rewards. Using food as a reward—particularly candy and sweets—can train children to think of food as a reward, which can grow into an unhealthy attitude toward food. Children willing to work harder for food than for rewards like stickers or hugs tend to be more overweight. That doesn't mean you can't ever offer candy as a reward or celebrate something with ice cream, but when it becomes the norm, it can become a long-term source of extra calories.

Screen Time. The more kids watch TV, the heavier they are, an effect found at as little as 1 hour a day. But it's not because of inactivity, the reason most people think. Playing a video game and using a computer are also sedentary activities, but these behaviors haven't shown the same risk of obesity. One reason watching TV and movies increases weight gain is that kids eat while they're watching, and they eat mindlessly, so they don't always realize how much they've eaten. It's very easy to overeat, and the more exciting or distracting the show, the more people tend to eat. (Although, background TV, though not the best idea for other reasons, isn't linked to weight gain.) The effect starts young too. An analysis of 12 studies of children ages 2 to 6 found they increased their calorie intake and decreased their fruit and vegetable intake with as little as an hour of TV watching.

The other reason is advertising: kids see a sugary cereal or sports drink commercial and they want it, at that moment and later. In one study, kids shown cartoons and given a snack ate 45% more if they saw food commercials with the cartoons. Fortunately, the rise of on-demand TV and subscription services makes commercials easier to cut out. Limiting what children eat, or disallowing eating where the TV is, or offering only healthy foods like apple slices and carrots as "TV snacks" can all offset the weight-gain risks of screen time.

Insufficient Sleep. Another way screen time cuts into kids' health is by interrupting their sleep, as we discuss. Study after study after study finds that getting too little sleep is linked to gaining too many pounds for people of all ages, and the strongest effects come from having TVs in the bedroom. Even getting 1 hour less than the recommended 10 to 11 hours nightly for ages 2 to 5 bumped up waistlines in young kids. One study of preschoolers found 4-year-olds who slept fewer than 9.5 hours a night were about 35% more likely to have obesity. One reason is that kids eat more when they're awake longer (in one study, it was too much milk at night), but there's also evidence that poor sleep messes with two hormones that control appetite: leptin (which tells us we're full) and ghrelin (which tells us we're hungry).

Drinking Calories. Without question, water is the healthiest choice to drink, but the options and temptations for other drinks are endless, and children who regularly drink sugar-sweetened beverages—whether it's soda, sports drinks, or sugar-added juices—have a 17% to 20% increase in their overall daily caloric intake. In one long-term study of 9,600 preschoolers, 2-year-olds who drank at least 1 sugar-added drink a day were heavier (and 1.4 times more likely to have obesity) than their peers by age 5. One piece of good news is that sugar-free, artificially sweetened drinks don't carry the same risks: secretly switching out a sugary drink for a sugar-free one meant gaining 2.25 fewer pounds and 35% less body fat in an 18-month study of 600 kids ages 4 to 11. What about milk? Counterintuitively, research finds that substituting skim or 1% milk for whole or 2% milk doesn't help reduce weight gain. In fact, a couple of studies have found the opposite: children drinking skim or 1% milk gained more weight than those drinking fattier milk. Possibly, the children drinking whole milk felt more full, making snacking less appealing.

Family Meals. Multiple studies have found that eating together as a family at the table, especially at dinner, is linked to a lower risk of obesity and various other healthy habits, such as eating more fruits and vegetables. But it's about more than just eating together. The children whose families kept the TV off during family meals also consumed fewer chips and less soda in one study, and another found staying at the table until everyone was finished was linked to a lower BMI in boys. A more intensive study that videotaped family meals found that warm family dynamics, enjoyment at the table, positivity from parents, and healthy talk about food (calling it "yummy" and not moralizing about food) reduced the likelihood children would be overweight. It seems the social dynamics, the healthy attitudes toward food, and meals cooked from scratch all play a role in reducing weight gain.

Size Matters. The sizes of packages, portions, spoons, plates, bowls, cups—all these make a difference. Serving sizes are most intuitive: the more you serve, the more gets eaten. One study gave children ages 2 to 9 either single servings or double servings, and kids at all ages ate almost a third more when given the double servings, regardless of their weight or their mothers' weight. Kids also asked for (and ate) about twice as much cereal when using a large (16-ounce) bowl than when using a small (8-ounce) bowl in a different study. And first graders given adult-size bowls and plates (double a child's size) served themselves bigger portions and ate 50% more than when they used child-size dishware. Similar findings about cups, plates, and spoons consistently show that bigger means eating more, and those calories don't get offset that day or the next. Even doubling a package's size increases how much is eaten from it by 18% to 25% for meal foods and 30% to 45% for snack foods. (Interestingly, this is even true with non-food items, such as shampoo, detergent, and dog food. The larger size might "normalize" using a large amount or might convey a perception of abundance.) So always have your child eat at their play kitchen, and you'll keep the serving sizes small, right?

But the size issue goes both ways: when McDonald's shrank the size of their Happy Meals' french fries, children's overall calorie intake dropped too. Specifically, their fat and salt intake decreased while their protein intake doubled because the company simultaneously promoted milk instead of soft drinks. (They also added apple slices, and these changes interestingly correlated with an increase in apples and decrease in ice-cream orders among parents too.) And doubling servings might be a way to encourage kids to eat more of the good stuff. In one study, doubling children's servings of fruits and vegetables with pasta led them to eat 43% more fruits—except the fruit was applesauce, so that's not a huge surprise. They didn't eat any extra broccoli or carrots, but they did eat less pasta than when they had a standard serving of applesauce.

Even the shape of dishware can influence how much kids consume. Taller containers look like they contain more than short, wide containers with the same volume capacity. In one study, teens poured and drank almost twice as much juice or soda when using short, wide glasses than when using tall, narrow glasses that held the same amount. Even experienced bartenders, told to pour a single 1.5-ounce shot, poured more liquor into short, fat glasses than into tall, thin ones. (Now you know which glass to ask for on date nights.)

The "CAN" Framework

Social psychologists have known for years that simply educating someone doesn't motivate him to change his behavior alone. If it did, every smoker would quit, and we would all exercise 5 times a week and ditch the daily sodas. Instead, our behavior is dictated by thousands of daily decisions we're constantly making, often without conscious intention, using mental shortcuts we discuss in the cognitive traps section on page 305. Not many areas offer parents as rich an opportunity to manipulate those decisions than eating behaviors in the home. Experiments have found that the average person thinks she makes about two dozen decisions about food each day, but really we make a couple hundred. It's just the vast majority of these are unconscious decisions related to serving size, the utensils and plates we use, how long we end up eating, where we sit, who we eat with, and so on. We don't think of these as decisions about food, but they all influence how many calories we ultimately take in. We discussed how much size matters, but just to drive home how much education and knowledge can be outwitted by the subconscious, one of our favorite studies involved 85 nutrition experts at an ice-cream social. Those given a larger bowl served themselves nearly a third more than those using a small bowl, and using a larger serving spoon increased the amount of ice cream they scooped for themselves by 15%. And those were nutrition experts!

But parents can become the wizards behind the curtain by using the CAN approach advocated by Brian Wansink: make healthy food "convenient," "attractive," and "normative," or the normal choice. This idea is based on dozens of studies showing that more convenient and more attractively presented food is consumed more often and in greater quantities, regardless of whether it's vegetables or candy. And as social creatures, we imitate what we see and do what we perceive to be "normal," consciously or not. If everybody else is having dessert, you're more likely to order one. If no one else orders a drink besides water, you're likely to skip the cocktail too. And anyone who has hidden chocolate from themselves knows all too well that out of sight is out of mind—but it's harder to ignore the choice sitting right in front of you.

Making the healthiest options in your home the easiest, the most visible and convenient, the best looking, and the most typical will guide your child's diet toward a healthier one overall. For example, when a school cafeteria moved fruits from plain bowls in a dim corner to colorful bowls front and center under bright lights, fruit sales doubled. The home equivalent would be keeping fruit in a colorful, fun bowl on the counter or table. You don't need to take away favorite foods—in fact, a different study found that removing chocolate milk from the cafeteria altogether resulted in lower overall milk sales, more wasted white milk, and fewer students eating school lunches. Forbidden "fruit" is more attractive, so don't make the high-calorie treats off-limits, just less accessible and more infrequent. (That's why gorging on Halloween candy once a year isn't a big deal.) But make the healthy stuff what's "normal": a different study increased the proportion of white milk in the cooler from 10% to 50% of all the milk options available, and white milk sales nearly tripled.

These three elements—convenience, attractiveness, and normalcy—interact in both positive and negative ways. (It's the convenience of a cookie jar that makes the cookies disappear quickly.) On our website at

TheInformedParentBook.com, we've described various study findings related to these ideas and how those findings might be applied at home.

Sugar and Spice Aren't Always Nice

The way we think and talk about food has become almost mythical in recent years. Gluten or sugar is "evil," and organic is "pure." In reality, we need a good balance of just about everything, barring any allergies or conditions such as celiac disease. Evolutionary nutrition theories posit that our innate enjoyment of sugar ensured we got enough energy (high in sugar means high in calories) in times of food scarcity and that our learned preference for salt helps us balance our electrolytes.

But in today's society, there's no shortage of sugar or salt for most Americans. If anything, we have to work hard to avoid consuming excess salt and sugar, especially if relying on processed and prepackaged foods rather than fresh fruits and vegetables and meals made from scratch. Unfortunately, this extends to our children as well. For example, researchers assessed the sugar and sodium content of more than 1,000 infant and toddler foods in grocery stores in 2012. The infant foods fared pretty well: all but 2 of 657 infant vegetables, dinners, fruits, dry cereals, and ready-to-serve mixed grains and fruits were low in sodium, defined as fewer than 140 milligrams per typical serving, and the majority had no added sugar. Still, about half the mixed grains and fruits contained added sugar and got more than a third of their calories from sugar. The toddler foods fared far worse. A third of the 72 toddler dinners assessed contained added sugar, and 72% of them were high in sodium, defined as more than 210 milligrams per typical serving. Most of the toddler cereal bars, breakfast pastries, and fruits had added sugar, as did the snacks, desserts, and juices for infants or toddlers.

Why does this matter? Emerging evidence just in the past decade has revealed two insights into how our brains react to food. One discovery is that the taste preferences we develop early in life follow us, affecting what we like as adults, how much we eat, and, consequently, our health. The other is that brain scan studies have shown the impact sweetness has on the brain, and most of us absolutely love it. The brain responds to sugar and other sweet tastes (including artificial sweeteners) the way it responds to cocaine, though less intensely: it stimulates the reward center of the brain, which also controls our cravings. A handful of studies on obese adults have found their craving and reward responses in the brain are stronger than those in healthy weight individuals, lending some support to the theory that sweet foods can become addictive.

Nearly a quarter of children ages 2 to 5 are overweight or have obesity in the United States, a number that climbs to a third of those ages 6 to 19. Federal guidelines recommend that no more than 5% to 15% of total daily calories comes from added sugar, and US children ages 2 to 5 average about 13%. Both increased sugar intake and obesity increase insulin resistance and the risk of type 2 diabetes. Between 2001 and 2009, type 2 diabetes among US youth increased 30%. Meanwhile, the IOM recommends no more than 1,500 milligrams of sodium per day, but about 80% of children ages 1 to 3 consume more than that daily. High sodium intake leads to high blood pressure, which can lead to heart disease.

None of this means sugar or salt is "evil." It's unclear whether the brain distinguishes between the natural sugars of fruits (fructose) and the added sugars in a Snickers bar (usually sucrose), but our kids would be in pretty poor shape if we tried to cut out all sugar from their diets. Without fruits, nutrient deficiencies would cause other health problems. Plus, sugar tastes good, and taking it all away removes a lot of the pleasure of eating, also not a healthy attitude to instill in children. Rather, as with so many other aspects of parenting, the key is moderation, and picking battles well.

Deciding How Vital Vitamins Are

Supplements for Children

Walking through any aisle of a natural foods store might send you the message that no one can have too many supplements. These aisles also usually feature a children's section, with an array of options from acidophilus to, yes, zinc. Research suggests, however, that children might need very limited intervention in the way of supplements, primarily iron and vitamin D.

Let's start with vitamin D. It's trendy: deficiency in it is being blamed for everything, and supplements are flying off the shelves. This vitamin is present in some foods (organ meat, egg yolk, oily fish—all the child favorites) and added to others ("vitamin D fortified!"), but we can process it for ourselves as long as our skin is exposed to ultraviolet light (there is nothing, nothing under the sun, it seems, that's all good or all bad for you, including the sun). Regardless of how we acquire it, we have to process it in our bodies by way of the liver and the kidney before we can use it. How do we use it? We need it to take up calcium from our diet, a component that is critical for building our bones, which are in a constant state of turnover and rebuilding. We also need some calcium in our blood, and vitamin D helps with that. In addition, vitamin D plays a role in many other processes, from cell division to inflammation to immunity. Determining vitamin D levels usually involves measuring the intermediate that results after the first step of processing in the liver, a molecule known as 25-hydroxy vitamin D, or calcidiol. According to the US NNIH, a scientific consensus about which levels are optimal has yet to be reached, but it's clear that anything below 30 nmol/L (12 ng/mL) leaves a child at risk for the bone disease rickets and an adult at risk of osteomalacia, or bone softening. The cutoff for "normal" is open to some interpretation, but 50 nmol/L (20 ng/mL) or above is considered adequate for good health. Above 125 nmol/L (50 ng/mL) has been, according to the NIH, linked to potential adverse effects, especially at levels over 150 nmol/L (60 ng/mL).

While several studies have found "alarmingly" low levels of vitamin D in many US children, how those studies have defined "low" has varied considerably. Consider a 2009 study published in *Pediatrics* that evaluated blood levels of 25-hydroxy vitamin D in a nationwide sample of about 5,000 children ages 1 to 11. Based on their findings, if expanded to the entire population, at least 1 in 5 children is deficient in vitamin D when the 50 nmol/L cutoff was used. If the authors used a higher cutoff of 75 nmol/L, more than two-thirds of the children had deficient 25-hydroxy vitamin D levels. In addition, 25-hydroxy vitamin D levels were most likely to miss this higher threshold in 8 out of 10 Hispanic children and 9 out of 10 black children. But were they really deficient?

A sufficient vitamin D status according to current AAP guidelines is 21 ng/mL. The AAP recommendation is that all children from infancy onward have a minimum daily vitamin D intake of 400 IU to avoid rickets and stunted growth, but the IOM and the Endocrine Society recommend 600 IU per day for children ages 1 to 18 years. They also recommend supplementation for infants because enough might not be mobilized into the breast milk (and women aren't excluded from the latest epidemic of vitamin D deficiency). Vitamin D deficiency associated with breastfeeding has been confirmed in several studies. A 2012 study published in *Pediatrics* looked at vitamin D levels in 4-month-old breastfed infants who also were receiving 400 IU of vitamin D supplementation daily during the winter months. In spite of the supplements, the majority of these infants still had vitamin D insufficiency or deficiency.

Another study in *Pediatrics*, from 2010, found that more than half the 459 infants and more than a third of the 459 mothers in their study were vitamin D deficient, meaning that their levels were less than 20 ng/mL (50 nmol/L). Perhaps not surprisingly, maternal deficiency was a risk factor for infant deficiency (you can't pass something into your breast milk if you're deficient in it). Being born in winter bumped the risk by fourfold, and maternal BMI of 35 or greater increased risk more than threefold. Black infants had a more than threefold increased risk of deficiency. The authors also found that when the mother used prenatal vitamins in the second and third trimesters of pregnancy, the deficiency risk for the infants dropped by 70% and by 63% for the mothers if they took prenatals in the third trimester. However, almost a third of the women who took prenatals still had a vitamin D deficiency when they gave birth. A 2014 randomized controlled study in a population of New Zealand mothers and infants also found that prenatal and infant supplementation reduced the risk of vitamin D insufficiency (<20 ng/mL). Some special populations—preterm infants, children taking antiepileptic drugs—might need more supplementation.

As noted in the section on introducing complementary foods on page 206, iron deficiency becomes a concern as infant iron need starts its steep increase during the first year of life. Red blood cells need iron to grab oxygen molecules and transport them to tissues, and as infants grow, they need more oxygen and more iron. This mineral is critical to brain development, and deficiencies in iron can lead to motor and cognitive developmental delays. The current evidence-based recommendations are that infants up to age 6 months who are formula-fed receive iron-fortified formula and that children from age 6 months onward should be fed iron-rich foods (meats, iron-fortified foods). Drinking straight cow's milk is not recommended before age 1 year.

Why the problem with cow's milk? Milk is tricky. According to a trial of 1,311 Canadian children, milk intake boosted vitamin D level but decreased iron level. The authors of the study found that limiting intake to 2 cups (500 milliliters) seemed to hit the right balance of boosting vitamin D without inhibiting iron uptake. As with other studies, these authors found that children with darker skin had higher dietary requirements for vitamin D to maintain target levels, although "target" in that study was 75 ng/mL, higher than the current AAP recommended 50 ng/mL.

"My 4-Year-Old Has Never Eaten a Single Vegetable"

Emily's youngest son has never voluntarily consumed a naturally green food. He eats fruit. He'll eat raw carrots these days. But even as a baby starting on solids, he declined all foods that were green and most that were orange. The joke in their family was (and is) that given his steady and robust growth, he must photosynthesize. But what is it about foods—green foods, vegetable-type foods—that he dislikes so much?

Actually, in his case, it was worse than that for several years. He exhibits what is called neophobia, or a rejection of unfamiliar foods. As a result, in his first few years eating solid foods, he ate only five different things, none of them vegetables and only one of them a fruit. Now in grade school, he has expanded his repertoire and eats most meats and fruits and some breads and has an intractable sweet tooth. But vegetables, grains, even french fries? Nope. Emily would blame her parenting, but she has two older children who eat just about anything and always have, so what else explains this not-that-uncommon dislike of new foodstuffs?

In seriousness, neophobia is an immediate concern because it stresses parents and can lead to a tension-filled parent–child dynamic around a process—eating—that is required to stay alive. But in the long term, it holds some risk because it can lead to an unhealthy diet and nutritional imbalances.

So it might not be very comforting to learn that a lot of it might be in the genes. An interesting 2013 study of 66 same-sex twin pairs (identical twins and fraternal twins) used parent-completed questionnaires about food neophobia (there's a scale for that!) to see how common the tendency to avoid new foods is between twins. They found a very strong correlation between identical twins and food neophobia rating but no relationship at all between fraternal twins. Not surprisingly, being neophobic was also associated with refusing to eat offered foods, even foods offered repeatedly. Thus, the tendency to avoid new foods was linked to both genetics and to tensions between the parent and the child over feeding. As we noted in the section on breast- and bottle-feeding on page 84, feeding matters, as do the relationships around feeding. Some researchers consider the systematic avoidance of unfamiliar foods to be an adaptive behavior to protect against accidental poisoning, which lends credence to the genetics explanation. Even nonhuman animals have been documented in the practice.

The strong genetic input these results imply doesn't mean genes are the entire story, although they certainly are a big part of it. A variety of factors "feed" a child's refusal of foods, including the parent–child feeding dynamic noted earlier, what the child's friends or family are doing, the level of prompting and pressure exerted, and, simply, personal taste . . . and smell . . . and sensitivity to touch. For example, we have 30 or so genes that encode proteins that help us detect a bitter taste. Variants in those genes can modulate taste perception so that a food may completely lack a bitter taste to one person but be repulsively bitter to another. Taste is a sensory experience just like vision or hearing or touch. Just as one person's beautiful floral cologne is another person's noisome nightmare, a parent's fresh, delicious cilantro could be a child's soap-like mouthful.

The sense of smell might play a big role in food avoidance. Some research suggests that neophobes find many food smells to be less pleasant than non-neophobes do and even exhibit a sort of "protected sniffing" in such tests, as though to defend themselves against an unwanted onslaught of food smell. If even smelling the food creates a defensive behavior, imagine how the prospect of tasting something unfamiliar must feel. And some of that defensive behavior has been linked to a risk for social anxiety in children. That doesn't mean that food avoidance causes social anxiety but does suggest that children who tend to be anxious might show that anxiety in food avoidance. It's yet another reason not to make the problem worse by making food the center of a parent–child struggle.

Interestingly enough, those taste preferences, like most other traits we have, arise not only from our genes but also from internal and external environmental influences. Our experiences with flavors as we develop in the womb, experienced via amniotic fluid, shape our later preferences, according to a 2011 review. That might be one explanation (besides genes) for the results of a study of Australian mothers and their infants suggesting that a parent's food preferences might shape those of the child, findings that other studies confirm. For example, one study showed that a mother's consumption of anise during pregnancy primes newborns to have a preference for anise.

Beyond eating a wide range of foods during pregnancy and modeling an interest in food variety for your child, what else can the parent of a neophobe do? One consistent recommendation is repeated exposures to the food, without comment, pressure, or urging. One 2011 study that relied on self-report from 129 mothers found that children who breastfed exclusively for 6 months or longer had lower odds of being neophobic later. Children who received complementary foods before 6 months had higher odds. Worth noting, breastfed infants show a little faster adaptation to new foods, possibly because breast milk, like amniotic fluid in utero, exposes the child to a broader variety of flavors than does formula.

That emphasis on "no pressure" seems to be important; studies suggest that mothers who have anxiety about feeding (as described in Chapter 5) when their babies are 4 months old are more likely to be dealing with neophobes when those babies are 2 years old and that pressure to eat plays a role in that dynamic.

Of course, though, many neophobes outgrow their distaste for new foods and come to embrace mushrooms and onions and kale. Indeed, food neophobia usually peaks between the ages of 2 and 6 years, after which, presumably, a vista of colorful culinary delights awaits them. By adulthood, we're supposed to have outgrown it (although we all know some adults who still won't eat onions, mushrooms, or kale). And interestingly, in older age, we may revert a little, wanting only the foods that are familiar again.

Produce Aisle Showdown: GMO vs. Organic

Organic food is expensive, but the message that organic is better, conventional is bad, and genetically modified (GM) foods are the worst can lead to a weight of parental guilt that overwhelms pocketbook limitations. How much does that extra expense buy your family? In reality, results of most studies involving head-to-head comparisons of these classes of foods don't show huge distinctions among them or results compelling enough to justify guilt or shame if conventional foods are the best fit for your family's budget. We don't get into the comparative ecological or environmental effects of any of these approaches because that deep dive has filled entire books. For the sake of brevity, we have focused only on direct human health outcomes and nutrition. To be candid, with conventionally grown or GM foods, we don't find results that are alarming.

GM foods currently on the market in the United States are as follows:

- *Papaya:* This GM fruit was described as the "single-handed savior" of Hawaii's papaya industry (and now makes up 80% of its product), which was under dire threat from the ringspot virus— something that could have wiped out all papaya plants.
- *Zucchini:* According to a 2013 review, as of 2005, 13% of zucchini grown in the United States was GM zucchini, modified to resist three viruses. Its cousin, yellow squash, is also present in GM form in small percentages of yellow squash grown in the United States.
- *Canola:* Most of the canola (rapeseed plant) grown in the United States is modified for herbicide resistance. After processing, very little remains but the fats. GM canola was approved in 1996.
- *Corn:* As with canola, the vast majority of US corn, from 84% to 89%, is genetically modified, with modifications for resisting herbicide and insects; 75% of corn crops are modified for both. As with other oils derived from plants, after processing, very little remains in the oil but the fats. GM corn has been grown in the United States since the mid-1990s.
- *Cotton:* According to the 2013 review by Bawa and Anilakumar, 93% of cotton grown in the United States is genetically modified for herbicide and insect resistance. The US Department of Agriculture put that percentage at 91% in 2014 for the herbicide-resistant cotton and 84% for the insect-resistant form; 79% is modified for both. The food relevance of this fact relates to cottonseed oil, which is used in cooking.
- *Sugar beets:* This is a common source of sweetener in the United States, where almost all sugar beet crops are modified for herbicide resistance. The sugar extracted from this plant and used as sweetener is pure sucrose, which contains no other molecules (DNA, protein).

- *Soy:* Soybeans modified for herbicide resistance now make up 94% of soy grown in the United States, according to the USDA, but most brands of soymilk use non-GM soy.
- *Alfalfa:* A version of alfalfa is modified to resist herbicide.

According to the WHO, the main concerns regarding GM foods and human health are as follows:

Allergies. The WHO notes that conventional foods are not tested for allergenicity, although plenty of them certainly are allergenic (peanuts, strawberries, and eggs, for example). GM foods, however, are tested for allergenicity. According to the WHO, no allergic effects have been detected for GM foods that are currently available. The WHO information also notes that transferring genes from organisms that commonly cause allergies to organisms that don't is discouraged.

Gene Transfer. The WHO information cites a concern about gene transfer from foods that have been genetically modified, specifically transfer of genes used to modify the food to intestinal bacteria or cells of the body. They note that the likelihood of such a transfer is low and that the use of transfer protocols that don't involve using antibiotic resistance genes is encouraged, as transfer of this resistance to gut bacteria would be the primary concern.

Outcrossing. Outcrossing could happen when genes from GM plants escape the GM population and flow into conventional forms of the crop or into wild populations. According to the WHO, the primary concern is a transfer like this occurring from GM crops meant for animal feed into crops meant for human food.

The WHO notes that all GM foods on the market have undergone safety assessments performed by "national authorities."

No blockbuster findings causally linking GM foods and negative health effects are available. One study conducted by a group in France became infamous for its impenetrable data presentation, poor design, irrational outcomes, and apparent violation of animal ethics guidelines, but also is famous among groups opposed to or concerned about GM foods, because the rats in the study developed enormous tumors. That study, however, was retracted by the journal that published it, and the European Food Safety Authority and the Federal Institute for Risk Assessment in Germany both "slammed the paper," according to a 2013 *Nature* news article by Barbara Casassus describing the retraction. No published study has otherwise shown such alarming outcomes.

The question of buying organic food versus conventional food is also not as exciting or clear-cut as public debate might imply. No blockbuster findings of health-relevant differences have emerged for these two ways of growing food crops and food animals, either. Both methods involve the use of pesticides, but some studies suggest lower pesticide residues on organic crops. The caveat is that pesticide concentration isn't as important a consideration as which dose of pesticide produces negative effects. In addition, overall, pesticide exposure from consuming food grown via either method remains below limits set for safety. Some data suggest mixed results regarding level of antibiotic-resistant organisms in organic versus conventional foods, with both carrying microbes with increased resistance to some antibiotics. It's difficult to find any study reporting differences or favorable findings for either growing approach that don't have ties to industry—organic, conventional, or GM food—in some way. That doesn't make the results of any of them invalid, but given that huge revenue is at stake on all sides, it requires noting.

Regarding animals we eat, conditions for rearing animals used to produce organic foods are generally perceived as better for the animals, require that antibiotics and growth hormone not be used, and hold to feeding protocols that emphasize only organic feed. Some studies suggest a more desirable nutrition profile for organically grown beef compared to conventionally raised beef.

What We Did: Emily's first son didn't have a nonorganic food cross his lips for the first couple of years of his life. Her younger two sons received a mix of organic and conventional foods, with a trend toward conventional foods. Meat and dairy purchases are all still organic, as are soft-skinned fruits like strawberries and blackberries. She has never specifically excluded GM foods from their diets. Tara's family buys organic fruits and vegetables only if they're on sale and cheaper than conventional, but they try to eat organic meats. She has never excluded GM foods from her family's diets.

Attack of the Allergens: Milk, Wheat, Nuts, Eggs, and the Rest

Allergies are basically the immune system gone amok. Our immune systems are pretty amazing and sophisticated pathogen-fighting machines. But they can be a little too sophisticated for their own good sometimes: the symptoms we experience from allergies are a self-destructive response from the immune system overreacting to a substance it perceives to be an intruder but that really wouldn't have hurt us, such as pollen, peanuts, or penicillin. Unfortunately, the overreactive immune response can hurt us—in the case of severe allergies to substances like peanuts or gelatin, the response can even kill someone.

Just as the immune system itself is complex, so is the study of immunology, and we know far less about what causes allergies or how to prevent them than we do about many other medical conditions. What we've outlined here is the field's knowledge to date, but much of it is frustratingly inadequate. (Note: See page 250 for specifics on animal allergies.) Still, the way researchers investigate allergies in just the past decade has become smarter, not only taking into account parents' allergies but also looking specifically for reverse causality, where a conclusion mistakes X for causing Y when it's really Y contributing to X. For example, some evidence has linked longer breastfeeding to lower allergy risk, but it's not clear whether extended breastfeeding actually reduces allergy risk. Some studies have found that mothers choose to breastfeed longer after noticing any symptoms that might indicate an allergy in their child. This "reverse causation" might also account for why extended breastfeeding has been linked to a higher risk of asthma.

About the only thing clearly supported by the evidence is that children have a higher risk of allergy—eczema, food allergies, asthma, etc.—if their parents or siblings have one (though evidence doesn't support testing kids for food or other allergies preemptively just because their parents have an allergy). Similarly, the few factors researchers have identified as increasing allergy risk tend to apply primarily to these already-at-risk children, not to kids without a family history of allergies. Kids with 1 allergy are more likely to have another too. For example, someone with a food allergy is 4 times more likely to have asthma, more than 3 times more likely to have respiratory allergies, and more than twice as likely to have dermatitis. But misery loves company. A long-term Dutch study following nearly 200 people found more than half experience an allergic disease at some point from birth to age 26: a quarter had eczema, 14% had a food allergy, 17% had asthma, and 28% had respiratory allergies (such as pollens, molds, dust mites, animals, cockroaches, or other insects).

Here's the good news on allergies: there's not much evidence that eating any differently during pregnancy or breastfeeding influences your child's risk (regardless of how long you do or don't breastfeed). The most recent studies on breastfeeding have not found clear evidence that breastfeeding plays any role in development of wheeze, eczema, asthma, or food allergies. Nursing at least 4 months may delay eczema, cow's milk allergy, and wheezing, but it may not prevent these in the long run for kids already susceptible, and it has no effect on risk for kids not already at risk for allergies. Alternatively, using hydrolyzed formulas (partially or fully) instead of cow's milk formulas may reduce the risk of autoimmune skin conditions, or it may just delay their onset, but they're good substitutes for kids with a cow's milk allergy. Soy formula doesn't increase or decrease risk of any allergies.

Allergies vs. Sensitivities and Intolerances

Though often confused, food allergies and food sensitivities or intolerances aren't quite the same. For example, lactose intolerance doesn't directly involve the immune system and therefore isn't the same as a milk allergy; it's the body's inability to digest lactose (because of too little of the enzyme lactase) whereas a milk allergy involves an immune response to milk protein. How do you know it's a real allergy? The only surefire way to know is a challenge test with an allergist, but it's likely not an allergy if the child has previously eaten the food several times without incident. A food allergy involves an acute response usually within 2 hours (sometimes within minutes) of exposure to the food. Reactions can affect the eyes (red, teary), lips and skin (swelling, hives), respiratory system (sneezing, coughing, congestion, wheezing, chest tightness), gastrointestinal system (nausea, vomiting, reflux, diarrhea), and cardiovascular system (faster or slower heart rate, drop in blood pressure, dizziness, faintness). The severity of the reaction depends on the amount of food, how it was prepared, other foods eaten with it, the person's age and metabolism, and whether she exercised afterward. Exercise can increase risk of anaphylaxis, a severe reaction involving multiple organ systems that can be fatal, more often in teens and young adults. Delayed treatment with epinephrine (EpiPen), having poorly controlled asthma or another allergy, and being more than 20 minutes from a medical facility increase the risk of death or near-fatal reactions.

More than 170 foods have been identified as allergens for someone somewhere, but the big 8 are peanuts, tree nuts, eggs, milk, fish, shellfish, wheat, and soy. The ugliest of these is typically peanuts, the allergen most responsible for anaphylaxis and death and unfortunately the least likely to go away. There is no cure for food allergies—treatment is only avoiding the food—but many children outgrow food allergies by late childhood or adolescence, especially milk, eggs, soy, and wheat. (Fish and shellfish allergies, by contrast, are more likely to develop in adults and remain lifelong.) Trying to pin down how many people suffer food allergies is challenging, especially if relying on self-reported allergies. For example, in a study of 116 children with suspected cow's milk allergy, testing found only 40 of them actually had the allergy. The best estimate is a wide one: a review of the literature funded by the National Institute of Allergy and Infectious Diseases found food allergy affects more than 1% to 2% of the US population but fewer than 10%. Peanut allergies seem to hover around 2% in the most recent estimates, and cow's milk allergies have been pinned to about 2.5% (but up to 7.5%) of newborns, though most kids outgrow this by age 3. One study found about 80% of cow's milk–allergic children are also allergic to human milk.

Regardless of the precise numbers, all the research points to an increase in food allergies over the past several decades. The United States saw an 18% increase in food allergies between 1997 and 2007. Tree nut and peanut allergies in particular increased but have leveled off in the past decade. A proportion of this is likely due to increased awareness and diagnosis, but there appears to be a real increase as well, though it is unclear why.

Can We Prevent It?

When it comes to prevention, it's thought to be all about timing, but the magical window of opportunity, when the immune system is ready to ignore a new food instead of rebelling, isn't well defined and likely varies by food. Research conclusions have done a one-eighty in the past couple of decades on the relationship between food introduction and allergies, and guidelines are still literally all over the map: from Australia to Britain to the WHO, almost none are the same. It's finally been established that waiting to introduce potentially allergenic foods, the traditional wisdom for years, doesn't prevent food allergy and may even increase the risk. It's the Goldilocks principle: not too early, not too late. Too early is generally before 4 months old. Too late, again, depends on the food, but the longer it takes to introduce a food, the higher the likelihood of developing a food allergy. For example, waiting to give kids eggs until 12 months old tripled the rate of egg allergies in one study.

One long-term study on early feeding and allergies, published in *Pediatrics* in 2014, followed children from infancy through age 6 years and looked at the effects of exclusive breastfeeding and timing of solid food introduction on allergies. In terms of introduction of foods, they found no significant effect of timing of any food and probable food allergy. The authors do mention a lower rate of probable food allergies in children who had milk, eggs, or peanuts before 1 year of age compared to those who didn't, and they found the reverse link for soy, fruits, and cereals, but these associations were not significant. The only relevant factor they found was that exclusive breastfeeding up to at least 4 months old was associated with slightly reduced odds of developing a new probable food allergy, compared to no exclusive breastfeeding. But the authors suggested that the protection of breastfeeding might apply only to children who don't fall into the allergy high-risk category.

Bringing together data from a couple of studies, potatoes after 4 months, oats after 5 months, meat or wheat after 6 months, rye after 7 months, fish after 8 months, and eggs after 11 months were all linked to a higher risk of food allergies (particularly eggs, oats, and wheat). Introduction of peanuts and eggs shortly after 4 months has been linked to a lower likelihood of developing allergies to those foods, and introducing any foods by the fourth month seems to reduce eczema in kids already at risk. In fact, in August 2015, the AAP endorsed a policy of introducing peanut products between 4 and 11 months old, particularly in high-risk infants, because early exposure appears to result in an 11% to 25% absolute reduction in the risk of peanut allergy, or an 80% reduced relative risk. In one major study that contributed to the AAP recommendation, children ate peanut butter or another peanut product 3 times a week, starting before their first birthday. Delaying solids also doesn't seem to reduce the risk of asthma, seasonal allergies, food allergies, or other allergies to whatever is floating in the air, but a late introduction to potatoes, rye, meat, and fish has increased the latter.

Treating Allergies

Again, we don't have a cure for allergies. It's about avoiding the allergens and using epinephrine for severe reactions and antihistamines for milder ones. Avoidance is admittedly difficult, though. About half of all children with food allergies accidentally eat their problem food within 5 years, and three-quarters take a bad bite within 10 years. Those with peanut allergies accidentally ingest or inhale peanuts within 2 years of diagnosis—a good argument for keeping EpiPens handy everywhere your child goes and educating all care providers, relatives, friends, and airline attendants. Unsurprisingly, somewhere between 40% to 100% of deaths from food-related anaphylaxis resulted from eating food catered or prepared away from home, but having an emergency action plan in place has led to improved health outcomes. Still, nothing is guaranteed. Even with early and repeated epinephrine treatment, 12% to 14% of anaphylaxis-related deaths can't be prevented.

Ongoing research has been exploring immunotherapy to undo an allergy, and some findings show promise, but none of these are ready for primetime. (This means that if you read about a new study on reducing an already-established peanut allergy, it's probably not something you should try at home.)

Celiac Disease

Slightly different from a typical food allergy, celiac disease is an autoimmune condition involving a hypersensitivity to gluten, a protein found in wheat, barley, and rye. With food allergies, which involve histamine, the reaction to the offending food is usually pretty quick, but with celiac disease, the reaction is delayed 48 to 72 hours after eating the gluten. The reaction itself is also different: food allergies usually cause hives or other anaphylactic reactions, but a celiac body's response to gluten is to prevent it from absorbing food nutrients and to damage the small intestine's lining.

Celiac disease affects about 1% of people in the United States and is more common among non-Hispanic whites than other races/ethnicities. It appears to involve a genetic susceptibility, but there's also some evidence—albeit conflicting—that when a child first has gluten might affect whether she ever develops the disease. Most evidence shows that babies who first consume food with gluten early (before 3 or 4 months old) or, especially, late (after 6 or

7 months old) appear at higher risk for developing it. Several large studies and reviews have found that introducing gluten while a child is still breastfeeding appears to reduce the risk of celiac or possibly simply delay its onset (it's not clear which)—as long as kids aren't weaned quickly afterward. Lots of gluten at the time of weaning increased the risk in those studies. But the data can be contradictory on breastfeeding. One large study found a higher risk with introduction after 6 months old and among any babies who breastfed longer than 12 months. And a study in early 2015 followed 6,400 kids in Finland, Sweden, Germany, and the United States for 5 years and found that the average age when infants first had gluten (ranging from 4 months old to 7.5 months old) made no difference at all in whether they had developed celiac disease by age 5. Basically, there's a lot we still don't know.

CHAPTER 8

You, Your Child, and the Environment

On Chemicals and "Chemophobia"

Chemistry has its share of seemingly impenetrable terms and words whose parts are so unfamiliar, they actually create anxiety when we consider exposure to the chemicals they represent. After all, dihydrogen monoxide might sound like something you'd want to check on before ingesting it, but when you use a different symbolic representation for it, it's just water. We're familiar with water and we think of it as harmless, so that familiarity makes us comfortable. Of course, water isn't harmless. Drink too much, and you can die. Inhale it, and you can die. That familiar old dihydrogen monoxide isn't quite so harmless after all.

In the context of chemicals, fear of unknown symbols, even if they might represent relatively familiar things, is known as chemophobia. Some science communicators aren't terribly thrilled with the term "chemophobia" because it carries an element of mockery of people who find chemical words off-putting, anxiety-inducing, or difficult to understand. But it's come into common use, and there is a spectrum of chemophobia. On one end are those who believe the food manufacturers who play off the fear, buying their "chemical-free" foods. "Chemical free" is not possible. Chemicals are just molecules, which are made of atoms, and everything—even gluten-free brownies—contains chemicals. Obviously, that phrase is really shorthand for "does not contain ingredients with strange chemical names you might not understand."

Somewhere in between that end of the spectrum and chemistry PhDs who love their chemicals sit the rest of us, wondering what exactly epicatechin is and what it has to do with chocolate.

When it comes to chemicals, everything's got its dose or timing or route or combination thereof that makes it a poison or "toxin." Nothing is 100% safe. A very nice organic whole wheat flour may be great to ingest, but inhaling it will be unpleasant, at best. Salt, as necessary and safe-seeming as it is, can be deadly if ingested in large amounts. We don't look at the salt on our tables or the water in our bottles and think "chemical," but that's because our familiarity with them breeds comfort, not chemophobia. The best cure for any chemophobia you feel when you read alarmist articles or strong claims about "chemicals" in food, air, or water is to consider how much unfamiliarity feeds the fear. And then ask a chemist or a toxicologist. In our experience, they're pleased to see anyone showing an interest in their fields and in learning the facts and evidence about chemicals.

BPA: A Case Study?

BPA, or bisphenol A, is a compound that occurs in hard, clear plastics (polycarbonate plastics, carrying the number 7). It also occurs in the lining of food cans and is present in some dental sealants. In the 1990s, studies in animals started yielding results suggesting that exposure to BPA could influence a number of outcomes as a result of disruption of signaling pathways involving steroid hormones. A growing list of possible effects from the metabolic to the reproductive led to its being banned by the FDA in 2012 for use in baby bottles and sippy cups.

A 2013 review of BPA, published in *Fertility and Sterility*, cites 91 studies linking BPA to human health, with 53 of those appearing in the preceding year. That sounds like a mountain of compelling evidence. And human studies, most of them population-based (epidemiological), have found correlations between BPA levels in urine or blood and outcomes like obesity or high blood pressure; however, because correlation means only a mathematical relationship and not a cause-and-effect association, the relevance of these findings has been unclear, and controlled trials are hard to come by.

They are not nonexistent, though. In one recent randomized trial, the study authors, a team in Korea, gave participants soy milk from cans that contained BPA in the lining or from glass bottles and then took blood pressure measures. After drinking 2 bottles of soy milk from glass bottles, the participants had low urinary BPA. After drinking 2 cans of soy milk, however, the participants had very high urinary BPA, 16 times the level of those drinking from glass. Under both conditions, blood pressure fell, by 7.9 mmHg in the glass bottle group but by only 2.9 mmHg in the can group. This outcome was widely reported as a 5 mmHg increase in blood pressure, but what it really represents is a less-steep decrease (or, as the authors put it, it's an increase after the systolic blood pressure is "adjusted for daily variance"). Soy milk is associated with reduced blood pressure, so the implication is that the BPA interfered with that beneficial effect of the soy milk. The 60 study participants were older women, and a few had high blood pressure, but overall, they were a healthy group. Other studies have found similar bumps in BPA urinary levels after people consumed foods from cans.

The relevance of BPA in the urine isn't entirely clear, but this measure has been linked to obesity in children. In a 2012 cross-sectional study in which the authors write that they controlled for many relevant variables, including caloric intake, urinary BPA values in the highest three-quarters were linked with increased prevalence of obesity. For example, 10% of children in the lowest quarter of urinary values were obese whereas about 20% of those in the second, third, or fourth quarters of values were. Why the obesity rate would plateau at 20% even as urinary BPA values increased is unclear. What the authors could not control for is whether children who are obese tend to eat foods that have more BPA in them or if having more body fat translates into having more stored BPA. In 2014, the FDA ruled that BPA in food packaging is still safe. It has been used in linings of food cans since the 1960s.

What about how infants and children handle BPA compared to adults? Some studies had initially suggested that younger mammals metabolize the chemical less readily, with the implication that it might then persist in and affect tissues. However, studies with nonhuman primates suggest that young primates are as metabolically efficient in dealing with BPA as adults are.

In terms of early life effects, the bucket of research looking at embryonic, fetal, and newborn exposures is huge and heavy, but the vast majority of studies are correlational. As an example, a 2014 study looked at the relationship between urinary BPA levels in women in their second and third trimesters and then at levels in the children from these pregnancies when they reached age 1 and age 2 years and followed the children's height to age 5 years. These authors found no significant relationships with BMI and only an association between BPA levels in early childhood and accelerated growth. If growing a lot means eating a lot, and eating a lot possibly means more BPA ingested, then that correlation involves some pretty significant confounders. The adjustments the authors made for diet are a little messy because, as they note, they originally designed their diet-related questions to evaluate exposure to environmental chemicals, not to assess nutrient intake.

When considering BPA and potential effects on the brain, which many parents might want to know, the evidence base for correlations in people is lacking. A little over a dozen studies, almost all involving rats and mice, looked at the association of cognitive end points and BPA exposures. The findings are variable and, as the metabolic differences between rodents and people in the BPA context make clear, possibly not translatable to people. One 2011 study looked at the influence of BPA and phthalates, another plasticizer of suspect effects, on childhood social impairment as it relates to autism spectrum disorders. They found a correlation with phthalates, six of which have been severely restricted in the United States from use in children's toys or toys children can put in their mouths, but found no significant associations with BPA exposure, as determined by urine values from women in their third trimester of pregnancy. A 2012 study involved examining associations between dental restorations (which contain BPA) and cognitive outcomes. The study was a randomized safety trial to compare results with two types of dental restorations in children, and one of the types contained BPA, which can leach out. But the authors also performed an additional analysis for neuropsychological outcomes and found no significant associations with either type of dental restoration and intelligence, achievement, or memory test scores.

A very recent study, published in January 2015, took a different approach to BPA. The authors performed a correlational study, as most BPA studies are, but in this case, they added a causal element and made their study interspecies, as in they looked at several different species: humans, sheep, rats, and mice. For humans, they looked at the association between maternal and cord blood BPA values from 24 pregnant women and their babies and a marker of oxidative stress. Oxidative stress results from an imbalance toward having too many damage-causing oxygen species in tissues. These molecules work with the immune system and are normally present, but when they go into overload, the result can be tissue damage and inflammation.

The researchers found correlations between BPA levels and levels of the oxidative stress biomarker. When they gave pregnant rats, mice, or sheep BPA at levels that represent human exposures, they found the same correlation between BPA levels and the biomarker. The fact that controlled administration of BPA turned up the same relationship as the human correlational study suggests a real biological association between the BPA exposure and the increased oxidative stress biomarker. This work is the first to take this approach, and more work will undoubtedly follow to see if the findings can be replicated and confirmed.

Overall, the BPA picture is primarily correlational or offers results from rodent models. You might think that following the ban and that with the introduction of substitutes for BPA, consumers could rest easy. Unfortunately, the substitute compounds may not be any better than the BPA we have already known for more than a half century. A 2015 paper published in *Fertility and Sterility* reported that two of the substitutes, bisphenol S and bisphenol F, already in use as alternatives, mount strong competition with BPA for causing adverse effects in human testes cells and rodent cell cultures. We may be seeing the start of another confusing, sprawling, correlational evidence base all over again.

Bug Off: DEET and Other Mosquito Repellents

It's estimated that no living creature on earth has caused more deaths (besides humans) than the mosquito. From yellow fever to malaria to West Nile virus to dengue fever to various forms of encephalitis, mosquito mommies have left a devastating impact on humanity. Fortunately, most of these diseases are no longer threats in the United States, but West Nile returns every summer to some degree, and dengue fever has occurred in parts of the South. In 2012, a total of 5,674 people contracted West Nile virus, of whom 286 died. And it's not just mosquitos: more than 19,000 people have contracted Lyme disease every year since 2004. Even if children don't catch a disease from a bug bite, they can suffer allergic reactions, and the itching can lead to scarring or skin infections, such as impetigo.

The two chemical compounds that show the greatest effectiveness in warding off mosquitos and other critters are DEET and picaridin. Neither is 100% effective, but both are pretty good at keeping blood-sucking arthropods at bay, and they are the most common active ingredients in US mosquito and tick repellents.

So these keep the mosquitos away—but at what cost? Both DEET and picaridin have been approved for use on all children, with no lower age restriction. Based on the available toxicological data, both chemicals have low acute toxicity, and normal use of both should not present a health concern to the general US population, including children, as long as the label directions are followed. For instance, a 20% picaridin product should not be applied more than twice per day to adults or children. The effectiveness of both DEET and picaridin appears to last 3 to 7 hours, though up to 25% DEET has been necessary to last the longer duration.

But there are some worrisome studies out there on DEET and picaridin—until you dig a bit deeper. A 2001 study reported extremely rare instances of DEET exposure "causing" encephalopathy (brain disease or swelling), seizures, and—in 3 cases—death in children. The authors of that study noted that "surprisingly, [mortality] did not correlate with the concentration of the DEET liquid used, the duration of skin exposure, or the pattern of use," casting some doubt on whether DEET caused all the incidents. And these 18 cases were the only ones recorded worldwide. Five of the cases involved oral DEET exposure, though all 3 deaths followed skin exposure (and a lot of it over long periods of time). In a more recent review of DEET, the authors wrote about these cases that "the role of DEET in either the illness or deaths was and remains purely speculative." Despite the use of the term "DEET-induced encephalopathy," they wrote, it's never been shown how DEET might have physiologically caused those incidents, and there is not enough evidence to say it did.

In another review in 2014, the researchers found no evidence of severe adverse events linked to recommended DEET use in animal testing, observational studies, and randomized trials. Their main takeaway came down to a risk–benefit analysis: "The theoretical risks associated with wearing an insect repellent should be weighed against the reduction or prevention of the risk of fatal or debilitating diseases including malaria, dengue, yellow fever and filariasis (a roundworm infection)." Millions of people use DEET each year, and the risk of seizures like those cited in the 2001 paper, if even caused by DEET, is very, very low. The EPA estimated in a 1998 review of DEET that the risk of seizures is about 1 per 100 million users, equivalent to 3 people in the entire United States each year if every resident applied repellent with DEET. That's literally several thousand times lower than the risk of contracting a disease via mosquito or tick bites, some of which can cause fever, seizures, and coma.

The CDC has even urged women who are pregnant or breastfeeding to use repellents containing DEET to limit the risk of transmitting West Nile virus to the fetus, and researchers have found no negative effects among women exposed to DEET during pregnancy, though there was some evidence of DEET in the cord blood of some study participants.

Meanwhile, a 2008 assessment of DEET and picaridin risks found that risks increase if more than 40% DEET is used on children under age 12, if 25% DEET is chronically used (daily or several times a week) on children under 12, or if a product containing more than 15% picaridin is chronically used on children 17 and younger (infrequent use showed no risk).

What about alternatives? Electronic devices that supposedly repel insects don't work, and citronella candles are only mildly effective if you sit directly in their plume of smoke. Research into essential oils has shown some promise, but the only one actually registered with the EPA that comes close to DEET's effectiveness is oil of lemon eucalyptus, which is comparable to lower concentrations of DEET, around 6.65% to 15%. There's a small amount of evidence that 2% soybean oil may be similarly effective.

Children and Medication

More than half of all drugs approved by the FDA lack labeling for children, which could mean instructions for use or simply a label stating that children shouldn't receive that drug. The situation is far better than it was nearly 15 years ago, when more than 80% of drugs had no pediatric labels, but there is still a ways to go before guidance for medication is more clearly available in black and white, based on research, rather than requiring parents to rely on only doctors' clinical experience. What we'll cover here are just a handful of very general medication-related issues that most parents will encounter. We do not provide specialized or detailed information on medications or specific medical conditions.

Coughs, Colds, and Respiratory Infections

Lots of things can be challenging about parenting, but one of the worst might be staying up with your coughing, sneezing, stuffed-up, miserable child and feeling like there's nothing you can do to help. If the problem is bacterial, antibiotics will take care of it, but most often these bugs are viruses, and even a "simple" cold can mean a week of misery for the whole family. Unfortunately, children under 4 should not take the cough and cold meds that we adults can dose up on—nasal decongestants (pseudoephedrine, phenylephrine), antihistamines (diphenhydramine, brompheniramine, chlorpheniramine), cough suppressants (dextromethorphan), or cough expectorants (guaifenesin)—or at least not without a doctor's guidance. Not only can these medications cause serious harm, especially in children under 2, but a large Cochrane Review in 2014 of admittedly not-great studies didn't find strong evidence that these treatments work for cold and cough symptoms in children anyway.

So what can you do? If your child is at least 1 year old, you can head to your kitchen and pull out the honey. For coughs, a number of studies and a Cochrane Review found honey worked better than no treatment, a placebo, or diphenhydramine. (It didn't work better than dextromethorphan, but that shouldn't be given to kids under 4 without a doctor's advice.) Infants under 1 can't take honey, though, because of the risk of a bacterial infection from botulism. Yet one small study found something interesting when researchers gave coughing children ages 2 months to 4 years old a teaspoon of agave syrup, an extract from a cactus that's similar to honey but safe for children under 1. They compared the agave syrup to a placebo (grape-flavored water) and no treatment for one night. The next night, all the parents reported improvements in the cough, but the kids who got the agave syrup had a slightly better improvement . . . and so did the kids who got the grape-flavored water. So the agave syrup worked, but only as well as the placebo. But it was better than nothing. So that's something.

What else might help? There's some evidence for the benefit of cool-mist humidifiers, but warm-mist ones might worsen symptoms. Vapor rubs on a child's chest may help but shouldn't be used for children under 2 or those at risk for seizures. Using saline drops and nasal suctioning helps with stuffiness (even if this experience is rarely fun for parent or child). Children's acetaminophen and ibuprofen (but not aspirin, which has been linked to a serious condition called Reye's syndrome) can treat fever, aches, and pain when used at the ages and doses recommended by the manufacturer (pay attention to labels—concentrations vary!) and ideally under the advice of a doctor.

Et tu, *Tylenol?*

For a good 10 to 15 years, more and more studies started to find an unsettling link to children's use of acetaminophen (brand name Tylenol)—development of childhood asthma symptoms. Study after study would find that kids were 2 or 3 times more likely to develop asthma between ages 5 and 9 if they used acetaminophen before their first birthday, and one of the requirements for causation, a dose-dependent relationship (more acetaminophen, higher risk of asthma), was present as well. Soon, it appeared antibiotics showed a similar association with developing asthma and a similar dose-response effect. Finally, around 2010 or 2011, researchers started asking the question they probably should have been asking all along: Is there something else that's the common link between asthma and use of acetaminophen and antibiotics? Something like, say, more respiratory infections in infancy? Sure enough, as researchers started to revisit their data sets and more studies were conducted and systematic reviews were analyzed, it emerged that the same kids who were taking more acetaminophen and antibiotics were also the same kids having more respiratory infections than average before they were 2 years old—and respiratory infections early in life are known to increase the risk of asthma. Two large reviews of the evidence in 2013 and 2014, one looking at 64 studies and the other looking at 11 studies, assessed the quality of the studies and their findings after taking into account children's frequency of respiratory infections. And they found that the link between asthma and both acetaminophen and antibiotics was not the medication but rather the reason children were taking the medication (what researchers call "confounding by indication")—the respiratory infections.

Not only are these findings reassuring—there is no evidence now to support the concern that using acetaminophen or antibiotics in infancy will increase a child's risk of asthma—but this tale offers two other valuable insights. First, this is how science works. It's a process of gradually testing hypotheses, narrowing the research questions, and seeking alternative possibilities before drawing any definitive conclusions. No study standing completely on its own is worth much without others that replicate its findings or test its possible limitations. Second, be wary of the headlines. For years, many of these studies led to headlines scaring parents out of using Tylenol when their child was in pain for fear that they would increase their child's risk of asthma—unnecessarily.

Homeopathy and the Placebo Effect

Homeopathy follows the logic in the expression: "Hair of the dog that bit you." In short, the idea is that you take a teensy amount of something that causes symptoms similar to what you're experiencing. Got bitten by a dog with rabies? Place a single hair from the rabid dog on the wound to try to cure it. (They really used to do that.) Sound a bit irrational? Well, that's what homeopathy practitioners claim: taking the tiniest amount possible of something that supposedly causes the symptoms you don't want and diluting it to a microscopic dose will cure your symptoms. Any treatment effect from homeopathic medicine amounts to that of a placebo: you feel better because you expect to feel better even if the substance you took has no active ingredients that would treat your symptoms.

When water containing the tiniest drop of the agent that causes a malady has been diluted 100,000 times, for example, that equates to a 6X or 3C homeopathic dilution. Homeopathic practitioners claim that the remaining substance contains the "memory" of whatever causes the problem. Place a drop of that water in a pill, and that's your homeopathic medication. Although practitioners claim that the greater the dilution, the *stronger* the therapeutic effect supposedly is, no chemistry or evidence supports this concept. The only difference between a homeopathic solution and water is the imagination.

The good news is that your imagination can be pretty powerful, so for problems like headaches, general stomachaches, fatigue, and maybe some lower back pain or other relatively minor complaints, the placebo effect works. No, there's nothing in the homeopathic medication that actually treats your symptoms, but if you think it does and you feel better, it doesn't matter all that much. What matters is if the problem isn't mild but something more serious that requires medical treatment. If a parent uses homeopathy to treat an ear infection that worsens and actually requires antibiotics, the harm (aside from draining your wallet) is in delaying necessary treatment, which can lead to a worse situation. Furthermore, medications labeled "homeopathic" may contain other active ingredients that could cause harm or interact with other medications.

What's So Essential About Oils?

At the time we wrote this book, a search of "essential oils" in PubMed pulled up a little over 4,600 results. The vast majority of these involved animal studies, Petri dish studies, or uses in food science (killing bacteria on lettuce, for example). Just under a dozen evaluated essential oils as mosquito repellents, and a couple hundred involved aromatherapy (mostly for stress, anxiety, and coping during stressful medical procedures, such as chemotherapy or childbirth). What didn't we find? Any studies that showed essential oils can effectively treat asthma, acne, gastrointestinal disorders, autism, arthritis, influenza, urinary tract infections, yeast infections, diabetes, blood clots, ear infections, eczema, constipation, Alzheimer's, tuberculosis, menopause, cancer, low libido, Hashimoto's disease, multiple sclerosis, fever, or Ebola virus. The popularity of essential oils has exploded in recent years, and they have plenty of uses, from cleaning supplies to, yes, aromatherapy to ease a mild headache or anxiety. But they should not be ingested, especially by children, unless there is evidence they can treat a specific condition and a physician can support the use. (There is preliminary evidence that peppermint oil, for example, can treat irritable bowel syndrome, but it also should never be used with a child under 3. It can cause rashes, and doses greater than 1 gram per kilogram of body weight can be deadly.) Studies with essential oils can be challenging because they are not standardized, and it's difficult to tell what caused a particular outcome. (Again, the placebo effect can be powerful.) Furthermore, more than a half dozen of those PubMed results involved essential oil poisonings in children, some with serious consequences. A number of oils, including clove, wintergreen, and oregano, for example, are blood thinners. In general, essential oils should not be used topically with children under 2. Some oils used with a diffuser may help with fussiness, coughs, headaches, anxiety, or slight nausea, but there is scant evidence to support these uses, and parents should never assume diffused oils are necessarily harmless.

The Mellowing Effects of Melatonin

Some children experience more problems than others when it comes to falling asleep or getting sufficient sleep even if parents follow a strict routine every night. This challenge can be especially true for children with developmental conditions, such as ADHD or autism spectrum disorders. Melatonin is the hormone that tells the body it's time to sleep and helps regulate the body's internal clock. It's closely tied to light exposure, which is why watching TV or using computer screens or tablets before bed can make it harder to fall asleep, because the blue light can interfere with the brain's release of melatonin. Research has shown melatonin can be effective in treating jet lag, in training the circadian rhythms of blind people, in treating children's migraines, and in reducing some children's seizures because of its antiepileptic properties. But it has also been shown to reduce the time it takes for children to fall asleep, particularly children with autism or ADHD who have sleeping problems. In a systematic review of nine studies involving autistic children, melatonin helped them fall asleep faster and stay asleep a little longer (anywhere from 45 to 70 minutes longer on average), improving daytime behavior, even though it did not reduce how often they woke up in the night. A similar smaller review found comparable effects in children with ADHD, ages 6 to 14. Side effects in all these studies were mild (headache for a day or two) or nonexistent, and no studies have identified serious side effects or problems with long-term use (although most studies are short term, except one that tracked two dozen kids for 18 months). Most of these studies used doses of 2–5 milligrams. In studies lasting as long as 3 years, no long-term effects of chronic melatonin use have been found.

The Hygiene Hypothesis:
The Help and the Harm of Playing in the Dirt

Put simplistically, the phrase "hygiene hypothesis" represents the concept that parents in developed countries in particular keep their children too clean—their houses are too clean, their bodies too free of infection thanks to vaccines, their guts too devoid of immune-system-challenging microbes and parasites. The upshot, goes this simplistic version, is that the part of the immune system that infections and parasites challenge fades into the background from disuse and makes way for the allergic and self-attack side of the immune response. This shift in the balance, according to this idea, has resulted in the increase in allergies and autoimmune diseases of recent decades. This hypothesis emerged in the late 1950s. In support of it, researchers cite increased prevalence of allergies and of autoimmune diseases like multiple sclerosis and type 1 diabetes (formerly known as juvenile onset diabetes) and the fact that rates of both increase in migrant families, sometimes even in a single generation, once they move from a developing to a developed country. Other factors are possible explanations for these findings, however.

The concept that too much hygiene can be problematic has led some to turn to parasite exposure to treat diseases like asthma and gastrointestinal immune disorders like Crohn's, with mixed outcomes. All such studies involving people are very small, making any firm conclusions difficult. The rage for probiotics also traces in part to this concern about a "too clean" environment leaving our guts devoid of "old friends" (that's really what the researchers call them) in the form of our microbiotic ecosystem inside of us. But results of probiotic studies and various end points are also mixed, and if the bacteria in these supplements do make it to our intestines, as bacteria, they might be capable of some unexpected behaviors.

As a parent, you will make many choices balancing risks and benefits, good and bad outcomes. Allergy and asthma are miserable, at the least, and can be life-threatening, but the risk of developing either is minimal compared to the risks associated with infectious diseases against which we vaccinate. Hard data and large studies regarding the role of diseases or microbes in allergy, asthma, and autoimmunity are still lacking, so what is the evidence-based parent to do? A couple of immunologists Emily talked with once had some pretty simple parenting advice when it comes to children and hygiene: "Let 'em play in the dirt," on the premise that a little dirt might give a child's immune system a good workout and won't do much harm either way.

Inflammation and Children

Inflammation has become a byword for "not good for you" in recent years. But the reality is that inflammation is good for you quite often: it's the way your body fights acute injury and disease and gets you back to health. It's a nonspecific response, one in which the body marshals several general defenses against the injury or invasion. Fever, specialized cells, and specific molecules (called cytokines) all kick into gear to take on the invader or call a repair-and-defense team to the site of injury. Part of this reaction involves making the blood vessels leakier to allow immune system cells access to the site of injury or invasion. The upshot is a pretty inhospitable environment for microbes (an overheated host, killer cells) and a gateway to healing and fighting off local infection in the case of a wound. That's all good. Indeed, the AAP guidelines about fever, a systemic manifestation of inflammation, say that parents should focus on making the child comfortable, not fever free, because fever is often beneficial. Brain damage, which is usually a parent's greatest fever-related concern, seldom occurs with fevers under 107.6 degrees Fahrenheit, according to the NIH.

But as with chemicals, when it comes to inflammation, the dose makes the poison. A little inflammation can be a good thing, keeping you healthy and sometimes going into action so subtly that you don't even feel that bad. But if the inflammatory response ratchets up too high or goes on too long, those cells and molecules that facilitate defense and healing can become a liability. An example is the body's response to viruses that result in what are known as hemorrhagic fevers. The body's extreme response to the viruses is one factor in the high fatality rates with these diseases, as the body produces an excess of inflammation-related molecules and damages its own blood vessel lining (the endothelium). Levels of molecules involved in the rapid inflammatory response are generally higher in patients for whom the diseases are fatal.

> As with chemicals, when it comes to inflammation, the dose makes the poison.

In the case of hemorrhagic fevers, the dose of inflammation is acute and overwhelming. But in other diseases, the dose can be low but cause damage because of the length of exposure. The damage to the endothelium that builds up silently over time in blood vessels is an example of the effects of chronic, low-grade inflammation, and the disease it causes is atherosclerosis, or hardening of the arteries. Inflammation that isn't shut down in a timely way but persists also can result in collateral damage to nontarget tissues.

In addition, the inflammatory response can be inappropriate in terms of when it happens, not just how much or how long. Allergy is the inflammatory version of a false alarm, when the body shifts into gear and releases floods of histamine. This release causes an acute inflammatory response that includes leaky blood vessels and the action of immune system cells and inflammatory molecules and, at its most extreme, can lead to anaphylaxis. In some cases, the body triggers inflammation systemically with no known trigger and causes tissue damage; these diseases are "autoinflammatory" disorders, such as Behçet's disease, a systemic inflammation of the blood vessels that can affect the joints, nervous system, and digestive tract.

Some diseases carry a hereditary component, a risk factor you and any biological children can't do much about. But diet and lifestyle behaviors are risk factors for chronic inflammation, and these can be under your control. At the top of most lists of these factors is smoking, including exposure to secondhand smoke. Stress and obesity are also risk factors, as is a lack of exercise. Interestingly, too much exercise can also raise your risk for chronic inflammation. A diet rich in plants and varied natural colors, in addition to favoring whole over processed foods, is listed in many sources as a way to fend off inappropriate inflammation.

Cats and Dogs and Turtles, Oh My!

Cat and Dog Allergies

Allergies are no fun. If there were concrete steps you could take to reduce the risk that your child would develop allergies, it's probably safe to say you would take them. But would that include getting rid of your "child" before you had children—such as your dog or cat?

If the question were whether you would get rid of a pet who had bitten your child, especially multiple times, the answer may be a bit simpler: these tend to be more serious injuries, and they may indicate a developing pattern of behavior. But the research on how pets do or don't affect the allergies risk is far shakier. The question involves two unproven theories: the allergen hypothesis, which initially suggested that exposure to allergens can sensitize individuals but has now flipped to suggest early exposure can build a tolerance, and the hygiene hypothesis, which suggests that not having regular exposure to lots of germs in childhood can increase the risk of allergies because the immune system doesn't develop fully.

The problem is that both of these hypotheses are incredibly difficult to test. The development of allergy conditions is complex and not entirely understood, potentially involving many different interacting factors. The only clearly established risk factor is having a family history of allergies. There are no trials in which families are randomly assigned to own a pet or not own a pet, a study that's unlikely ever to happen. And we cannot raise kids in laboratories, which would allow sufficient control of environmental factors. So we're stuck making sense out of incomplete observational studies, which involve so many other variables that it's tough to determine what is or isn't contributing to (or preventing) allergies. Dozens of studies have explored whether dogs, cats, rodents, and birds are linked to asthma, eczema, wheeze, hay fever, and other forms of allergies, but even in high-risk children—those with a family history of allergies—the research is equivocal. In fact, families with a history of allergies are already less likely to have pets, so it's not possible to entirely account for that confounder, which can make it look as though not owning a pet is linked to allergies. Furthermore, allergy risk would depend on types of pets and breeds, how much exposure the children have to the animals, whether the animals are indoor or outdoor, what pets nearby neighbors might own, the geographical area and environmental allergens, the children's genetics . . . and so on.

But we can still have a look at what has been found to date, keeping in mind a couple of important caveats. First, studies differ a great deal in how they measure family history and children's outcomes as well. Second, most infrequent wheezing—a sign of allergy—in children younger than 6 will eventually go away on its own. Third, the variables each study does control for vary almost as much as the number of dog breeds out there.

One analysis of 11 European studies found a small amount of evidence to show that having a furry pet in a child's first 2 years reduced his sensitization to allergies in the air—that is, making it less likely he would develop allergies. Another older analysis of 32 studies found cats decreased asthma risk while dogs increased it. But then, one large, much more recent meta-analysis of 21 studies found owning dogs or pets in general, though not necessarily cats, reduced the risk of a type of eczema as much as 25%. (See what we mean?) The only thing resembling a consensus is that owning a dog when a baby is a newborn appears to slightly decrease the risk of some allergies, eczema and/or asthma, but the effect is weak, it mostly applies to those without a history of allergy, and there are still many other factors that could play a role.

The extent to which owning a dog or a cat can reduce allergy risk, then, is still uncertain, but the good news is that the most recent studies, especially long-term ones, don't find owning a dog or a cat in early childhood *increases* a child's risk of developing allergies. A different question is whether being born into a dog- or cat-owning home might play a role in allergies later on, when children grow up and get a dog or a cat on their own. It appears that owning a dog or a cat in early childhood might slightly decrease this risk, but the effect is again weak.

If a child does end up being allergic to dogs or cats, there are a variety of hypoallergenic breeds that might work (though there's no such thing as a 100% non-allergenic dog or cat). Or, if a child develops an allergy to a beloved furry creature who is already a part of the family, then the deliberations about what to do should involve an allergist. Aside from these situations involving known, diagnosed allergies, about the only consensus on pets and allergies is that concerns about future allergy development should not be a factor in whether to get or give up a pet dog or cat.

Dogs and Biting

What do dogs and sharks have in common? Deaths from dog bites are almost as rare as shark attacks (which are rarer than humans being struck by lightning), but this rarity means nearly every incident makes the news—making them seem more common than they are. Only 33 people died from dog bites in 2010, for example, compared to more than 3,700 drownings and more than 33,000 poisonings. However, that doesn't mean you should be complacent about the coexistence of a child and a dog. When Tara brought home her first son from the hospital, her long-haired Chihuahuas were curious about this odd intruder who weighed about as much as they did. As he grew, trouble inevitably brewed as he became a bit too curious about their tails and ears, but the combination of her watchful eyes on him and her dogs' training long before he was conceived have prevented any incidents. Emily brought her sons into situations of similarly experienced dogs and adult humans. The most important part has been knowing what's likely to lead to causing a dog to become aggressive. One survey of about 800 dog owners found that many did not know that certain factors or situations could put kids at risk for bites. Some of the misconceptions were that puppy training could completely eliminate the risk of biting (nothing is 100%), that family dogs bite only if teased or hurt (affectionate petting or hugging can lead to bites if a dog feels frightened or threatened), and that bites result from "asserting dominance" over children (a debunked myth). Another misconception is that it's safe to leave a sleeping baby alone with a family dog, yet most fatal attacks of infants occur from a pet in the home, often while the baby is sleeping. One tragic case study reported on 3 infants, all under 3 months old, who were mauled by the family dog when left unsupervised in electronic swings.

One study found the most common trigger for bites to younger children or children familiar to the dog was "resource guarding," in which the child was approaching, touching, or reaching for a dog while it was eating or chewing a bone or toy—almost half of kids familiar to a dog were bitten while the dog was guarding its food. The second most common trigger was causing the dog pain, intentionally or not, such as hitting the dog or stepping or falling on him. Yet every dog in that study (111 dogs) had either a behavioral or medical abnormality upon further assessment, so it was likely that at least two factors led to the bite.

Another study found younger children were more often bitten in their home during positive interactions, such as petting or hugging, with a familiar dog whereas older kids were more often bitten by unfamiliar dogs outdoors. The highest-risk age group for any bite was under 2 years old—precisely the age of kids who understand least how to avoid causing a dog pain or fear. (This same study found that the pit bull terriers involved in bites were more than twice as likely as other dog types to be unfamiliar to the child.) The authors pointed out four guidelines based on what they had learned from analyzing 200 bite incidents:

- Stationary dogs (including lying down) should never be approached by children.
- Any nearby item (sometimes including a parent) to a dog could be considered "high value" and worth defending.
- Even "benign" touching might cause a dog to react defensively if the dog is hurt or fears being hurt.
- Some social interactions are viewed differently by dogs and humans, such as hugging, which can feel threatening to dogs.

What about the role of a dog's breed? An oft-quoted study conducted by the CDC, the American Veterinary Medical Association, and the Humane Society found that more than half of fatal dog bites over two decades were attributed to pit bull–type dogs ("pit bull" is not an actual breed) and Rottweilers, but that finding did not mean these dogs presented a greater risk than other breeds. Breed identification can be subjective and wasn't available in all cases, and dogs are frequently crossbred. Further, the data were based on news accounts, which may bias which breeds were mentioned since a pit bull attack grabs more headlines than a Chihuahua or Pomeranian attack (though those happen too). There is also no way to accurately track multiple incidents from a single dog so that one particularly aggressive poodle isn't counted as five different dogs.

In reality, it's almost impossible to link bite risk to particular breeds: there is no centralized reporting for either bites or breeds, and it's difficult to accurately estimate ownership rates of breeds, whose popularity as family pets rises and falls. A long look across the research shows that bites from a particular breed have increased as popularity of that breed has increased. When cocker spaniels are popular, cocker spaniel bites are more common. When German shepherds are popular, German shepherd bites are more common; Emily still has a facial scar from a German shepherd bite she sustained as an infant, but then she went on to grow up with German shepherds around her much of her life. But it's tough to know how many total cocker spaniels or German shepherds are in the population at any specific time, and without knowing that, it's impossible to figure out an aggression rate for any particular breed. Obviously, we'll see more bites from Rottweilers if a lot of people own them, and obviously we'll see fewer bites from greyhounds when there are fewer of them around. Meanwhile, if dogs trained to fight, such as pit bull types, are the ones involved in bite incidents, that tells us nothing about dogs of the same type brought up to be family pets.

Research to date has found that the five primary interacting factors influencing a dog's likelihood to bite are hereditary, early experience, socialization and training, medical and behavioral health, and the victim's behavior. Even if breed could be isolated as a factor—which has not been shown—it would be low on the list. It's true that a larger dog's bite can generally induce more serious injuries simply because it's bigger, but small dogs can cause serious injury too, especially if they meet some of the characteristics already associated with bites. Perhaps the most comprehensive study of dog bite–related deaths, published in 2013 by the *Journal of the American Veterinary Medical Association*, analyzed all the factors associated with the dog bites over 10 years. They identified 7 factors common among the situations, and 81% of the cases involved at least 4 of these factors—but breed wasn't one of them. The 2 most common—each involved in 85% of the cases—were unfamiliarity between the victim and the dog and a dog that had not been spayed or neutered. The other factors included not having an able-bodied person present to intervene, the victim not being able to defend himself (age or disability), the dog not being a family pet, past owner mismanagement of the dog, and owner abuse or neglect. Older dogs and dogs trained using punishment were other factors among pets, but puppy classes reduced the risk of aggression. One final conclusion of this study was that "it would be inappropriate to make assumptions about an individual animal's risk of aggression to people based on characteristics such as breed."

Salmonella *Risk*

Your child plays with a toad found in the yard. Your son's preschool classmate brings in a baby chick for show-and-tell at Easter time. Your daughter excitedly moves her hand along the scales of a boa constrictor at a street fair. Every one of these scenarios has something in common with raw cookie dough: the risk of *Salmonella* poisoning. When your pets (or other animals your children encounter) go beyond dogs and cats, it's important to recognize the illnesses animals can bring into the home. *Salmonella* is a big one because the risk is greatest with reptiles and amphibians. That doesn't mean you have to get rid of your prized iguana or your 25-year-old boa constrictor, but keep them out of reach from the kids and don't bring the pet (or its tank, if it has one) into food prep areas. Be sure kids wash their hands if contact with the animals does occur.

After a *Salmonella* outbreak, it can take months or years to determine the source. For example, an outbreak caused by African dwarf frogs spanned 2008 to 2011 because it took that long for epidemiologists to piece together the source of the infection (the frogs) and then the common factors in the frogs. Almost a third of the 376 individuals who got sick—mostly children—were hospitalized, but none died.

Salmonella can also exist in mammals, such as kittens and gerbils, hamsters, or other rodents, but mammals usually show symptoms of infection, so avoid pets that look particularly quiet, tired, or sickly (or that have diarrhea or weeping eyes or runny nose). Baby chicks, on the other hand, can shed the bacteria from their feathers without being affected at all. Every spring, health departments see a new wave of *Salmonella*-related sickness because of the popularity of chicks at that time of year. Other kinds of birds and hedgehogs are also well-established carriers of *Salmonella*.

A variety of other illnesses can also be caused by pets, such as lymphocytic choriomeningitis virus (LCMV) in pet rodents. Typically, wild mice are the most common carriers of LCMV—a good reason to set traps or clean up droppings—but hamsters have transmitted the virus to humans as well. However, with this infection and others from animals, soap and water are the best methods of prevention. That and keeping an eye on small children, since kissing a frog is more likely to give your little princess an infection than a prince.

Kids and Guns: Avoiding Avoidable Tragedy

Including a section on firearms may seem an unusual choice for a book such as this, but it's one of those areas where the research is greatly misunderstood or simply not taken seriously. It's also one of the areas where evidence is spottiest due to restrictions on firearm-related research for many years in the United States, thereby requiring us to use some studies older than those in most other sections. Yet the dearth of research and the ignorance of what the data reveal are tragically costly. Since Newtown, when school shootings have been better publicized, many parents' top worry about guns relates to school shootings, perhaps because parents feel the least amount of control over preventing such an incident. But the odds of a child age 5 to 18 being killed at school is not far off from the odds of dying in a shark attack. Only 1 in 3.1 million people die of shark attacks, and in 2009–2010, the odds of a child dying in a school shooting were about 1 in 2.5 million (compared to 1 in 16,000 for car accidents).

The real danger is gun accidents and suicides in the home. It's almost impossible to know precisely how many children die from accidental gun injuries each year because of inconsistent data collection methods across the United States, but even the most modest measures show it's at least a couple hundred a year. And those don't include nonfatal injuries to children, numbering in the thousands annually.

Just about all of these deaths, however, are preventable. Firearm policy is particularly contentious in the United States, but it is impossible to dispute comparisons of US firearm injuries with those in other high-income countries—the United States leads by a long shot. Firearm suicide rates among children ages 5 to 14 are 8 times higher, and unintentional firearm injuries are 10 times higher in the United States than in any other high-income country. The presence of a firearm in the home is particularly linked with suicides because youth suicides are usually impulsive, firearms are the most lethal of suicide methods (90% death rate, compared to hanging, the second most lethal, at 83%), and second suicide attempts after an incompleted one are rare and usually unsuccessful. Therefore, how an attempted suicide turns out depends largely on whether a child has access to a gun.

For toddlers and preschoolers, however, the concern is generally more about risk of gun accidents. Although it's a no-brainer, the safest way to prevent a gun accident in your own home is simply not to have a gun. But many choose to have guns for various reasons, and your child likely spends some time in other people's homes, whether you are with them or not. An estimated one-third of parents with children under 18 own guns—including one-third of parents with kids under 4.

The next safest option, then, is keeping any guns in the home unloaded and locked up, with the ammunition stored separately and also locked up. A study from 2005 found that keeping guns unloaded—both handguns and long guns like rifles and shotguns—cut the risk of child- and teen-firearm suicide or unintentional gun injury by 70%, and keeping them locked cut risk by 73%. Both locked and unloaded? An 84% reduced risk. In other words, among 100 children hurt or killed by an unlocked, loaded gun, 84 incidents would not have occurred had the gun been locked up and unloaded. That study involved only a little over 100 incidents that were compared to nearly 500 gun-owning homes without an incident, but it was well-designed and accounted for differences in geography, child's and gun owner's ages, and household income and education. Another decade-old study found that equipping guns with a magazine safety, a loaded chamber indicator, and a personalization device—allowing only the owner to use it—could have saved almost 500 lives in 2000.

Yet one study found that 1 in 5 gun-owning parents with children under 18 stored their gun loaded, and a third stored their gun unlocked (including parents with children under 12 in the home). And 8% had at least 1 unlocked, loaded gun in the home. One reason these parents may store their guns unlocked and/or loaded is cognitive dissonance—they incorrectly believe that they are an exception to the statistics for one reason or another.

For example, in a study of rural and urban Ohio residents, almost 90% of respondents believed their children—no matter how old they were—wouldn't touch a gun they found, and half of these said their kids "knew better" or were "too smart" to touch a gun. Only 12% of the 122 gun owners in that survey stored guns locked and unloaded, primarily those with a higher income, a bachelor's degree, or kids ages 5 to 9. The authors suggested that parents' "unrealistic expectations of children's developmental levels and impulse control" might affect how the parents stored their guns and whether they addressed gun safety with their kids.

Similarly, in another survey of about 400 parents in Atlanta, three-quarters thought their child would leave a gun alone and/or tell an adult if they found a gun. Among the 28% who had children ages 4 to 12 and owned a gun, three-quarters thought their kids could tell the difference between a toy gun and a real gun, and a quarter thought their child could be trusted around a loaded gun. In another study among about 200 gun-owning parents in rural Alabama, more than a third of the parents who said their kids didn't know where the guns were kept and one-fifth of parents who said their kids had not handled the gun were contradicted by their children. In fact, 73% of kids under 10 knew where their parents' gun was stored, and these statistics weren't affected by whether the parents kept their guns locked up or whether they had ever talked about gun safety with their children.

What all this research tells us is that many parents, whether gun-owning or not, have unrealistic expectations about what their children will do and what they're capable of when it comes to finding a gun. We know the expectations are unrealistic because of the research looking specifically at what children do when they find a gun even if they have received gun-safety training.

Only a handful of studies have looked at this, but their findings are consistent. One involved observing 64 boys, ages 8 to 12 and split into groups of two or three, for 15 minutes in a room that contained two brightly colored water guns and a .380 caliber handgun in drawers. Three-quarters of the boys found the gun, and half overall handled it. Half of those who handled the gun, or a quarter of the whole group, pulled the trigger with enough force to discharge it. Whether the boys' parents thought their kids were interested in guns or not was unrelated to which boys picked it up or pulled the trigger. About half the boys who found it were uncertain whether it was real or a toy, but even some of those who knew it was a real handgun played with it and even pulled the trigger. Moreover, 93% of the boys who handled the pistol and 94% of those who pulled the trigger said they had received some kind of gun-safety instruction, whether it was from police officers, teachers, or family members.

In another study, 24 pairs of preschoolers were left in a room with a two-way mirror, with two toy guns (a large silver cowboy gun and a black cap gun) and two disarmed handguns (a .38 caliber and a .22 caliber). Afterward, in identifying each of the four guns as real or toys, the children made an average of more than one mistake, more often mistaking a real gun for a toy. Two weeks later, after a 30-minute gun-safety presentation to the families, the children were observed again. The presentation made little difference to how much they played with the real guns, and those who still played with the guns the second time said they did so because the child with them encouraged it or else they figured it was fine because they didn't get in trouble the first time. Almost half the participants' parents owned guns, and four children told the study authors they had played with their parents' gun without their parents' knowledge. Kids who had access to their parents' guns or had handled their parents' guns (with or without permission or supervision) were more likely to play with the guns in the room—even if they knew the gun was real—and more likely to show aggressive behavior. The same author of this study found in a different one that guns seem to hold an allure even to boys with little apparent interest in them and that children's attitudes and behaviors around guns don't match up.

What about more formal gun-training programs? One of the most popular gun-safety programs for kids is the National Rifle Association's Eddie Eagle program, but only two peer-reviewed studies have assessed its effectiveness, comparing it to a different behavioral program or no program at all. Both studies found the same thing: the kids could repeat back what they learned in both trainings, and the children receiving the behavioral training better demonstrated safety skills in supervised role-playing—but neither group showed the safety skills when placed in real-life situations.

Finally, the most elaborate study compared two groups of boys and girls ages 4 to 7: one group of 34 kids received a week-long in-depth firearm-safety program that also covered conflict management, making good decisions, and resisting peer pressure. The 36 others received no training. Then the children were paired up: one-third untrained, one-third trained, and one-third with children from each group. When the pairs played by themselves in a room containing a hidden black toy cap gun and a real semiautomatic pistol, at least one child in each pair found at least one gun, and half the boys played with it. Only one child among those who didn't play with it left the room to tell an adult. Not only did the week-long safety program have no effect on children's willingness to play with the guns, but 72% of the kids who went through the training played with the guns, compared to 45% of the children who didn't receive training and played with the guns, and 47% of kids in mixed pairs. In fact, 15 kids who initially said, "Don't touch that!" during the experiment touched the gun.

Again, the kids made mistakes trying to determine whether the guns were real or toy, more often mistaking the real gun for a fake one, and knowing a gun was real didn't stop kids from playing with it. There were no differences among the kids in terms of who pulled the trigger, who played more aggressively, or what their parents expected they would do, but children of gun-owning parents were more likely to play with the gun or say it was okay to play with guns. The authors suggested that children at these ages were too cognitively immature to comprehend the lessons in the gun-safety program—past research has shown they have a hard time identifying a dangerous situation and taking actions to prevent an accident—and that their curiosity may overcome their judgment, making it hard to use strategies they've learned even when they've practiced them.

The research therefore shows that children under 12 cannot be trained to leave a gun alone or practice gun safety. The only prevention that has been shown to work, aside from not having a gun in the home, is keeping firearms unloaded and locked up. But even if you do this in your own home, an average 1 in 3 parents of your children's friends likely own guns, and research shows many of them don't lock up their guns or keep them unloaded. While ownership varies by geography, socioeconomic status, and other factors, it's almost certain that your child will eventually be in a home with a gun. The only way to know if they're locked up and unloaded is to ask.

Air Pollution: What We Can't See Can Hurt Us

You might be surprised to learn that over the past couple of decades, air pollution in general has declined. However, as anyone who lives in an urban area can tell you, the air still gets thick. At some point, you might wonder what the risks of these airborne molecules from exhaust and industry carry for your child.

Obviously, conducting randomized controlled air pollution trials on pregnant women and children isn't ethical, so most of the studies look at cohorts of pregnant women or children based on where they live and what the inferred exposure to air pollution might be. In some cases, the way air pollution values are derived starts with high-level data measures, which then are put through some serious number-crunching to get at a value that can be used to examine correlations. The problem with any air pollution studies is that almost no one—not pregnant women, not children—spends their entire day in the same area or even outdoors. A child who lives in a suburban area away from freeways but who attends school near a freeway may have a real-life air pollution exposure that is very different from what models based on her home address would indicate. The same applies for a pregnant woman who works indoors in a busy downtown but walks out for lunch every day and to and from her transport and the office. All these factors are worth keeping in mind when considering air pollution studies and their results.

For this section, we looked primarily at systematic reviews of different outcomes as they relate to outdoor air pollution during pregnancy or during early childhood. And we note that as bad as the air might seem in some parts of the United States, in many areas of the world, it's far worse. Also, a note on jargon: the hazy air you see on a "Spare the Air Day" arises in part from the presence of tiny particulates made up of metals, soil and dust particles, acids, and organic chemicals in the air. In air pollution studies, these are treated in terms of their size, either 10 microns or 2.5 microns, which is relevant to the physical limitations on their ability to access certain tissues. Particles that are bigger than 2.5 microns but smaller than 10 microns are "inhalable coarse particles," according to the EPA. As that term implies, these particles can make their way through respiratory passages and into the heart and lungs.

Examples of these kinds of particles are the dust and other matter kicked up from roadways or from industries such as sawmills. "Fine particles" are the 2.5 micron size or smaller particles that give air a hazy look, and according to the American Lung Association, these can penetrate into the tiniest airways of the lungs. They result from combustion and are present in smoke from fires and in exhaust from cars and industry. And even smaller particles, nanoparticles, clock in at less than 100 nanometers; diesel exhaust is one source of these ultrafine particles. While the size of particulates can affect their ability to enter tissues, other factors like chemical interactions affect this ability as well. The effects of these particles on tissues typically show up as tissue inflammation, which explains their strong association with cardiovascular disease.

The EPA sets standards for this kind of pollution, and nationally, the United States manages to stay below those standards for 2.5 and 10 micron particulate matter. The current trend for both kinds of particles, from 2000 to 2013, is downward, with a 34% decrease in that time period nationally. In different regions of the country, that trend also is a downward one, but some areas of the United States are doing better than others, and many still hover above or on the edge of exceeding the EPA standards. You can find daily updates and regional data on air particulate matter online at Epa.gov/airtrends.

Now on to the data. A 2013 review of air pollution exposure and outcomes for newborns notes that the link between exposure to air pollution and increased infant mortality is a consistent finding in studies from around the globe. These authors speculate at some possible causes for this link but note that results for lower birth weight are more mixed. One such study of lower birth weight, a retrospective study of pregnant women and their newborns, found that exposure to either 2.5 or 10 micron particulate matter above median levels was associated with lower birth weight. In addition, for African American women and their children, the odds for very low birth weight were more than 3 times greater with exposures above median levels, a risk that was twice that of the overall population with the same exposure. One 2010 meta-analysis of 20 articles concluded that there is an association between 2.5 micron particulate matter exposure and preterm birth, with a 15% increase in risk with each stepwise increase in exposure. In another meta-analysis, published in 2011, the authors crunched the numbers from 10 observational studies and found increased odds of congenital heart defects with increasing exposures to different air pollutants, including 10 micron particulate matter.

Air pollution has been strongly linked to negative effects on cardiovascular health, so it makes sense that research would turn to its effects on high blood pressure in pregnant women. A 2014 review of this subject covered 17 papers that assessed various types of pollution, including 2.5 and 10 micron particulates, and factors such as whether a pregnant woman lived near a highway. Most of these studies found an association between air pollution exposure and increased risk for pregnancy-related hypertension, and the meta-analysis confirmed increased risk for each individual pollutant measured, with the exception of carbon monoxide. The risk increase wasn't dramatic, based on their analysis, with incremental increases in 2.5 micron particles, for example, leading to a 47% increase for any pregnancy-induced high blood pressure disorder (gestational hypertension or preeclampsia) and 30% increase for preeclampsia alone.

And what about the children? The authors of a 2013 review of studies examining how air pollution causes damage suggest that the effects of air pollution on children begin in the womb, arranging or "programming" the cardiovascular system toward the path of asthma and other lung disease through oxidative stress, or an imbalance that tilts toward an overabundance of molecules that can cause significant cell damage. Some research in animals suggests that the effects of these molecules in utero can lead to lasting changes that result in later disease. These molecules are an important and normal part of the immune system armory, but as with many components of the immune system, too much of a useful thing can end up causing disease. It's not clear, though, whether those molecules are present because of the air pollution or because of the disease it causes.

Air pollution has also been associated with cancer, and a 2014 review of nine studies examined its link with childhood leukemia. The analysis indicated that being exposed to air pollution from residential traffic was associated with a 53% increase in the risk of childhood leukemia, but prenatal exposure was not associated with any increased risk. To put that into perspective, as readers of this book likely understand by now, increased risk doesn't mean inevitability. For example, 1 in 100 children is born with some genetic condition, such as Down syndrome, which is associated with an increased risk for childhood leukemia. Even with that risk factor, however, only 1 in 8,000 of these children will actually develop the disease.

One reason for the interest in looking at causes of childhood leukemia is that no one is quite sure what causes it. The same applies to childhood asthma, which is on the rise, with the steepest increases occurring among African American children, according to the CDC. A number of explanations have been proposed to explain the increase, including rationales based on the hygiene hypothesis discussed on page 247, but given the association with the lungs, pollution is an obvious candidate. Many studies, however, focus on air pollution as a trigger for asthma attacks rather than as a cause of asthma itself. Studies that do look at air pollution exposures and asthma home in on indoor air pollution factors, like those associated with dust mites, mold, roaches, and pets, which may sensitize a genetically predisposed child and lead to allergic reactions and asthma. Particulates related to dust mites and cats are especially strongly associated with this chain of events.

As far as outdoor or ambient pollution goes, a 2010 study tracked the hospital records of 37,401 British Columbian children relative to their locational air pollution exposures in utero and in infancy. These authors found significant associations between asthma diagnosis and early life exposure to pretty much everything, including carbon monoxide and 10 micron particulate matter. But the odds increases for asthma seem small—8% to 10% at most. Asthma rates among the study participants were 9%. These findings are purely correlational and rely on air pollution data that have gone through several layers of massaging to be usable in the analysis. In other words, it's not definitive. Add to that a very recent study from Johns Hopkins University that looked at factors influencing asthma rates among 23,065 children and found that where the children lived (urban or rural) was not associated with their developing asthma, but household poverty was, as was being African American or of Puerto Rican descent. The role of air pollution in that demographic pattern is unclear, but living in the presumably more polluted city was not a factor.

Great, you may be thinking, but what can I do? You have to breathe. In the United States, many urban areas take air pollution measures daily and predict when particulate matter will exceed the standard. These days, often designated with some catchy phrase like "Spare the Air Day" or "Ozone Action Day," are a guide for anyone who needs to keep tabs on when particulate matter levels exceed the standards. And obviously, it's never a good time to stand around inhaling car exhaust if you can help it.

The Water We Drink

Water has, throughout history, been both our greatest ally and our greatest nemesis. We can't live without it, but plenty of the worst bugs imaginable—polio, cholera, amoebas, botulism, giardiasis, E. coli, Salmonella, hepatitis A, rotavirus, and more—have made their way into our bodies through water. In the United States, we've been fortunate to have some of the highest quality water standards in the world so that most of these diseases are a far-off memory (we no longer die of dysentery, unless we're playing the Oregon Trail) or a headline in a foreign newspaper. A greater concern these days relates to industrial contaminants dumped into the water supply by factories. For example, a retrospective study of 2,000 pregnancies among women living in Cape Cod, Massachusetts, found twice the risk of stillbirth and 1.4 times the risk of placental abruption among pregnant women who had been exposed to tetrachloroethylene, a contaminant in the vinyl lining of asbestos cement pipes in that public water system from the 1960s through the 1980s. Fortunately, these situations are rare, but unfortunately, we have to rely on scientists and the media to identify these problems before they can be addressed.

Overall, however, the water available to us is pretty safe. Two federal agencies regulate the sources of the vast majority of water that most people drink: the EPA for municipal tap water supply and the FDA for bottled water. FDA regulations require bottlers to process, bottle, hold, and transport water in sanitary conditions, to ensure the water sources and the water in bottles is free of harmful bacteria and chemicals, and to regularly test both. That said, not every single bottle of water gets tested, and contaminants do get into some, but they are almost never in levels that could cause harm. A review of 46 brands of bottled water sold in the United States primarily found low amounts of various minerals—some actually contain nutrients needed in daily intake, such as calcium, magnesium, and sodium—but nothing that would raise concerns. Spring water brands tended to have higher levels of most substances than purified or distilled brands, but all the copper, zinc, magnesium, aluminum, lead (yes, lead), chromium, antimony, phosphorus, calcium, sulfate, chloride, and nitrates found were in levels well below EPA drinking water standards.

US tap water almost anywhere is some of the safest water you can drink. When preparing formula, store-bought nursery water rarely offers any benefit over what comes out of your tap. Well water, however, may be riskier. An estimated 15 million households rely on wells for their water supply in the United States. Well water is more susceptible to ground contamination from fertilizer, pesticides, failed septic tanks, urban runoff, and other potentially concerning substances. These wells do need to be checked regularly, and the EPA or local departments do periodically check wells that serve large numbers of people. Those serving fewer than 25 people remain unregulated, however, leaving checking up to the individuals who use it.

What concerns most people about water is fluoride, a mineral that has polarized various communities since Grand Rapids, Michigan, became the first city in the world to fluoridate its water, in 1945. The mineral's history is actually fascinating: a young dentist named Frederick McKay arrived in Colorado Springs to open a practice in 1901 and discovered that loads of residents had severe brown stains on their teeth, some so bad it seemed chocolate permanently mottled them. A study at the time found the stains among more than 90% of children born there. Even more bizarre, however, these brown teeth seemed impervious to decay. What McKay was seeing is now called fluorosis, resulting from high levels of fluoride that interact with the mineralization of teeth while they're forming under the gums, but it took more than 30 years (and several other towns' residents with the stains) to discover the cause was fluoride in the water supply. By then, the National Institutes of Health's Dental Hygiene Unit had taken up study and determined by the late '30s that most people would not develop fluorosis with water fluoride levels of up to 1 part per million.

But the resistance to decay with fluoride was intriguing, and in 1944, the City Commission of Grand Rapids decided to participate in a citywide experiment by fluoridating its drinking water. A decade later, cavities among nearly 30,000 schoolchildren there had dropped by 60%. Today, more than 200 million Americans have fluoridated water (usually this means adding fluoride, but it can also mean reducing fluoride levels in areas where fluoride occurs naturally in greater amounts). Yet, since the beginning, conspiracy theories have proliferated about the "dangers" of fluoride. In reality, the evidence base on the benefits and low risks of fluoride really couldn't be more solid. Large-scale studies and systematic reviews have consistently found that exposure to low levels of fluoride reduces tooth decay and cavities. One such review in 2008 scanned more than 5,400 articles and winnowed them down to 77 papers that met the authors' criteria. They concluded, "Fluoridation of drinking water remains the most effective and socially equitable means of achieving community-wide exposure to the caries [cavities] prevention effects of fluoride. It is recommended that water be fluoridated in the target range of 0.6–1.1 milligrams per liter, depending on the climate, to balance reduction of dental caries and occurrence of dental fluorosis."

Fluorosis is the only scientifically established risk of water fluoridation and usually occurs because children get fluoride from other sources simultaneously, such as swallowing toothpaste. In a few areas of the country, fluoride naturally occurs at levels above 2 mg/L, so if you live in these areas, children should use a different drinking water source until their adult teeth fully come in. Because fluorosis affects teeth while they're still forming, those teeth that have already broken through the gums can't develop it. Still, even among children who do develop fluorosis, most cases are so mild only a dentist would notice. A study in 2010 found that only 5% of the US population had mild cases of fluorosis (barely visible stains). Another 2% had moderate cases, and fewer than 1% had the kind of severe staining McKay saw in the early 20th century.

Other risks can result from excessive fluoride, but none that can come from standard water fluoridation. An extremely rare (in the United States) crippling condition called skeletal fluorosis can damage the bones but requires about 8,400 mg/kg of fluoride exposure. For a 55-pound child, that means 200,000 milligrams of fluoride, or drinking approximately 200,000 liters of fluoridated water, something that would kill a child if he could somehow manage to drink that much in a day (much less retain all the fluoride, since the body clears it out in a week or so anyway). There are also concerns that fluoride might affect the neurological, endocrine, or digestive systems, but it would require well over 4 times the amount of fluoride present in drinking water. There is no evidence for any effects at lower amounts.

If you research fluoride online, however, you are bound to come across a now-infamous "China study" that had alternative health sites up in arms when it was published in 2012. It's become the cherry-pick of choice among antifluoridation activists because it's a systematic review and meta-analysis of studies conducted by Chinese researchers on "developmental fluoride neurotoxicity." The first line of its conclusion sounds sobering indeed: "The results support the possibility of an adverse effect of high fluoride exposure on children's neurodevelopment." Yet no one seems to read the conclusion's second line: "Future research should include detailed individual-level information on prenatal exposure, neurobehavioral performance, and covariates for adjustment." Those last three words are crucial: the authors did not control for other factors that might have affected their results. Here's what they did: they reviewed only papers involving children in China and one group in Iran, already making their findings potentially less relevant for US children. But China has not fluoridated its water since 2002, and most of the children in the studies lived in rural areas with naturally occurring high levels of fluoride, ranging from 2–10 mg/L. Meanwhile, the "control" (comparison) children in the study were also exposed to fluoride—about 0.5–1 mg/L, or right about the amount of US fluoridation standards. The authors found the children with the high fluoride exposure had lower IQs and other poorer neurocognitive outcomes than the control children, who, again, were exposed to approximately the same levels as US children. Further, the authors did not take into consideration any other environmental contaminants the children might have been exposed to, such as arsenic or lead. (It's entirely plausible that areas with high levels of naturally occurring fluoride also have higher levels of other minerals and metals.)

So, no, this China study offers no evidence that fluoridated water is harmful to US children. Meanwhile, if there is a fluoride conspiracy, it's worldwide: a 2013 review estimated that 370 million people in 27 countries drink fluoridated water (including European ones, despite a bizarre misconception that the EU banned fluoride), plus 50 million others who drink water in which fluoride naturally occurs. And they seem to be doing fine.

CHAPTER 9

⚜

This Is Your Child's Brain on Screens

Tablets, Smartphones, and Other Mobile Devices

Almost three-quarters of kids under 8 years old in 2013 had used a mobile device for something at least once, whether it was watching videos, playing games, or using other apps. By the time you read this, that rate will no doubt be higher. And the numbers of kids regularly using smartphones, tablets, and similar touch-screen devices is increasing too: from 2011 to 2013, the proportion of daily users under 8 increased from 8% to 17%. Again, by the time you read this, those numbers will seem quaint. Like TV use, smartphones and tablets are neither inherently good nor inherently bad. How they affect children depends entirely on the kinds of apps they're using (and whether they're age-appropriate), how long they use the device, and whether parents are involved or monitoring use. Surveys have found playing games tops the list of activities children do with mobile devices, followed by taking or looking at photos, listening to music, watching videos, and, well, actually calling someone. More than half of children using these devices don't need an adult's help: they figure out how to swipe, tap, and exit apps pretty quickly on their own or after just watching mom or dad a couple of times.

Unfortunately, research into apps and learning is incredibly thin. Limited research shows children can develop and practice literacy skills, number knowledge, and spatial skills, such as with puzzle apps or tangram sorts of shape games, and more likely we'll see an explosion of research in this area soon. Until then, we know as much as we know about educational TV programming: quantity and quality matter, but quality is hard for parents to assess on their own. Common Sense Media is a fantastic resource that continually updates its website based on current research and parent reviews. What constitutes "a lot" or "a little" or "just right" will also have to wait for more research, but the most important thing for parents to keep in mind is that children get a balance of all activities: engagement with adults, interaction with their peers, activities that enhance fine and gross motor skills, and experience with print media.

An emerging area of study where we actually have some research, however, is nighttime use. As with TV and computers, smartphones and tablets emit blue light, the wavelength most likely to interfere with the hormone melatonin, which tells our brains to sleep. One study on e-books found using one before bed reduced adults' melatonin release and pushed back their circadian rhythms (internal body clocks). Another 2015 study found children who slept near a small screen (such as a smartphone) got about 20 minutes less sleep compared to those who didn't. So even if a child is learning by completing a farmyard puzzle, doing so in the half hour or hour before bedtime may make falling asleep tougher.

Mobile Devices Before Age 2

In 2013, more than a third of children under 2 years old had used a mobile device, compared to just 1 in 10 kids only 2 years earlier. For years, the AAP has recommended no screen use for children under 2, and the evidence backed that up as long as TV was the main screen in kids' lives. But now that smartphones, tablets, and similar mobile devices have entered the scene, new research is suggesting flexibility is the name of the game for infants and toddlers. After all, who would argue that using a videophone app to talk to a parent deployed overseas was a bad thing for an 18-month-old? The problem is that it will take years for the evidence in this area to build, and much of it may be out-of-date by the time it's published. So we'll discuss the little that we know and a lot of what we don't know.

We know there is no evidence showing benefits for kids under 2 using a mobile device by themselves. Again, maybe as apps become more sophisticated and more research is done, this will change, but for now that's the state of the evidence. One reason mobile devices may offer limited solo learning experiences relates to children's "transfer deficit," their difficulty in transferring information and learning something from two-dimensional media compared to three-dimensional live experiences. For example, in one experiment, toddlers ages 2 to 2.5 either watched a live person hide a stuffed dog through a glass window or else watched it on a TV monitor. When the kids entered the room themselves, only half the children who watched the monitor found the stuffed dog compared to nearly all the children who watched the live demonstration.

However, repetition of two-dimensional experiences can reduce that deficit, and it's well established that children learn through engagement and interaction with adults. If a smartphone is part of that interaction, especially if the activity involves repetition, it's possible that kind of use carries benefits. One potential double-edged sword of mobile devices for the littlest kids is distraction. They've been used to distract kids as they get anesthesia for surgical procedures, and they can be valuable in other situations to distract a child, but using them for distraction too often may interfere with how children learn self-regulation. No evidence has shown this—it's an open question—but some have called for study in this area. It's also unclear whether mobile use might increase the risk of attention problems in children, something that has been seen with very early exposure to TV but which seems more connected to *not* doing other activities rather than anything about TV programming. Yet touch-screen devices offer quite a bit that TV does not, something even many traditional toys do not: interactivity (the device prompts a child to do something and then responds), personalization, and progressive learning (moving up through levels). Both traditional toys and touch-screen devices can be highly portable, can promote interaction between a child and an adult, and can react to something the child does (such as a jack-in-the-box). TV offers none of these things. (Books, by the way, offer all of them.) So it's entirely reasonable that mobile and touch-screen devices could promote as much learning as many traditional toys do, such as blocks or musical instruments, but we just don't know yet. If nothing else, using interactive apps instead of passively watching TV is definitely a step up for kids under 2. After all, consider the following ways apps and mobile Internet use might promote learning and engagement with an adult and the world:

- Playing games or puzzles together
- Reading e-books together
- Creating multimedia projects like collages
- Looking up information to answer a question about the world
- Taking photos
- Connecting with faraway family members
- Creating a predictable routine (using timer and alarm apps)

The Screen as Classroom

A long, robust history of research shows that technology can play a positive role in learning, and that extends to TV and, more recently, to apps. One of the coolest studies in recent years even took a peek at kids' brains while they watched *Sesame Street* and saw the areas related to different skills, such as language development and cognitive abilities, show signs of activity when the show's content matched those skills. *Sesame Street* was, unsurprisingly, a good choice for this experiment. The show practically single-handedly sparked research into the potential for educational TV, and a number of studies have identified positive effects from it, especially on children from lower-income homes. One long-term study even found that the positive effects from *Sesame Street* on academics and social skills lasted for years into school. Yet other programs (albeit less studied) don't always have the same influence— quality matters. Effective educational programming shares several common elements: keeping story lines in logical order (no flashbacks), having a logical ending, repetition (within the show and then re-watching the show itself), and fun elements of fantasy (animated objects, puppets, etc.). These kinds of programs, as well as those that specifically incorporate language learning into them (again, *Sesame Street* blows all the others out of the water), have been shown to help children with literacy development, reading skills, and early number skills.

When it comes to social interactions, the bulk of research finds that, even with TV programming, kids imitate what they see. If they see friendly playing or peaceful resolution of conflicts, they are friendlier and less aggressive when playing with other kids afterward. When they watch someone practicing altruistic behavior or self-control, children tend to exhibit more altruism and self-control themselves. Shows promoting diversity, such as

Sesame Street, and not stereotyping people also appear to have moderate positive effects on children's attitudes and beliefs, especially when paired with discussion afterward. These potential benefits start somewhere between ages 2 and 3. Besides *Sesame Street*, other shows known to have positive effects, both in literacy and social skills, include *Mr. Rogers' Neighborhood*, *The Electric Company*, *Arthur*, *Blue's Clues*, *Reading Rainbow*, and *Barney & Friends* (though our children would have watched that purple dinosaur over our dead bodies). Disney and Nickelodeon also do a decent job with preschool programming, though the effects are more mixed once school-age hits.

However, children's brains don't appear ready to start learning from all this programming until around age 2 (for the same transfer deficit reason we discussed in the section on mobile devices, on page 271). A study that compared how well children learned vocabulary from a person in front of them versus from a children's program found that kids under 22 months didn't learn anything from the TV program. Another similar experiment found that only kids 17 months and older learned words by watching an educational DVD 6 times over 2 weeks. And a review of all the research through 2010 found that kids even through 24 months have a hard time learning from TV, whether it's language skills or social skills or anything else, even though it's not clear why.

E-books and Mobile Devices

There's good news with e-books: they're associated with the same literacy development as print books—with some caveats. Less is more. The more an e-book resembles a print book and the less interactivity it has, the more benefit a child derives from it, especially when reading it with an adult and interacting with that adult. Reading e-books with more bells and whistles, kids were less likely to point to pictures or words or to talk about the story, some of the very skills that enhance literacy. Parents should treat e-books exactly the same way they treat print books, with the same level of engagement and focus on the story, if they want to reap the same benefits.

Although researchers are only just starting to publish findings on kids' ability to learn from smartphone and tablet apps, the early results are promising. One study tested children's vocabulary after playing two apps, Martha Speaks and Super Why. Both led to an increase in vocabulary scores for children ages 3 to 6. However, as we noted before, a strong enough evidence base has not yet built up to establish what makes a high-quality learning app.

Presumably, apps with more of the elements we mentioned previously—reactivity, interactivity, personalization, progressive learning, and promoting interaction with an adult—will have a higher likelihood of teaching children something, but more research is needed.

TV: The Good and the Bad

Television is nearly inescapable in the lives of children. Even if your home doesn't have a TV, your child's playmates probably have TVs, and many restaurants, bowling alleys, doctors' waiting rooms, and other locations your child will visit have them. In and of itself, television's ubiquity is neither good nor bad. If your kid is watching *Sesame Street* in the pediatrician's waiting room, she is probably learning and it's a worthwhile distraction while you wait. If the TV at the car dealership shows five ads for McDonald's while you're getting a tire rotation, you may be less thrilled. But regardless of where TV pops up in your child's life, her home environment will play the biggest role for the first several years, so it helps to know what research has uncovered about watching the boob tube.

On a typical day, American children ages 8 months to 8 years are exposed to nearly 4 hours of background television, and for younger children, background television has very clear negative effects. A study of 3-year-olds found that direct TV exposure and household TV use were linked to childhood aggression even after taking into account spankings, the child's neighborhood, mother's depression, parenting stress, and other factors. But the greatest concern is language development.

One study found each additional hour per day of watching baby DVDs or videos led to a significant drop in language development scores among infants ages 8 to 16 months but not among toddlers ages 17 to 24 months, regardless of whether parents watched with the children or not. Earlier findings explain why: while infants and toddlers played with toys in the presence of a parent, researchers had a TV program on for half the play period. One study used a baby video and the other an adult program, but the results were the same: parents spoke less to their babies and interacted less with them while the TV was on even though the parents focused on their children nearly the entire time and the babies focused on the toys and ignored the TV.

Another study found each extra hour of TV for 2-year-olds predicted poorer vocabulary skills, number knowledge, engagement in the classroom, and gross motor skills when they entered school at age 5 even after considering other contributing factors. (Interestingly, they were also bullied more.) Other studies have found similar results, though at least one found that the effects were at least modest enough that analyzing the numbers in different ways could show a positive, negative, or neutral effect on language development.

> Nothing replaces human interaction.

Here's what that all means: background television at any age reduces interaction and has no positive effects, regardless of what's on. For children under age 2, no programming or videos offer much benefit. Nothing replaces human interaction. Somewhere around age 2 or 3, however, the balance tips: well-designed educational TV can start to offer benefits to children. Non-educational content, however, is linked to poorer academics and behavior by the time school rolls around.

Advertising

The plain truth is that marketing works, so if ads promote junk food or smoking, kids find it attractive, but if they promote how awesome broccoli is, that may increase kids' interest in broccoli. Of course, nobody makes ads about the awesomeness of broccoli, or much else that's healthy, so there isn't as much research to see if it actually does work both ways equally effectively. But we know brands drive food choices, healthy or not. A 2014 experiment tested how well children recognized milk and apples from McDonald's and Burger King, and the kids recognized all but the Burger King apples pretty well. In another experiment, children thought the exact same foods tasted better if they were led to believe it came from McDonald's. A large IOM review looked at the whole of research in this area and found food marketing definitely influences children's food preferences and how much they eat—which more research has shown can affect their waistlines. Of course, marketing works only if your kids see it. Broadcast channels tend to have more food advertising than cable channels (though the poor quality of the food is the same), whereas on-demand programming often has no commercials at all.

Screens in the Bedroom

About 1 in 5 babies, 3 in 10 toddlers, and 2 in 5 preschoolers have televisions in their bedrooms. And there is nothing positive to come from that as far as research has found. Even if kids have plenty of other physical activity, even if they play team sports, and regardless of how much other screen time they have, having a TV in the bedroom is strongly linked to being overweight across all income and educational levels—independent of parents' weight. Why? Both too little sleep and poor-quality sleep are strongly linked to obesity, and kids with TVs in their rooms stay up later to watch TV. Further, the blue light from the TV can delay their body's release of melatonin, so it's harder for them to fall asleep even when the TV is off. Some research has also shown it's harder for them to settle and sleep after watching TV because of the excitement in the shows themselves; but regardless of the mechanisms, all the effects are the same: less sleep, more weight gain.

The Violence Connection

One recent survey revealed that 90% of pediatricians believe that violent media exposure increases aggression in children, and various polls have revealed that anywhere from 70% to 80% of Americans believe that media violence contributes to "some or a lot" of real-life aggression and violence— and the research clearly bears this out. Mountains and mountains of research from the past six decades have consistently found the same thing over and over: violence in the media contributes to children's aggressive behavior, real-life violent acts, desensitization to violence, nightmares, bullying, depression, difficulty sleeping, reduced empathy, and fears of getting hurt. The findings hold true for the youngest children up through late adolescence.

Yet violence permeates every aspect of our media, including children's shows. Any parent who has helpfully warned another to skip the first 5 minutes of *Finding Nemo* or to hold off on letting their toddler watch *The Lion King* will attest to Disney's maddening fascination with killing off parents. A tongue-in-cheek (but well-conducted) study published in a British medical journal's 2014 Christmas edition found that important characters in children's animated films died 2.5 times more often in 45 top-grossing children's animated films than in a comparison group of 90 top-grossing adult dramas. And these weren't peaceful deaths: murder occurred 2.8 times more often in the kids' flicks!

All this violence seeps into children's subconscious in sometimes surprising ways, having as much ability to shape behavior as people in real life do. Superheroes are fun, but when heroes repeatedly use violence as an acceptable way to resolve conflict, children learn that violence is a valid way to solve problems. When children are used to seeing film and TV characters, both the bad guys and the good guys, carrying guns, it increases the fascination and acceptability of weapons and can even glamorize their use for personal power. When women and minorities are repeatedly the victims of violence, this pattern reinforces sexist and racist beliefs and behaviors in the real world and in our children's brains.

Perhaps the most significant effect of children's exposure to media violence is an increase in aggression, found in hundreds of real-life experiments, lab experiments, cross-cultural studies, and long-term studies in children, teens, and young adults. How strong is this evidence? The AAP statement on media violence compared the strength of the association between media violence and aggression to other established health associations: the link is stronger than that "between calcium intake and bone mass, lead ingestion and lower IQ, and condom nonuse and sexually acquired HIV infection, and nearly as strong as the association between cigarette smoking and lung cancer."

Some may argue that the steady decline in violent crime in the United States and the well-adjusted lives of adults who grew up watching *The Lone Ranger* contradict these findings. Yet media today is more violent, and more realistically so, than in the past. A 2014 study of violence and firearm use in films found that movie violence has more than doubled since 1950, and gun-related violence has more than tripled since 1985. One study assessed 5 G-rated and 51 PG-rated movies and found a third of them showed characters with firearms. Although 64% of the characters were police officers, soldiers, or similar characters, a quarter were criminals, and 12% were other characters, such as parents or cowboys. No studies suggest that watching violent media in childhood will cause children to go on pillaging rampages when they're older, of course. Rather, the media exposure leads to an increase in short-term aggressive behavior, aggressive thoughts, and aggressive emotions and a higher long-term risk for getting into fights, spousal abuse, and other interpersonal violence (and, yes, the long-term studies suggest the link is likely causal). Viewing violence can lead to desensitization and a normalization of violence as a valid tool for dealing with problems. It also taps into already existing aggressive thoughts or ideas and increases an individual's arousal, which triggers an automatic tendency to imitate the behavior. One study found 3- and 4-year-olds who had watched programs with violence showed more antisocial symptoms, more attention problems, and poorer overall academic performance later, in second grade, even after adjusting for their original level of aggressiveness.

Finally, fearing the monster under the bed or the bogeyman in the closet is probably as much a rite of passage as losing a tooth, but when children start believing in monsters in real life, it can affect their mental health. Media violence, real and fictional, has been linked to anxiety, depression, post-traumatic stress disorder, nightmares, and social isolation. Television coverage of events such as school shootings, disease outbreaks, terrorist attacks, and environmental disasters can increase stress and anxiety. Studies of children's physical and mental health after the 9/11 attacks found that more than a third of children reported at least one symptom of distress related to watching 9/11 coverage on TV, with greater effects for those who watched more TV in the days immediately following the attacks. Similar effects were seen for watching coverage of the Boston Marathon bombing.

CHAPTER 10

Development and Its Derailments and Delays

Developmental Screening and Milestones

In the United States, more than 1 in 10 children has a developmental delay of some kind, but half these children fly under the clinical radar for years. Because the best window of opportunity for addressing delays is typically in earliest childhood, a missed red flag can also mean a missed or delayed chance for the most effective intervention. For this reason, your child's doctor should be making developmental assessments at every well-child visit, following standard guidelines.

There are all kinds of lists available online regarding expected developmental milestones at different ages and stages; for example, the CDC has plenty of information available as part of its "Learn the signs. Act early" campaign. With that ready access, we don't want to be repetitive here and have provided only a quick overview in the box on page 282. But what you might not find with these online lists is the steps in the process of identifying when a child has missed a milestone.

Your child's visit to the pediatrician will typically follow a pattern that starts with surveillance, in which the clinician runs through a short milestone checklist and observes the child. It's in your child's interest for you to identify and retain a pediatrician who comes to know your child's developmental trajectory, because in addition to asking you about concerns you might have, the pediatrician will also monitor your child's developmental trajectory over time. It's also important for you to communicate any concerns you have to the pediatrician—don't worry about coming across as a worrywart.

According to the AAP algorithm (the process clinicians step through in making a diagnosis) for monitoring for developmental delays, the pediatrician should always ask the parent about concerns and keep a developmental history of the child that is based on observations of the child and keeping accurate records. Any red flag that this surveillance turns up—concern from the parents or from the doctor—should lead to some screening to see if referral is needed. In addition, the AAP algorithm states that children should receive a routine developmental screening at ages 9, 18, and 30 months. An autism-specific screening is also recommended at the 18-month visit.

Research supports the recommendation that pediatricians should go beyond surveillance as a first step and use a screening tool routinely at well-child visits, because surveillance by itself is not sufficient for detection. Clinician judgment on its own can perform only slightly better than just selecting children by chance, with one study showing that this approach would have missed 45% of children eligible for early intervention. That's probably not surprising considering that a clinician might see the child for 15-minute bursts every few months at most. Tools that parents complete are generally more useful than those that involve child responses.

Among the various screening tools pediatricians might use, their success rate in identifying problems that are present ranges from 68% to 88%. Their ability to identify that no problem exists when no problem exists ranges from 70% to 88%. Interestingly enough, when two of these tests, the parent-completed PEDS and ASQ, were compared head-to-head in a 2009 study of 60 children, they showed only fair agreement with each other that was statistically no better than if they agreed by chance, suggesting that these tests either capture different features of development and one or the other might miss some subpopulation of children with a developmental delay.

SOME COMMON DEVELOPMENTAL MILESTONES UP TO AGE 3 YEARS

Caveat: As with all things parenting, your mileage may vary.

- *Around 6 months:* Turns head at hearing name called, briefly sits without support, smiles, plays peekaboo
- *Around the 1-year mark:* Waves bye-bye, pulls to standing, might say "dada" or "mama"
- *18 months:* Follows pointing and also points, uses several words, walks
- *2 years:* Uses short phrases, can point to named objects, follows one-step instructions
- *3 years:* Uses sentences of 4 to 5 words, climbs, engages in pretend play, copies parents and peers

If You Give a Kid a Book

The past decade or so has seen an explosion of DVDs, flash cards, tablet and smartphone apps, and overall "systems" to teach your baby to read. They seem to be selling the idea that reading is a straightforward linear process of recognizing letters, attaching sounds, building them into words, and—voilà!—comprehension. Alas, it doesn't work that way. Reading is one of the most complex cognitive tasks we ask our brains to do, and it brings together a wide range of interacting skills that takes years to develop. A handful of studies have directly assessed some of the programs that claim to teach babies to read. One of the best designed ones randomly split up 117 babies, ages 9 to 18 months, and assigned the intervention group to use a program involving DVDs, word and picture flash cards, and word books for 7 months. Then they comprehensively assessed both early literacy skills, such as knowing letter names and sounds and decoding words, and conventional reading, including vocabulary and reading comprehension, in both groups. Even though the parents of the babies using the reading program perceived benefits and had confidence in the program, their infants showed no greater abilities in any literacy, speech, or related areas after 7 months of the program than babies who had no exposure to the program. All other studies on similar systems, though not typically as rigorous, have found similar results. In short, no, your baby can't read, and these programs won't change that.

What does help children eventually become successful readers is surrounding them with an environment as rich as possible in words and books. One long-term study, for example, found that 60% of the differences in vocabulary among 8- and 9-year-old children was explained by how much language they were exposed to at home before they were 3 years old.

These activities specifically support literacy:

Lots of Talking. Starting in infancy, the more words children hear, the stronger their verbal development, but this talking needs to come from real people—not the radio or TV—and the more the speech is directed at the child, the stronger his language development becomes. One study found children who experienced more "child-directed speech" had bigger vocabularies by age 2 than those who overheard speech but were directly addressed less often.

Books, Books, Everywhere! Numerous studies have found that children's reading ability correlates with how many literacy resources they have at home. When kids are young, just handling books (even if that means chewing them) is considered an "early literacy behavior," as is talking about pictures or imitating what's seen in a book. A meta-analysis of 99 studies of reading from preschool through high school found "print exposure" explained 12% of the differences in preschoolers' and kindergartners' oral language skills.

Storybook Reading. Reading aloud to your child starting from the early months is one of the single most influential things you can do. As children get older, discussion through open-ended questions, such as what your child thinks will happen next, why something happened, how a character feels, or even what's already happened, offers additional benefits. An analysis of 11 studies found that having children retell or act out a story they've read supports reading comprehension, expressive vocabulary, receptive language (understanding what they hear), and overall early literacy development. And don't despair if your child wants to read the same book all the time: repetition builds familiarity and may encourage kids to try reading that book on their own later.

Discipline Without Endangerment

The goal of discipline is twofold: in the short term, to stop or prevent a specific behavior, and in the long term, to socialize a child, to teach him self-control, caring for others, and how to be a moral, ethical, empathetic citizen. A large body of research has investigated disciplinary methods and children's behavior, but it's a huge, messy field. Many factors interact, and we can hit only the highlights here. First, however, make sure whatever behavior you are trying to get from your child is developmentally appropriate. Your pediatrician and a variety of other books can be helpful resources to ensure your expectations for your child's behavior are realistic.

Unless you've been graced with perfect, magical children, discipline, which comes from the words "to teach," is necessary to raise healthy, well-adjusted children. "Permissive parenting," or letting kids do what they want without consequences, tends to decrease children's compliance and increase their antisocial behaviors. A working discipline system requires both a positive parent–child relationship and strategies to reward and strengthen positive behaviors and to discourage negative behaviors.

The positive relationship begins the moment your child arrives in the world as you develop routines, respond to your baby's needs, and provide a secure and loving environment. The stronger a child's attachment to her parent, the more a parent's approval matters. Around age 3, the average child starts being able to reason, and usually by 4, children have developed cognitively enough that negative reinforcement may be effective. But until a child can developmentally understand consequences to her behavior, supervision and redirection or distraction are most effective for preventing children from hurting themselves or getting into something they shouldn't. Spanking, time-outs, and similar methods won't work (more details on these in a moment), but they will upset, frighten, and confuse your child.

Researchers have also identified other components that promote the development of self-regulation in children generally, starting with a loving, warm, affectionate home environment with a positive emotional tone and opportunities for play. This includes giving children attention for positive behavior, removing attention for negative behavior, maintaining consistent daily routines, and using consistent responses to children's behavior. Discipline methods must also be consistent and occur immediately after an undesired behavior each time it happens.

Parents must also help children gradually learn to internalize their motivation for a behavior: kids must understand why it's right to do something or wrong not to and then want to comply because they want to avoid the natural consequences of the behavior. One way this internalization happens is through modeling. Children are the greatest imitators, so they will mimic and eventually internalize behavior they see. The stronger their attachment to a person, the more they imitate that person's behavior. So modeling the behavior you want to see (and not doing what you don't want to see) is one of the strongest ways to influence children's behavior.

Moral internalization grows from a child's development of empathy—he doesn't want to hit the dog because he knows it hurts to be hit. Kids are also more receptive to their parents' wishes when they physically and emotionally feel good. If children are angry or in pain, they may resist or even retaliate against what their parents want. And finally, kids have to know what they did wrong to fix it. While it sounds obvious, parents need to clearly, calmly verbalize in age-appropriate language what a child did wrong and what they should have done. Rambling lectures, shouting, smacking without an explanation, and so on just don't work if a child has no clue how he messed up or what he should have done instead, and these parent behaviors can undermine the parent–child relationship.

Then there are the things that interfere with internalized morality and development of self-control: guilt, anger, fear, and erosion of the bond between parent and child. If children are not attached to their parents, they don't identify with them, so they don't internalize their parents' (or society's) values, leading them to do what they want instead.

Praise and Reprimands

What generally encourages good behavior is what you'd expect: giving children regular positive attention, listening to them, helping them use words to express their feelings, letting them (and helping them) make choices (and understand consequences), praising them for good deeds, ignoring minor misbehavior to discourage it, and, again, modeling the behavior you want them to emulate.

But for most kids, providing that framework doesn't prevent all inappropriate behavior. A recent meta-analysis of 41 studies looked at whether different positive and negative verbal and nonverbal responses to children reinforced good behavior and decreased inappropriate behavior. Nearly every study showed that reprimands and negative nonverbal responses, such as narrowed eyes, crossed arms, or a "look," decreased bad behavior. However, the verbal reprimands were calm and firm without being harsh—harsh verbal responses upset kids and can actually decrease their willingness to follow instructions—and the findings supported using time-out or removing privileges to back up reprimands and "looks." Other research finds reprimands are effective when stated simply and targeted to specific behaviors. If they're used constantly or willy-nilly, or especially during time-out, they lose effectiveness. All these—verbal reprimands, negative emotional expressions, time-outs (more on these shortly), and removing privileges—worked regardless of whether praise and positive reinforcement existed.

Meanwhile, verbal praise alone had mixed results. Across all ages, from 1 to 10, sometimes it worked, sometimes it didn't. In general, praise worked better for kids who already tended to be compliant as opposed to those already prone to breaking the rules or misbehaving. Even when praise did work, it didn't work as quickly as reprimands (negative verbal responses) did. Praise appears to work best within an overall warm relationship, particularly when paired with nonverbal responses, such as hugs, smiles, pats, and other physical affection, or with specific rewards, like stickers or bonus time.

Time-Out and Removal of Privileges

Both forms of negative reinforcement—removal of privileges and punishment—can be effective when done correctly. Children must understand what they did wrong and know the potential consequences ahead of time. The consequence must happen immediately the first time the behavior occurs and then administered calmly, consistently, and immediately to subsequent similar behaviors. Explaining why a behavior is inappropriate and why the consequence is occurring also effectively teaches children how to behave appropriately and comply with future requests. Sometimes, natural consequences (brief pain from an otherwise harmless fall after a warning not to jump or a broken toy) combined with a reprimand is sufficient.

But punishment and removing positive reinforcement aren't the same even though they're often conflated. For example, time-out used as "punishment" can lead to feelings of isolation and shame, which doesn't work very well. But when time-out is used as removal from a loving, fun environment that the child wants to be a part of, it's far more effective and not harmful. Dozens of other studies have found it ranging from 25% to 80% effective.

So what about all those popular articles saying time-out doesn't work and hurts kids? Well, time-out doesn't work when it's done wrong. "Time in" has to be awesome—a positive, encouraging environment—for time-out to work. If a kid's environment is negative, boring, or otherwise unpleasant, then time-out becomes positive reinforcement: your child gets attention and won't stop his behavior if time-out is better than the alternative.

Time-outs also work best as a long-term strategy, which means introducing them can initially lead to an increase in children's outbursts or temper tantrums. When a parent calmly ignores this reaction, it fades, and time-outs become effective; but if a parent indulges the child, either continuing to talk to her or physically interacting with her, the child is getting attention and has little reason to begin complying. What if a child doesn't stay in time-out? One study found an effective solution: remove the toys or activities he might enjoy and stop interacting with the child. When the child asks for a specific item or activity he can't get on his own, he does't get it until he has served his time-out time. (If repeatedly using time-outs doesn't work, research suggests they can become harmful, which means intervention with a professional may be warranted.)

How long should time-out last? Plenty of sources suggest 1 minute per year of age, but there's little evidence to support that rule. Some studies have found that 1 minute is generally too short to work but that 4 minutes works for kids ages 3 to 6. Other studies have found contingencies work better: a child can be released when she has not acted out for a certain amount of time, or else the clock is reset.

There is no evidence that time-outs done properly hurt kids, decrease their brain volume, or increase loneliness and feelings of rejection. That's presuming, however, that time-outs are conducted with little fanfare, especially if in social environments. If the time-out is being used as a shaming tool, it's less likely to be effective. Certainly children may feel temporary loneliness, because that's the point; but if "time-in" is so cool that they want to be a part of it, then they will learn to behave so that they always get to spend time-in. Further, time-outs are effective for long-term compliance. When children are behaving, parents are generally warmer and more affectionate, which increases attachment and children's desire to behave well for its own sake. It's the virtuous cycle instead of the vicious one.

Spanking

Perhaps the most important thing to keep in mind about the research on spanking is that it's incredibly messy, and very little can be said definitively, starting with the definition itself. When does corporal punishment stop being "reasonable" and become abuse? Most of the research draws this line by including only practices that don't result in significant physical injury, such as spanking or slapping. Though vague and problematic, this definition offers a sense of what we're talking about in looking at the research.

Another challenge is that most studies are observational, and nearly all come from reported behavior from parents and children, so data reliability varies greatly, and it's very difficult to show that spanking actually causes a particular outcome rather than being correlated with it. Some of the long-term studies do address which direction an effect occurs, and theoretical research fills in the gaps about how spanking could cause outcomes, but the only definitive way to prove causation—a randomized controlled trial—would be unethical. Further, since the relationship between a parent and a child is so complex, the single factor of spanking being in a parent's discipline toolbox is unlikely to completely dominate a child's outcome, and studies cannot account for every single one of the almost infinite variables that could also play a role. If nothing else, more than 90% of Americans have been spanked as children, and there's almost nothing we could say is true of all those individuals.

But we do know that spanking increases the likelihood of some outcomes, depending on numerous factors: How often and how severely is a child spanked? Is spanking done in a moment of desperation or anger? Or is the parent calmly following through on an established practice the child has learned to expect in response to misbehavior? (The former may be more likely to make kids fearful or angry toward their parents.) Is spanking the only tool the parent uses, or is it combined with reasoning, time-out, removing privileges, and other discipline methods? In fact, one major shortcoming in the research is that these questions often aren't considered in studies. Even though corporal punishment could involve a single swat to the bottom with a hand or a switch made from a tree branch used repeatedly, many studies simply ask parents whether they've ever used corporal punishment without distinguishing between the types or frequency. We use "frequently" or "infrequently" to describe spanking here, but some studies define "frequently" as once a week and others as once a month or less. Then there are the differences in children themselves: their sensitivity, their perception, their temperament, their attachment to their parent, their cognitive development, and so on.

The largest study to date on spanking, published in 2002, was a series of meta-analyses on 88 studies over more than 6 decades on 11 categories of children's outcomes. The information that follows outlines what that meta-analysis found as well as others and more recent research, which largely confirms the pooled findings in that paper. In short, corporal punishment (primarily spanking/slapping, though other methods may be included) was associated with nearly a dozen negative outcomes. Nearly all the harms are dose-dependent: the more spanking happens, the more pronounced the effect. And nearly all of them have also been associated with even occasional spanking.

Noncompliance. About the only positive link with spanking was immediate compliance, but even this finding was weak. Initially, a smack might immediately stop an undesirable behavior, but the evidence doesn't show continued immediate compliance over time. Some studies even found decreased immediate compliance, and some didn't take into account children's baseline compliance with parents' directions in general (which makes those findings somewhat meaningless). But no evidence found that spanking works over the long term. Even worse, spanking can make other forms of discipline, including time-outs, verbal reprimands, and even positive reinforcement, less effective or take longer to work.

Decreased Quality of Parent–Child Relationship and Decreased Moral Internalization. Evidence shows that spanking can cause fear, anxiety, sadness, and anger in children and can directly interfere with infants' and children's attachment security to their parents, especially their mothers. Evidence also shows that children spanked for misbehavior have decreased moral internalization: they have lower long-term compliance, they don't feel guilty after misbehavior, and they don't willingly apologize or try to fix things up for those they hurt. And these two findings are linked. Remember we said pain might cause a child to resist her parents or retaliate? Spanking causes pain, and since we don't like pain, we do what we can to escape it. Sometimes that means not doing the behavior that leads to pain, but it can also mean avoiding the person inflicting the pain, and if a child withdraws from her parent or becomes less attached as a result of corporal punishment, that makes it harder for parents to socialize their children and help them internalize their motivations for behavior.

Finally, spanking on its own can't teach children to learn to have independent morality; all it can do is teach a child to avoid doing the behavior that led to the spanking. A long list of studies links corporal punishment to delinquency and antisocial behavior, but not all these adequately considered whether spanking caused kids to act out or whether kids who already acted out more got spanked more often, and their behavior continued into the teen and adult years. Most likely, both are occurring.

Poorer Mental Health. Harsh physical punishment is linked to depression and anxiety in children and teens, though these studies have tended to include frequent physical punishment that stops short of a legal definition of abuse, and many other relationship or environmental factors could play a role. It's less clear whether very infrequent spanking without an object, such as once a month or less, might affect children's mental health. In general, coercive discipline methods have been shown to decrease children's confidence and assertiveness and to increase their sense of humiliation and helplessness, but drawing a link between occasional spanking and adult mental health is still really shaky, especially given the many other factors that could affect these findings. Right now, there's no solid evidence to say infrequent spanking in childhood causes any mental health issues in adulthood.

Increased Risk of Domestic Abuse. Corporal punishment, including spanking, is on the same continuum as abuse and nearly always precedes it. That doesn't mean those who spank will eventually beat their kids, but those who physically abuse their children usually start with spanking. One study found that parents who spanked their kids were 7 times more likely to eventually assault them, such as punching or kicking. The big question, which researchers are still working to answer, is when corporal punishment transitions to serious abuse (as legally defined) and what factors cause that to happen. It's a stretch to say that a parent who was infrequently spanked as a child is more likely to abuse their kids, and no solid evidence supports that.

Reduced Cognitive Development. Only a few studies have looked at this, but they found that the more children are spanked, the slower they tend to develop cognitively, but none could show that spanking caused the slower development as opposed to the possibility that more slowly developing children may frustrate parents more and receive more spankings.

Increased Aggression in Childhood and Adulthood. There is no question that spanking and aggression in children are linked—it's one of the strongest findings. But there's a chicken-and-egg problem: Do children become more aggressive because they are spanked more, or do parents spank more aggressive children more often? For years, the answer eluded researchers because there are so many factors that affect aggression and a parent's decision to spank. But in recent years, several long-term, prospective studies have found that children do become more aggressive over time if they're spanked, even after accounting for a child's temperament and a wide range of other factors. One study involving more than 3,000 preschoolers found that increased spanking between ages 1 and 3 increased kids' aggression. At least one randomized controlled trial found the converse: when parents reduced their use of spanking, children's aggression decreased too.

The reason spanking leads to aggression isn't mysterious when considered logically. The great irony is that spanking often tries to teach what not to do with the undesired behavior itself: if a child hits someone else, and a parent hits the child as a punishment to discourage hitting, then the child learns that the way to get the behavior he wants . . . is to hit. The message that spanking is acceptable and effective is then ironically reinforced if spanking works.

What about the benefits of spanking? The answer there is straightforward. Not one study, regardless of size or design, has found a single long-term positive effect from spanking or any other form of physical punishment.

Toilet Training and Bed-Wetting

Expectations around toilet training are as related to culture and economics as they are to anything scientific. We'll leave the culture to you and your family and the economics between you and your day care provider (many require a certain level of toilet training for students) and address only the science here.

First of all, the ability to control bladder and bowel function in the day and night is a matter of developmental readiness, just like the ability to hold up your head or sit up or crawl. If the brain and muscles aren't having the appropriate chats yet about bladder or bowel control, no amount of cajoling and praising on the potty will be effective. For nighttime bladder control, in particular, the range of normal for age at gaining this milestone can go well over 5 years old, and nighttime dryness is the last milestone children usually reach on their toilet-training journey. About 20% of 5-year-olds still have "nocturnal enuresis" (nighttime bed-wetting), as do about 5% of 10-year-olds. One critical factor in a child's nighttime bladder control is production of an antidiuretic hormone that reduces urine production. If a child's not making enough of this hormone, no amount of training, bribery, or humiliation (please don't do that) will matter.

But urinating in a toilet during the daytime usually happens a lot earlier. The best way to tell that a child's reaching the milestone of "no more daytime diaper" is by noting the child's cues. Think about what you have to know and understand to use a toilet. Has your child mastered the basics of what's required? For example, can your daughter walk and sit and communicate to you that she needs to use the bathroom? Does she have the motor skills in place to pull clothes down and up or on and off, which often is the last toileting-related skill a child masters? Other considerations are her emotional maturity and level of independence. A child who seems developmentally ready and is showing the ability to stay dry for 2 or more hours during the day and waking up dry from naps might be a child who's ready to master the bathroom. Her brain also has to have matured the ability to "talk" with the bladder, sensing when it's full and controlling its function.

From the science, the key is not to rush, shame, or pressure the child. According to a 2008 publication, attempts to engage in intensive toilet training before a child is 2 years old hold no benefit, might create unnecessary and avoidable stress around toileting, and make the actual training period longer than it is when starting later. Keep in mind that "intensive" is defined as asking the child more than 3 times a day to use the toilet. The authors note that girls usually master toileting at a younger age than boys and that only 40% to 60% of children currently complete toilet training by age 3 years. Boys on average can go a complete night without a bowel movement by about age 25 months, whereas for girls the average is 22 months.

Constipation is not uncommon and can result when a child undergoing toilet training "holds it," out of fear or embarrassment. In addition, a child who readily urinates in the toilet but declines to have bowel movements in the toilet is more likely to be constipated as well, and experience painful bowel movements, causing more stress. An active approach to resolving constipation (for example, increased dietary fiber and sufficient fluids) can help resolve these not-uncommon issues. One randomized controlled study found that 22% of children exhibited "stool toileting refusal."

When is it time to worry about toileting and bed-wetting? Constipation always requires attention. If a child has been using the toilet regularly but starts to have accidents in the daytime, that can be a red flag for medical attention. The same applies for a child who's been dry through the night for some time but starts to experience bed-wetting episodes, or a child over age 5 who continues having daytime wetting.

IS IT ADHD/ADD?

ADHD/ADD is diagnosed in children based on meeting a threshold of behaviors that are present in the two categories of inattention and impulsivity/hyperactivity. According to the *Diagnostic and Statistical Manual of Mental Disorders 5*, behaviors have to have been present for longer than 6 months and show up in two or more settings (for example, school and home). In addition, they have to be a "clinically significant" problem, not just an annoyance to a teacher or parent, but something that interferes with the child's social, academic, or occupational functioning. And while everyone focuses on the hyperactivity part, children who are often in a distracted, "dreamy" state and are not very active at all might well fit the inattentive profile for this condition. A diagnosis usually cannot be made before a child is 4 years old, but because this condition has such a strong genetic component and is a neurodevelopmental one, it's very likely something that begins very early.

If you're wondering about behaviors to watch out for, that's a tough one when it comes to very young children. After all, they generally are highly active, emotional, not given to sharing, careless with belongings, and not so good at turn-taking in conversation or games. Impulsivity is also pretty common with very young children. So it might not be until a child reaches a certain age and is in a setting involving sharing, social interaction, and more controlled behavior that it becomes clear whether these childhood behaviors stand outside of the norm or fall in the range of typical. As with other neurodevelopmental conditions, sometimes we can't recognize a delay or absence of maturation until the time has come to expect it . . . and it's a no-show.

Early Childcare

Studying early childcare is complex because so many different interacting variables make it difficult to tease out all the contributing factors to a child's outcomes. The bulk of reliable data comes from the most comprehensive study on this topic, the Study of Early Child Care (SECC), funded by the National Institute of Child Health and Human Development. Researchers tracked more than 1,200 children from birth through early adolescence and conducted in-depth interviews with the families when the children were 1 month, 6 months, 15 months, 2 years, 3 years, and 4.5 years old, and then in first, third, and fifth grades. The children started at one of 10 research sites but now live in at least 38 different states, providing a good cross-section of the country. And the data collected in interviews and observations were incredibly thorough: family structure and size, parents' employment, family income, parents' mental health and social characteristics, parents' attitudes and beliefs about parenting and childcare, parents' sensitivity levels toward their children, the quality of the parent–child relationship, characteristics about the home (and whether it offered social and cognitive enrichment opportunities), and the child's behavior, social skills, cognitive skills, and academic achievement. About the only major weakness of the research is that not too many dads stayed at home with their children in this study, so findings tend to be mother-centric. Presumably many of the findings for staying home with mom would transfer to staying home with dad, but we don't know for sure because we don't have the data.

Putting that weakness aside, a couple of other insights are helpful to keep in mind:

- Effects apparently related to childcare were consistently modest. With all the other competing factors, in no area did childcare play a large role in children's outcomes. In fact, the effects were often so small that they contradicted one another, offset one another, or flipped at different ages (more behavioral problems at one age but fewer at another).

- Family factors, such as mom's and dad's sensitivity and parenting philosophies, socioeconomic status, and the home environment, more strongly influenced children's cognitive, language, social, emotional, and behavioral outcomes than childcare did—by a factor of 2 to 3 times.

- The quality of childcare matters—a lot. It can make the difference between stronger or weaker language development or better or worse grades than average years after the child has left childcare, and it plays a significant role in children's developmental progress, social skills, and behavior even after accounting for mothers' educational levels and overall parenting quality. The quality of the staff and the staff-to-child ratio particularly influenced the care children received, the SECC found. Better-educated caregivers with more child-related training are more stimulating, supportive, and organized and provide more age-appropriate experiences for children. A lower child-to-adult ratio and smaller groups lead caregivers to be more responsive and supportive to children, more socially stimulating, less restrictive, and less occupied with managing the children. Unfortunately, SECC found only 10% of childcare centers had "excellent" quality, and 60% did not frequently show "positive caregiving," but that finding is 15 years old.

Behavior and Social Skills

In general, the earlier a child starts childcare and the more time he spends there, the more likely it is that he'll have mild behavioral problems from about age 2 through the end of kindergarten. The effects started in kids who spent more than 30 hours a week in care and were highest in kids spending at least 45 hours a week in childcare. However, emphasis on the "mild" here with three other caveats: by third and fifth grade, these (small) effects had faded, this finding interacted with a child's temperament, and, again, higher-quality childcare decreased this effect (or entirely eliminated it in some studies). Plus, the more negative scores on behavioral assessments were not in the "at-risk" or "serious problem" range; they were just a tick above normal.

Despite the mild uptick in behavioral problems (which go away before third grade), several studies show that children who spend time in care away from their parents have stronger social skills and more self-confidence, manage challenges a little better, entertain themselves better, are more outgoing, and experience less stress in new situations. Wait—does that mean staying home with your kids produces socially incompetent, helpless hermits? Absolutely not. Again, these are big-picture views, and there is no way to remove the potential for selection bias. That is, parents with less socially competent kids may keep them home specifically because they struggle more in social situations or new experiences.

Cognitive Development

Findings on language and cognitive skills are mixed, probably because so many factors play a role. The SECC did not find major effects after they took into account all the other factors that might influence cognitive and language development. Other studies have found high-quality childcare (and preschool) leads to better academic performance in the early grades, but this effect is strongest for lower-income children (and even mediocre-quality care appears to help children from lower incomes). For those kids in childcare, children had stronger skills if they attended a place with opportunities for art, blocks, and pretend play and with more educated and trained caregivers (something parents can offer at home as well). In fact, caregivers' behavior predicted how well children did on standardized thinking and language assessments through the fifth grade even after considering how much time the child spent in care and a long list of family factors.

Family Relationships and Emotional Development

The only children with insecure attachments to their parents were those whose mothers were not sensitive at all to their children's needs, which probably would have happened anyway. In fact, high-quality care may enhance children's relationships with their parents in these situations. The SECC found the child–mother attachment relationship suffered if mothers were not sensitive to their child's needs and the child attended low-quality childcare, but the children of depressed (and presumably less sensitive) mothers had more positive relationships if their children attended higher-quality care.

Home Childcare vs. Day Care Centers

In general, the SECC and several other studies have found childcare centers had better educated and more professional caregivers and more child-oriented materials, but they also had larger group sizes and more structured activities such as "lessons." Family homes tended to have more time for casual learning and exploration—but also for watching TV. Over the long term, children who attended day care centers, as opposed to both home care with parents and home-based childcare, showed more independence from their mothers, better social skills with strangers, and higher scores on cognitive tests, including language and thinking skills from age 2 through third grade.

To Work, or Not to Work?

A couple of studies, including the SECC, specifically investigated differences among children whose mothers did or did not work outside the home (or from home but with full-time or part-time outside-home childcare). Bizarrely, the findings don't apply across all races, even after accounting for income differences. Basically, whether black mothers worked or didn't had no effect on their children's development. The data on Latina mothers are mixed and sparse. The picture is more complex with white mothers. White moms' kids showed no social, emotional, or cognitive differences overall if their mothers did or did not work full-time or part-time in a child's first year. But what's interesting is that a closer look shows negative effects in some areas for working moms' kids and positive effects in other areas. Children act up more at some ages, but then childcare gives them a boost in language and cognitive development, which in turn influences later behavior, and overall, the negatives and positives offset each other for a neutral effect. In short, the disadvantages and advantages of having a mom working outside the home seem to balance each other out.

Bottom line: nothing plays a bigger role than a child's home life and parents, including their parenting behaviors and beliefs. In the SECC, the children rated most competent and least problematic by their teachers had sensitive fathers who encouraged children's independence, mothers who believed in letting children decide their own activities and play, and parents who had a loving and emotionally intimate relationship with each other. (The SECC included little data about single parents or same-sex parents.)

HEALTH RISKS OF DAY CARE

If you do enroll your child at a childcare center, you might end up using a lot of sick leave for the first 6 months or so. Families with kids in day care lose an estimated combined 13 days of work a year for all types of infections. A meta-analysis of studies looking at illnesses among children in day care found a higher risk of upper and lower respiratory tract infections, ear infections, bronchiolitis, gastrointestinal infections, bronchitis, and pneumonia compared to their peers staying at home. The increased risk ranged from 1.5 times greater to about twice as high.

But there's good news. First, the illnesses are rarely serious. A Danish study of more than 1.1 million children over 15 years found that children in day care overall had only a 2% increased risk of hospitalization for gastrointestinal infection compared to children remaining at home. When compared by age, however, children under 1 year old were 44% more likely to have a gastrointestinal infection requiring hospitalization if they were in day care than if they were in home care. Second, the endless sickness does eventually end. One study found a 70% jump in serious infections among children under 1 year during their first 6 months of day care (the jump was lower for older kids), but by the time the kids had been enrolled for a year, their risk of infections was no different from children at home.

And finally, you're getting the inevitable out of the way early. A study in Quebec found that kids had higher rates of respiratory tract infections and ear infections at first. By elementary school, children who attended day care had 20% lower rates of respiratory tract infections and half as many ear infections. Basically, the immune system will get lots of exercise for the first several months after your child first begins regularly interacting with large groups of other children, regardless of whether that's childcare, preschool, or elementary school.

The Pain and Promise of Preschool

To what extent does attending preschool ensure children will succeed academically and beyond? This question has dominated early education policy discussions in the United States for decades, but all those debates and talking heads have done little to actually give parents any semblance of an answer or to provide any guidance on what kinds of preschool education benefits kids most. The confusion is not for lack of research. Dozens of experimental early education studies have been published since the middle of the 20th century, and a couple have amazingly followed children for more than 30 years to see how they fared in middle adulthood. A couple key insights from that research can be pretty easily summed up:

- The potential benefits of preschool include higher academic achievement in early elementary school, higher test scores, lower rates of grade repetition and special education, and higher levels of education overall.
- As household income and parent education go down, the positive effects of preschool education go up: children from lower income brackets reap the most benefit.

- As household income and parent education go up, the potential benefits of preschool level off: by the time we reach kids in the upper-middle to upper class, it's almost impossible to detect any effects from preschool.
- The quality of the preschool matters.

In short, it's easier to make bigger gains when you're starting with less in the first place. It's harder to gain much when you start out in a well-resourced home. A study in 2015 compared the cognitive abilities of 6,600 US kindergartners from across various socioeconomic backgrounds. The findings weren't at all surprising: children from the lowest income brackets had less computer use at home, fewer books at home, fewer expectations from parents that they would eventually attend college, and lower preschool attendance. But the most interesting aspect of this study was that the authors quantified the extent to which various factors contributed to children's cognitive performance. In comparing the highest and lowest scores in reading and math, consider the proportions each factor contributed to the gap in scores, in descending order:

- 18% was explained by the home learning environment: having been read to frequently; having a home computer; number of books, toys, and DVDs in the home; having visited the library in the past month; and how frequently the child played indoors.
- 14% to 15% was explained by parenting style and beliefs: positive interactions, parent supportiveness, expectations that a child will go to college, and rules about bedtime, food, and chores.
- 8% to 13% was explained by family background factors: family structure, household size, race/ethnicity, and mother's age.
- 6% to 7% was explained by early education: primary childcare arrangements, preschool attendance, and participation in extra-curricular activities.
- 4% to 6% was explained by health factors: mother's pre-pregnancy weight, prenatal smoking or alcohol use, mother's depression, any breastfeeding, low child birth weight, and child's health.

The only things that made less difference to the children's scores than preschool attendance (combined with childcare arrangements and extracurricular activities) were health factors. Meanwhile, the home learning environment dominated everything else. While these are the findings of just one study, they match up with those in dozens of other studies about the influence of the home and other factors versus preschool in children's development. They also explain why the difference between a middle- or upper-income child who attends preschool has little edge over a middle- or upper-income child who doesn't attend preschool. The overall learning environment at home plays about 3 times a greater role in children's later achievement. From infancy onward, the two strongest influences on children's cognitive and language development are responsive caregiving and regular language-rich interactions with caregivers, both of which parents in middle- and upper-income homes are often more able to provide. Also important to children's development is a variety of hands-on and direct experiences. It's a lot easier to read about and understand gardens, farms, and forests when a child has visited one.

Regardless, many parents want to know more about that last point: What does a "high-quality" preschool education look like? Once you separate the wheat from the chaff and focus only on the best-designed, longest-running, most comprehensive early education studies, a pattern emerges. High-quality early education includes three major components:

- Educated teachers with a low teacher-to-student ratio
- Highly interactive and language-rich activities among the children and the teacher
- Child-centered and play-based curricula

What's interesting about the last component is that the significance of it doesn't always reveal itself until years later. For example, one study of 68 kids who started preschool in the 1960s found that kids receiving direct, teacher-centered, academic preschool instruction and kids receiving a play-based curriculum had similar academic achievement for a decade. But around age 15, those who had attended the more academic-focused preschool started getting into trouble more than twice as often as the other children, though the study's small size makes it hard to generalize.

Acknowledgments

Emily acknowledges the people who made parenting, writing, and science an intersectional triad in her life. You know who you are.

Tara cannot enumerate all the ways these individuals helped her, but she thanks them all, for their parts big and small, in reading over sections, helping with research, brainstorming ideas, watching her children, and otherwise providing the essential support that enabled her to finish this book: Jessica Atwell; Suzanne Barston; David Bickham; her sister, Elizabeth Brown; Wesley Burks; Brad Bushman; Alice Callahan; Amber Cox; the "Crunchy Skeptics"; Colleen Curry; Tracy Dahlby; Dennis Darling; Liz Ditz; Beth Drummond; Yoni Freedhoff; Bobby Ghaheri; Amanda Jo Greep; Bailey Hall; Jocelyn Hybiske; her lactation consultant, Kathy Ireland; Clay Jones; Elias Kass; Ellie Lee; her editor, Marian Lizzi; Jason Luchtefeld; Rose Maioli; Adam Malcolm; Anne Gaskill McKibben; Bill Minutaglio; Rachel Moon; Melinda Wenner Moyer; her agent, Eric Nelson; Janie Oyakawa; Tiffany Pleasant; Holly Scheer; Cigal Shaham; Michael Simpson; Anna Spreichinger; Kelly Strutz; Matt Valentine; Jennifer Waggoner; Brian Wansink; Alice West; and her sons' pediatrician, Marion Willemsen-Reid. A special thank-you goes to her parents, Bob and Sue Haelle; to her amazing research assistant, Summer Slevin; and to the one person without whom the book could never have been a possibility, her partner and husband, Darrell Morehouse.

Appendix

Making Sense of Scary Headlines

No doubt this book will be picked apart by experts, real and imagined and self-appointed. We sifted through incalculably huge amounts of data, but we still could not read the entire literature base (or summarize every single thing we read). Rather, we tried to give an overview with the recognition that every person is individual. Every bit of research has limitations, and looking at the whole has limitations as well. In fact, this reality is partly at the heart of this book. Few answers are etched in stone or absolute. We can say a precious few things with certainty: vaccinating children has very low risk and effectively protects children from disease. Spanking has no long-term positive outcomes and has a range of possible negative ones. Feeding children is a good idea; how you do it matters a lot less than that you do it. The point is that the evidence—often a moving target in itself—is one tool that must fit into the bigger picture of our lives. If you tried to live according to every single thing in the scientific literature, that would be akin to the ancient Greeks trying to follow every single edict of their constantly bickering gods and goddesses on Mount Olympus.

This book is not and cannot be definitive, but it is a starting place. We have tried to give you a sense of what's actually in those obscure, jargon-full studies that come out week after week. Still, science is not a collection of static knowledge. It is a process. In some cases, the science has reached a consensus, but there is always room for surprise, and there will always be opportunities to fine-tune what we've learned. It therefore helps to have some tools for assessing all the headlines you'll be reading. Be wary of extreme words, such as "breakthrough," "cure," and "game changer." Be wary of any outrageous claims, especially if they sound too good to be true or exactly what you want to hear. As often as possible, look at the original study. You may not be able to access the actual study, but you can look at the abstract. Here are questions to consider:

- How many people are in the study? Twelve? One hundred? Ten Thousand?
- What kind of study is it? Did the authors conduct a randomized trial or is it observational? Is it prospective (following people forward in time) or retrospective (asking people what they remember)? If it's a meta-analysis, what were the selection criteria, and did the authors adjust for all the other factors ("confounders") in the studies? (See our website, The InformedParentBook.com, for a breakdown of the different types of scientific studies and the relative strength of each one in terms of how real or reliable the findings are.)
- Do they report their findings in absolute risk or in relative risk? Relative risk compares two different absolute risks, and absolute risk refers to how many people will experience a particular outcome. So the absolute risk of a particular congenital anomaly might be 1 in 1 million, and taking some medication may increase the risk to 5 in 1 million. So, yeah, the relative risk is 5 times greater, but the absolute risk remains 5 in 1 million.
- What are all the other factors that could account for the outcome that happened, and did the authors consider all the possibilities? How important are the ones they didn't consider?
- Is there actually a biological mechanism for something to happen? Maybe eating peaches is correlated with a higher risk of having a cesarean section, but is there any way that eating a peach can actually directly contribute to the risk of a cesarean section?

This is just a start, but hopefully this book has provided you with strategies for viewing new research and especially the news skeptically and critically. A good journalist will include many of the answers to the questions on the previous page in the story, but not all stories out there are written by good journalists. Read critically and consider the possibilities, but also pay attention to what the consensus of the evidence shows.

A Note on Our Research Rationale and Criteria

In writing this book, we had to draw a few lines. In some cases, the literature on a specific topic numbered in the thousands of publications. In others, including areas that are pretty important to women's health, the studies were quite sparse. To streamline our presentation as much as possible, we focused where we could on the results of systematic reviews and meta-analyses. For example, we have frequently cited Cochrane Reviews; these are systematic reviews that themselves undergo peer scrutiny of their design and process and then evaluate any papers they include using a standardized grading hierarchy and assessing publication bias. We also tried to stay with the most recent publications we could find because 20-year-old or even 10-year-old studies might not reflect modern investigational tools or practices. Where we cite single-trial studies, we sought randomized controlled trials or cohort, epidemiological, or observational studies with large populations as the best evidence.

We did occasionally wander outside the above-described parameters, especially when the literature on a specific subject was very limited. While PubMed certainly was our go-to database for searches, we also mined reference citations, university-maintained databases, and other sources, and we also frequently discussed interpretations with people with expertise in a specific area. Much of what we researched and found could not be included in the book out of consideration for space and our own determination to be as concise and useful as possible for the reader.

Cognitive Traps: Biases, Thinking Errors, and Logical Fallacies

We already told you in the introduction a bit about the pitfalls we encounter when we attempt to assess evidence. We're all subject to bias (and believing you're not is, yep, a type of bias). Although overlap exists between the two, it's important to recognize the difference between scientific bias and the kinds of psychological bias we're all subject to. Scientific bias arises from the peculiarities of a study's methodology. It's impossible to design a study that isn't at risk for some kind of bias, and we'll address just two types in particular.

Throughout the book we discuss "confounding factors" or "confounders." These are characteristics or factors in a study that might influence the results even though they're not what's being studied. For example, studies have shown that the children of women who had a couple of drinks each week during pregnancy have better grades than women who didn't drink at all during pregnancy. But women who have only a couple of drinks a week also tend to be women with higher incomes and higher education. What's more likely: a couple of glasses of wine during pregnancy makes kids smarter, or having parents with higher education and more money leads kids to make better grades? If researchers did not adjust their calculations to remove the bias created by income and education as confounders, the results would not be reliable. Even then, "residual confounding" effects can remain, but at least the authors have done due diligence in zeroing out the effects as much as possible.

Another way to reduce bias is to conduct "double-blind" randomized controlled trials. In a trial testing a medication against a placebo, for example, double-blind means the participant doesn't know if she's getting the medication or the placebo, but neither does the person giving it to her. As highly social creatures, humans pick up on the slightest social cues in a person's voice, expression, or demeanor, and if either person knows they're getting a fake pill, that knowledge can influence the way the experiment turns out. A double-blind design removes that potential for bias. Of course, not all trials can be double-blind. One reason alternative and complementary therapies are difficult to assess is the difficulty of "blinding" someone to real or "fake" acupuncture or aromatherapy. It's very difficult to rule out the placebo effect—the belief that you got better simply because you received a treatment—so these studies are usually rife with bias.

But then there's our psychology, a whole branch of which focuses on something called heuristics. These are mental shortcuts that enable us to make sense of the world around us. It would be impossible for us to assess every single thing we see, hear, smell, taste, touch, and even think at every second—we would go mad from overstimulation. So our brains developed shortcuts that help us process information more quickly and make snap judgments. This survival mechanism makes life livable. The problem is that it can also lead to entrenched thinking, decision-making, and behavior over time or when those mental shortcuts override rational thought. When you've been doing something one way for a decade, it's hard to change even when evidence for a better way is staring you in the face.

We've discussed the biggest of these pitfalls already—mistaking correlation for causation, confirmation bias, overreliance on the anecdote, and Dunning–Kruger (see page 95). But if you're wondering how and why the brain falls into these traps, see the more in-depth discussion on our website along with a list of other biases and logical fallacies that can trip us up in the pursuit of evidence-based truth. Meanwhile, we urge all readers to use the information in this book to make the decisions that are best for them and what they know and understand about their children. We hope it serves as your factual resource in the face of the relentless messages about "how you should be doing it" and "what you're doing wrong" that no parent can escape in the modern age.

Index

Accutane (isotretinoin), 35
ACE (angiotensin-converting enzyme)
    inhibitors, 35
acetaminophen (Tylenol), 36–37, 198,
    244–45
acid reflux, 35
acupuncture, 27, 31, 67, 72
adoption, 17–19
advertising, 276
age of parents, 1–2
airplane travel, 50–51
air pollution, 261–65
alcohol, 41–48, 146–47, 190
allergies
    to animals, 250–52
    food allergies, 212, 228, 230–35
    and hygiene hypothesis, 248
    medications for, 35
    and pacifiers, 165
alpha-fetoprotein, 25
American Academy of Pediatrics (AAP)
    on allergies, 212
    on Apgar scores, 121
    on breastfeeding, 130, 201
    on circumcision, 77–78, 79, 80
    on cloth vs. disposable diapers, 83
    on cosleeping, 188
    on electronic devices, 271
    on feeding schedules, 167–68
    on fevers, 249

on formula, 204–5
on iodine insufficiency, 4
on media violence, 278
on milestones, 281
on mother–baby contact, 130
on parental gender, 16
on shaken baby syndrome, 161
on solid foods, 207
on spoiling children, 167
on vitamin D, 222
on vitamin K shot, 124
amniocentesis, 21, 23–24
amniotomies, 70
anemia, 4, 6
anencephaly, 24
anesthetics, 71
anger crying, 155–56
animals, 250–56
antibiotics, 35, 244
antidepressants, 30–31, 33, 35, 37–38, 154
antiepileptics, 35
antihistamines, 28
anti-nausea drugs, 28
Antivert (meclizine), 28
anxiety, 29, 30–31, 72
Apgar scores, 120–21
aspirin, 34, 36, 59
assisted reproductive technology (ART),
    14–15
asthma, 244, 248, 252, 263, 264–65

About the Authors

Emily Willingham, PhD, is a compulsive writer and biologist and the parent of three sons whom she loves beyond measure. Her writing has appeared in online outlets including *Forbes*, the *New York Times*, *Scientific American*, *Slate*, *Discover*, and others. She probably asks "Why?" more than her children do.

Tara Haelle is a mother of two adored sons and a journalist whose work has appeared in *Forbes*, *Scientific American*, *Slate*, NPR, the *Washington Post*, *Wired*, *Parents*, and her parenting blog, *Red Wine & Apple Sauce*. She has been a writer, teacher, photographer, loquacious talker, and insatiable asker of questions for as long as she can remember.

For notes and further information, visit TheInformedParentBook.com.